New and Emerging Technology in the Treatment of the Upper Extremity

Editor

JEFFREY YAO

HAND CLINICS

www.hand.theclinics.com

November 2012 • Volume 28 • Number 4

ELSEVIER

1600 John F. Kennedy Blvd. • Suite 1800 • Philadelphia, Pennsylvania 19103

http://www.theclinics.com

HAND CLINICS Volume 28, Number 4
November 2012 ISSN 0749-0712, ISBN-13: 978-1-4557-4824-2

Editor: David Parsons

Hand Clinics (ISSN 0749-0712) is published quarterly by Elsevier Inc., 360 Park Avenue South, New York, NY 10010-1710. Months of publication are February, May, August, and November. Business and Editorial Offices: 1600 John F. Kennedy Blvd., Ste. 1800, Philadelphia, PA 19103-2899. Customer Service Office: 3251 Riverport Lane, Maryland Heights, MO 63043. Periodicals postage paid at New York, NY and at additional mailing offices. Subscription price is $368.00 per year (domestic individuals), $583.00 per year (domestic institutions), $184.00 per year (domestic students/residents), $420.00 per year (Canadian individuals), $666.00 per year (Canadian institutions), $500.00 per year (international individuals), $666.00 per year (international institutions), and $243.00 per year (international and Canadian students/residents). Foreign air speed delivery is included in all *Clinics* subscription prices. All prices are subject to change without notice. **POSTMASTER:** Send address changes to *Hand Clinics*, Elsevier Health Sciences Division, Subscription Customer Service, 3251 Riverport Lane, Maryland Heights, MO 63043. Customer Service (orders, claims, online, change of address): Elsevier Health Sciences Division, Subscription Customer Service, 3251 Riverport Lane, Maryland Heights, MO 63043. Tel: 1-800-654-2452 (U.S. and Canada); 314-447-8871 (outside U.S. and Canada). Fax: 314-447-8029. E-mail: journalscustomerservice-usa@elsevier.com (for print support); journalsonlinesupport-usa@elsevier.com (for online support).

Reprints. For copies of 100 or more of articles in this publication, please contact the Commercial Reprints Department, Elsevier Inc., 360 Park Avenue South, New York, New York 10010-1710. Tel.: 212-633-3812; Fax: 212-462-1935; E-mail: reprints@elsevier.com.

Hand Clinics is covered in *MEDLINE/PubMed (Index Medicus), Current Contents/Clinical Medicine, EMBASE/Excerpta Medica,* and *ISI/BIOMED.*

Printed and bound by CPI Group (UK) Ltd, Croydon, CR0 4YY

Transferred to digital print 2012

Contributors

GUEST EDITOR

JEFFREY YAO, MD
Associate Professor of Orthopaedic Surgery,
Robert A. Chase Hand and Upper Limb Center,
Stanford University Medical Center, Redwood
City, California

AUTHORS

CAMERON BARR, MD
Resident, Department of Orthopaedic Surgery,
Stanford University Medical Center, Redwood
City, California

REENA A. BHATT, MD
Attending, Department of Plastic Surgery, The
Miriam and Rhode Island Hospitals, Warren
Alpert Medical School of Brown University,
Providence, Rhode Island

ALAN T. BISHOP, MD
Professor of Orthopedics, Division of Hand
Surgery, Department of Orthopedic Surgery,
Mayo Clinic, Rochester, Minnesota

PAOLO CABITZA, MD
Full Professor, Università degli Studi di Milano,
IRCCS Policlinico San Donato, Piazza
Edmondo Malan, Milan, Italy

CATHERINE CURTIN, MD
Assistant Professor, Division of Plastic
Surgery, Robert A. Chase Center for Hand and
Upper Limb Surgery, Stanford University,
Stanford, California

SHAUNAK S. DESAI, MD
Robert A. Chase Center for Hand and Upper
Limb Surgery, Stanford University, Stanford,
California

SCOTT FLIEGER, MBA
Fletcher Allen Healthcare, South Burlington,
Vermont

JEFFREY B. FRIEDRICH, MD
Division of Plastic Surgery, Department of
Surgery; Department of Orthopaedics,
University of Washington; Harborview Medical
Center, Seattle, Washington

VINCENT R. HENTZ, MD
Emeritus Professor of Surgery and
Orthopaedic Surgery, Robert A. Chase Center
for Hand and Upper Limb Surgery, Stanford
University, Stanford, California

JERRY I. HUANG, MD
Department of Orthopedic Surgery and Sports
Medicine, University of Washington; University
of Washington Hand Center, Seattle,
Washington

DAVID B. JONES Jr, MD
Fellow, Division of Hand Surgery, Department
of Orthopedic Surgery, Mayo Clinic,
Rochester, Minnesota

JASON H. KO, MD
Clinical Fellow, Hand and Microvascular
Surgery, Department of Orthopaedics and
Sports Medicine, University of Washington,
Seattle, Washington

SCOTT H. KOZIN, MD
Clinical Professor, Department of Orthopaedic
Surgery; Chief of Staff, Shriners Hospitals for
Children, Temple University School of
Medicine, Philadelphia, Pennsylvania

STEVE K. LEE, MD
Associate Professor of Orthopaedic Surgery, Hospital for Special Surgery, Weill Cornell Medical College, New York, New York

D.J. MASTELLA, MD
Combined Hand Surgery Fellowship Program, University of Connecticut, Farmington, Connecticut; Hartford Hospital, Hartford, Connecticut

ROWENA MCBEATH, MD, PhD
Hand Surgery Fellow, The Philadelphia Hand Center, P.C., Thomas Jefferson University Hospital, Philadelphia, Pennsylvania

ALLAN MISHRA, MD
Adjunct Clinical Associate Professor, Department of Orthopaedic Surgery, Stanford University Medical Center, Menlo Medical Clinic, California

A. LEE OSTERMAN, MD
Professor, Hand and Orthopaedic Surgery, The Philadelphia Hand Center, P.C., Thomas Jefferson University Hospital, Philadelphia, Pennsylvania

MIN JUNG PARK, MD, MMSc
Instructor, Department of Orthopaedic Surgery, Perelman School of Medicine, University of Pennsylvania, Philadelphia, Pennsylvania

T.J. PIANTA, MD
Combined Hand Surgery Fellowship Program, University of Connecticut, Farmington; Hartford Hospital, Hartford, Connecticut

VINCENZA RAGONE, MEng
Biomedical Engineer, IRCCS Policlinico San Donato, Milan, Italy

PIETRO RANDELLI, MD
Assistant Professor, Università degli Studi di Milano, IRCCS Policlinico San Donato, Milan, Italy

MARK REKANT, MD
Assistant Professor, Department of Orthopaedic Surgery, Thomas Jefferson University, Philadelphia, Pennsylvania

PETER C. RHEE, DO
Fellow, Division of Hand Surgery, Department of Orthopedic Surgery, Mayo Clinic, Rochester, Minnesota

TAMARA D. ROZENTAL, MD
Assistant Professor, Department of Orthopaedics, Harvard Medical School, Beth Israel Deaconess Medical Center, Boston, Massachusetts

ADAM B. SHAFRITZ, MD
Associate Professor of Orthopaedic Surgery, College of Medicine, University of Vermont, Burlington, Vermont

ALEXANDER Y. SHIN, MD
Professor of Orthopedics, Division of Hand Surgery, Department of Orthopedic Surgery, Mayo Clinic, Rochester, Minnesota

STEVEN S. SHIN, MD, MMSc
Director of Hand Surgery, Kerlan-Jobe Orthopedic Clinic, Los Angeles, California

TAZIO TALAMONTI, MD
Resident, Università degli Studi di Milano, IRCCS Policlinico San Donato, Milan, Italy

JIN BO TANG, MD
Professor and Chair, Department of Hand Surgery, The Hand Surgery Research Center, Affiliated Hospital of Nantong University, Nantong, Jiangsu, China

RAYMOND TSE, MD, FRCSC
Assistant Professor, Division of Plastic Surgery, Department of Surgery, University of Washington; Medical Director, Brachial Plexus Program, Pediatric Plastic Surgery, Seattle Children's Hospital, Seattle, Washington

ANDREW J. WATT, MD
Department of Orthopedic Surgery and Sports Medicine, University of Washington; University of Washington Hand Center, Seattle, Washington; Division of Plastic Surgery, Stanford University, Stanford, California

A.H. WONG, MD
Combined Hand Surgery Fellowship Program, University of Connecticut, Farmington; Hartford Hospital, Hartford, Connecticut; University of Miami Plastic Surgery Residency Program, Miami, Florida

REN GUO XIE, MD
Associate Professor, Department of Hand Surgery, The Hand Surgery Research Center,

Affiliated Hospital of Nantong University,
Nantong, Jiangsu, China

JEFFREY YAO, MD
Associate Professor of Orthopaedic Surgery,
Stanford University Medical Center, Palo Alto,
California

DAN A. ZLOTOLOW, MD
Associate Professor, Department of
Orthopaedic Surgery; Attending, Upper
Extremity Center of Excellence, Shriners
Hospitals for Children, Temple University
School of Medicine, Philadelphia,
Pennsylvania

Contents

bony defects. The consistent, robust vascular anatomy and the versatility to function as either a thin, flexible periosteal or corticoperiosteal graft or as a structural cortico-cancellous graft have made this graft a valuable option for addressing recalcitrant nonunions. The rationale, indications, vascular anatomy, and surgical technique of harvesting these grafts from the medial femoral condyle are presented.

suture-free nerve repair is one development that can potentially improve functional nerve recovery and the outcomes of upper extremity reconstruction.

Modern imaging techniques applied to the pediatric glenohumeral joint have advanced understanding of the anatomic changes that occur secondary to muscular imbalance after brachial plexus birth palsy. A better understanding of the progression and timing of glenohumeral dysplasia has also increased awareness and vigilance of this problem. Early detection of glenohumeral joint subluxation is now possible, allowing for prompt treatment with closed, arthroscopic, or open joint reduction with and without tendon transfers. Dynamic ultrasound imaging, Botox, and arthroscopic techniques have expanded treatment options, providing minimally invasive methods to successfully manage glenohumeral joint dysplasia.

Dupuytren disease (DD) is a benign, generally painless connective tissue disorder affecting the palmar fascia that leads to progressive hand contractures. Mediated by myofibroblasts, the disease most commonly begins as a nodule in the palm or finger, and can progress where pathologic cords form leading to progressive flexion deformity of the involved fingers. The palmar skin overlying the cords may become excessively calloused and contracted and involved joints may develop periarticular fibrosis. Although there is no cure, the sequellae of this affliction can be corrected. This article focuses on the role of collagen in DD and the development of a collagen-specific enzymatic treatment for DD contractures.

Digital tendon repair is one of the most common issues in hand surgery and also one of the most vexing. A repair must withstand the forces imparted on it during early motion. Common clinical scenarios that challenge the hand surgeon are flexor tendon injuries in zone II, zone I, and extensor tendons. Repair of tendons that have flat morphology present a particular challenge to achieving a strong repair while maintaining the native tendon shape. This article evaluates modern tendon repair techniques. Early clinical experience using such methods have shown clinical success of improved motion and no known ruptures.

Nerve transfers have been performed for many years, but the technique is further developing and gaining increased recognition as a time-tested procedure. The original operations are continually modified to treat a wide variety of peripheral nerve injuries, and yield reliable results. In addition, nerve transfers can be used in conjunction with tendon transfers or nerve grafts in order to best treat a specific patient's set of deficits. This review of nerve transfers briefly discusses the evolution of the technique, general principles, some specific transfers, post-operative rehabilitation, and their place on the reconstructive ladder.

HAND CLINICS

Preface

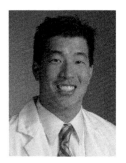

Jeffrey Yao, MD
Guest Editor

It is with great pleasure that I present the November 2012 Issue of *Hand Clinics* focused on New and Emerging Technology in the Treatment of the Upper Extremity.

Hand and Upper Extremity Surgery remains a constantly evolving discipline. Such as in many other specialties within medicine, technology and treatment modalities evolve continuously to meet the growing needs of surgeons and patients alike. As a result of these technological advances, patient care has improved vastly over the decades. Patients are staying in the hospital for shorter periods and are recuperating faster. Time lost from work and from play has steadily decreased with these improvements. While the fundamental pathologies we treat as hand and upper extremity surgeons have not changed much, the ways we treat many of them have seen significant change with time. Some changes are dramatic; some are subtle. Some are for the better; some are for the worse. Thankfully, the latter are the minority, and these changes are quickly identified and short-lived.

Competing factors play a role when evaluating new technology in the treatment of hand and upper extremity disorders in this day and age. These factors include equipment cost and marketing pressures from device companies balanced against the true benefit derived by our patients particularly when compared to older, potentially less costly and more "tried and true" modalities. Simply presenting a new tool to fix an old problem does not ensure its superiority over techniques that have been employed longer and have survived more scrutiny. It is our duty as clinicians and scientists to review new technology critically as it arises and to be able to differentiate appropriately between treatment modalities that are sound and will significantly benefit our patients from those that may simply be the result of shrewd marketing or may be a triumph of technology over reason.

I believe all the articles prepared for this volume of *Hand Clinics* have been thoughtfully prepared and researched and provide an objective view of each of the emerging technologies discussed. However, the reader should always keep in mind that with new technology, it is often difficult if not impossible to report high-level evidence from the beginning to support these techniques, as this type of data takes time to accumulate. Therefore, some of the topics discussed herein, while exciting and novel, are based on lower level evidence and the results and recommendations should be viewed accordingly.

I am eternally grateful to the authors of the following pages for their time and efforts to compile such thoughtful articles. I have learned an immense amount from these cutting-edge articles and I believe our readers will as well.

Hand Clin 28 (2012) xiii–xiv
http://dx.doi.org/10.1016/j.hcl.2012.09.001
0749-0712/12/$ – see front matter

hand.theclinics.com

I would also like to thank my many mentors, colleagues, trainees, and patients for their involvement in my continuous drive to challenge myself to look for better ways of treating patients with hand and upper extremity disorders, not necessarily to reinvent the wheel, but to improve upon it.

Last, I would like to thank my wife, Jennifer, whose unwavering support of my academic pursuits will never go unappreciated.

Jeffrey Yao, MD
Robert A. Chase Hand and Upper Limb Center
Stanford University Medical Center
450 Broadway Street
Suite C-442
Redwood City, CA 94063, USA

E-mail address:
jyao@stanford.edu

Bone Graft Substitutes

Reena A. Bhatt, MD[a], Tamara D. Rozental, MD[b],*

KEYWORDS

- Bone graft • Bone graft substitute • Bone substitute • Bone replacement • Autograft • Allograft
- Demineralized bone matrix • Bone morphogenetic protein • Distal radius fracture • Nonunion

KEY POINTS

- Preference is often given to autograft in the form of cancellous, cortical, or corticocancellous grafts from donor sites, such as the iliac crest and distal radius.
- Advances in surgical management and medical research have produced a wide array of potential substances that can be used for bone graft substitute.
- Any discussion on bone grafts and substitutes should begin with the goals of bone replacement.

Replacement of missing bone stock is a reconstructive challenge to upper extremity surgeons and decision-making with regards to available choices remains difficult. Preference is often given to autograft in the form of cancellous, cortical, or corticocancellous grafts from donor sites, such as the iliac crest and distal radius. However, the available volume from such donor sites is limited and fraught with potential complications. Advances in surgical management and medical research have produced a wide array of potential substances that can be used for bone graft substitute. Considerations in selecting bone grafts and substitutes include characteristic capabilities, availability, patient morbidity, immunogenicity, potential disease transmission, and cost variability. Recent decades have seen a market driven stimulus to use bone substitute products despite little comparative evidence for indications and safety. Each has associated benefits and potential negatives, and physicians must carefully weigh the risk/benefit ratio before making their selection. Any discussion on bone grafts and substitutes should begin with the goals of bone replacement. The following important properties are paramount for consideration for bone grafting, and ideally the graft should provide[1–3]

- Osteogenesis: grafts with osteogenic cells have the necessary synthetic machinery, osteoblasts, or progenitor cells able to survive the transplantation process to produce new bone.
- Osteoinduction: the environment of growth proteins necessary to induce differentiation of host progenitor cells to bone-producing cells. This is a complex process involving the mediation of multiple signaling factors, including the transforming growth factor (TGF)-β superfamily.
- Osteoconduction: a bioactive matrix that provides the appropriate framework for bony growth. This matrix supports and facilitates fibrovascular ingrowth, host progenitor cell migration into the scaffold, osteoblast attachment, and eventual manufacture of new bone. This passive ability depends on direct contact with exposed bony surfaces.
- Structural integrity: structural strength of the grafted material in compressive strength, and resistance to torsion and shear.
- Osteointegrative ability, the capability of the graft to integrate and bond to the host bone.

The authors have nothing to disclose.
[a] Department of Plastic Surgery, Warren Alpert Medical School of Brown University, The Miriam and Rhode Island Hospitals, 235 Plain Street, Bayside Suite 102, Providence, RI 02903, USA; [b] Department of Orthopaedics, Harvard Medical School, Beth Israel Deaconess Medical Center, 330 Brookline Avenue, Stoneman 10, Boston, MA 02215, USA
* Corresponding author.
E-mail address: trozenta@bidmc.harvard.edu

Hand Clin 28 (2012) 457–468
http://dx.doi.org/10.1016/j.hcl.2012.08.001
0749-0712/12/$ – see front matter © 2012 Elsevier Inc. All rights reserved.

hand.theclinics.com

AUTOGRAFT

The gold standard example of a substance that provides all of these factors is autogenous bone graft. For use in the upper extremity, autograft is most typically obtained from the iliac crest, proximal ulna, or distal radius. The Iliac crest, with its potential source of cortical and cancellous bone graft, is the current go to for autograft. These grafts are the benchmark to which allograft and substitutes are compared for in vivo performance.

Transplanted cancellous bone graft may have few osteoblasts, but contains predecessor cells that maintain osteogenic potential and therefore the ability to form new bone. The local graft environment also affords an enriched osteoinductive environment and one that is osteoconductive, but has little initial structural strength. Cortical graft, however, can assist in maintaining structural support while providing osteoconduction and some osteoinduction. Cortical graft provides strong structural support within the first 6 weeks after transfer, but is prone to fracture and prolonged osteointegration, resorption, and remodeling. Cortical and cancellous grafts should be stabilized with fixation during the healing process.

In addition to the iliac crest, autogenous bone graft may be obtained from the Gerdy tubercle of the tibia, distal tibia, the proximal ulna, and distal radius. Autograft is not in endless supply and may be associated with significant donor morbidity including pain, fracture, wound healing problems, hernia, injury to local nerves, blood loss, and abdominal perforation. A retrospective review of 239 patients showed an overall major complication rate of 8.6%, including infection, prolonged wound drainage, large hematoma, reoperation, pain greater than 6 months, sensory loss, and unsightly scars. The minor complication rate was 20.6%, including superficial infection, minor wound problems, temporary sensory loss, and mild or resolving pain.[4] Most morbidity for iliac crest harvest seems to be pain at the donor site, followed by sensory loss as shown in prospective and retrospective studies.[5,6] Harvesting autogenous bone graft is associated with increased operative time, hospital stay, and cost.[3] Furthermore, harvesting autograft is not possible in patients who have compromised iliac crest bone (undergone recent harvesting or fractures) or who may not have adequate volume available (patients with osteoporosis). Autograft fusion rates are also not universal, with reported failure rates between 5% and 35%.[7]

Bone Marrow

Bone marrow, a subset of autograft, is most useful for its osteogenic and osteoinductive capability. Bone marrow aspirate (BMA) may be obtained readily from the anterior iliac crest by a percutaneous route; BMA is highly cellular, allowing the acquisition of stem cells, with potential osteogenic aptitude, and growth factors that create an osteoinductive environment. Bone marrow is not an osteoconductive or structurally capable material, and has thus been used with demineralized bone matrix (DBM) carriers to take advantage of the osteoconductive properties of DBM. Bone marrow can be injected into bone defects alone or mixed with autograft as an extender.[8] BMA has also been used to supplement composite grafts: although the composite is osteoconductive, augmentation with BMA renders osteoinductive and osteogenic properties. In a prospective randomized trial, involving 18 medical centers, Chapman and colleagues[9] compared the use of BMA to supplement Collagraft composite graft with autograft in long bone fractures with internal or external fixation. The authors reported that composite grafts resulted in similar union rates and functional outcomes with fewer complications than autografts. Tiedeman and colleagues[10] studied the use of BMA, DBM, composite grafts of both, and autograft controls in a canine tibial nonunion model. The composite graft of DBM with bone marrow produced improved results compared with either agent alone and similar results to autograft.

There are multiple bone marrow aspiration sets available. One packaged harvesting system is Imbibe (Orthovita, Malvern, PA), which includes a Jamshidi needle and syringe.[11] The Healos bone graft replacement kit (Depuy, Raynham, MA) has bone marrow aspiration needles that are packaged with an osteoconductive matrix. Many of the companies that sell DBM also market bone marrow aspiration kits. The industry cost averages $375 per kit.[12]

ALLOGRAFT

Cadaveric allograft is a common choice for the upper extremity surgeon, but is limited in terms of the ideal bone graft characteristics outlined previously. The architectural foundation of allograft creates a natural osteoconductive scaffold for fibrovascular ingrowth, cellular attraction from the host interface, and eventual bony development. Allograft also demonstrates good osteointegrative capability at the host–recipient interface. By nature of allograft processing, osteogenic cells (osteoblasts and precursors) are largely unavailable. Although osteoinductive properties fluctuate depending on the preparation of the allograft, these grafts provide for variable structural support.

Allografts are available as fresh, frozen, or freeze-dried preparations. Fresh allografts are not routinely used because they may be quite immunogenic and are at greater risk for disease transmission; concerns or capabilities with storage also limit their use. Frozen allografts are primarily prepared by freezing, whereas freeze-dried allografts are prepared by freezing, then dehydrating to approximately 5% of water. Further processing of allograft can be performed with ethylene oxide or gamma radiation to make allografts safer with regards to immunogenicity and transference of viral particles, bacteria, and malignant cells. This processing, however, reduces the osteoinductive capabilities, structural strength, and bone incorporation. Gamma irradiation tends to affect the mechanical stability more, whereas ethylene oxide affects the osteoinductive capability. Frozen allografts are slightly more immunogenic and have a shorter shelf life than freeze-dried (up to 5 years if stored properly, versus an indefinite lifetime for the freeze-dried form) but freeze-dried allografts have less structural strength and osteoinductive capability. Frozen allograft may be used immediately after thawing, whereas freeze-dried forms are prone to microfracture and are weaker after rehydration.[13,14]

Allograft is available as cortical, cancellous, or corticocancellous graft. Forms include powder, chips, wedges, pegs, dowels, or struts. Allograft may be machined in custom shapes if necessary. Cancellous graft is traditionally incorporated by enchondral ossification through the allograft scaffold, with minimal initial strength that increases over time. In contrast, incorporation of cortical graft is by creeping substitution by way of intramembranous ossification, with initial inherent structural strength, which weakens with resorption, eventually strengthening with bony deposition and organization.[15]

These grafts are useful in many circumstances, especially in situations where inadequate donor autograft is available. Allograft bone is often used in distal radius and other upper limb fractures, where there is concern for poor healing potential (eg, patients with osteoporosis or who use tobacco), established nonunion, and fractures with extensive comminution. Cancellous allograft has been described in the treatment of bone voids after curettage, smaller nonunions, metaphyseal defects of tibial plateau fractures, and tibial pilon fractures. Cortical and corticocancellous allograft have also found widespread use in the management of nonunions of the femur and humerus, after tumor surgery, and for structural integrity with segmental bone loss. In these cases, allograft may be mixed with cancellous autograft to aid in the creation of an osteogenic and osteoinductive environment.[16]

Complications with allograft use include graft fracture, lack of integration with surrounding peripheral bone, and infection. Increasing mass of allograft is associated with increased risk of bacterial infection and nonunion. Transference of viral particles also is a potential concern.[2,17] Examples of allograft include allograft bone from Osteotech (Graftech, Magnifuse, and traditional allograft; Osteotech, Eatontown, NJ); Cornerstone (Medtronic Sofamor Danek, Memphis, TN); Allopure (Wright Medical Technology, Arlington, TN); University of Florida Tissue Bank; and Raptos, which is often mixed with DBM (Citagenix, Quebec, Canada). There are also composite products available, including Opteform (DBM Osteofil with corticocancellous allograft; Exactech, Gainesville, FL); Orthoblast (DBM with cancellous allograft; Citagenix, Quebec, Canada); and Dynablast (DBM and cancellous allograft; Citagenix, Quebec, Canada). The allograft derived from the Musculoskeletal Transplant Foundation, Lifenet, and Allosource dominates the current US market share of allograft. Allograft prices varies from the $150 range for smaller-volume graft with price increasing to thousands of dollars for larger-volume or newer combination products.

DEMINERALIZED BONE MATRIX

DBM is allograft that has been crushed to a consistent particle size and decalcified (demineralized). Subsequent refinements in processing are performed to reduce immunogenicity and disease transmission. The remnant maintains the trabecular collagenous organization of the original allograft. This organized scaffold serves as the osteoconductive component of the DBM. Removal of the mineral phase of the allograft improves the potential, albeit variable, availability of osteoinductive growth factors. The framework allows for new vessel ingrowth and the infiltration of mesenchymal and precursor cells, and eventual bone formation. The osteoinductive growth proteins available in the extracellular matrix induce mesenchymal cells to differentiate into bone-producing cells, but this ability is variable depending on storage, processing, and the inherent capability of the donor tissue. DBM does not impart significant structural integrity, but is useful for filling defects.[18]

Currently available DBM are produced with carrier vehicles, such as glycerol, starch, hyaluronic acid, collagen, and saline. Different forms on the market include moldable paste, putty, strips, gel, freeze-dried powder, and granules. Agents, such as DBM, are often mixed with harvested autograft or bone marrow to augment and improve bone healing and extend the volume of the autograft. DBM has also been combined with calcium sulfate or allograft products. These agents are widely used in filling bony defects after fracture (metaphyseal defects); nonunions in long bone fractures; bony cavities, such as subsequent to curettage of phalangeal cysts; and augmenting craniofacial reconstruction and arthrodesis procedures. DBM may be useful in distal radius fractures where there is concern for poor healing potential, such as in people with diabetes or those who smoke.

The primary negatives of DBM are lack of structural strength; concerns for reaction to certain carriers, such as glycerol; and possible disease transmission compared with standard autograft.[15,17,19] Sassard and colleagues[20] compared iliac crest autograft with a local autograft-DBM construct (Grafton, Osteotech, Eatontown, NJ) in posterolateral lumbar spinal fusion. Rates of fusion did not vary significantly between the two groups. Their results prompted the idea that Grafton may be a useful autograft extender. In the upper extremity, Hierholzer and colleagues[21] compared the use of Grafton DBM and iliac crest autograft in delayed union and nonunions of the humerus in a retrospective cohort series. Osseus union was 97% in the DBM group and 100% in the autograft group and mean time to union was similar in both groups. The autograft group had a 44% complication rate including prolonged pain or superficial infection. Their conclusion was that both were useful in delayed and nonunion of humeral shaft fractures, with a higher complication rate in the autograft group. With regards to distal radius fractures, nonunions are uncommon because this bone is typically well-vascularized. Small retrospective studies suggest that indications for DBM in distal radius fractures is limited to patients with poor healing potential, such as those with diabetes, those who smoke, patients with peripheral vascular disease, and those with autoimmune disorders.[22] It is difficult to make recommendations in upper extremity surgery secondary to the paucity of randomized clinical trials using these products; most published trials are animal studies or small retrospective studies.[23]

Commonly available DBM products include Grafton DBM and Xpanse (Osteotech, Eatontown, NJ); Dynagraft and Acell Connexus (Citagenix, Quebec, Canada); Optium DBM (Depuy, Raynham, MA); and Osteofil (Medtronics Sofamor Danek, Memphis, TN). Examples of composite DBM products include DBX (DBM plus collagen carrier; Musculoskeletal Transplant Foundation and Synthes, Paoli, PA); Orthoblast and Dynablast (DBM with cancellous allograft; Citagenix, Quebec, Canada); Opteform (DBM Osteofil with corticocancellous allograft; Exactech, Gainesville, FL); Allomatrix (DBM with Osteoset calcium sulfate; Wright Medical Technology, Arlington, TN); and Allomatrix Custom (DBM with cancellous bone graft; Wright Medical Technology, TN). The market leader in DBM products was the Musculoskeletal Tissue Foundation. It should be noted that many of these products are cross-listed by other companies. With market competition, costs of DBM have decreased but this product is still likely to be more expensive than allograft. DBM products range from $140 for 1 mL to more than $500 for 5 mL, with increasing price depending on volume and composition.[12]

BONE GRAFT SUBSTITUTES

To bypass donor site morbidity, volume availability, potential immunogenicity, and disease transmission, a variety of bone graft substitutes have been developed. No perfect substitute yet exists that embodies all the ideal qualities of autograft. Except for bone morphogenetic proteins (BMPs), these products do not routinely have osteogenic or osteoinductive capabilities unless mixed with autograft or BMA. Most of these agents have osteoconductive capability, creating a matrix for host cells to regenerate bone. They are also osteointegrative. The ideal bone substitutes are resorbable and have a strength profile similar to cortical or cancellous bone, but this remains variable among the different products. Cost is also highly variable. There are a multitude of compositions in the market and choice of substance depends on patient injury characteristics. These products are most useful in well-vascularized bony defects with good soft tissue coverage. Currently available products include mineral derived graft, cements, calcium sulfate, bioactive glass, and growth factors.

Minerals

Hydroxyapatite (HA) is the basic component of the mineral phase of bone. Its unstable crystalline structure allows for exchange of ions, thus its composition fluctuates between the mineral salt precursors calcium phosphate and tricalcium phosphate (TCP) in vivo. This is the basis behind the clinical introduction of the calcium phosphate salts, such as TCP and HA, in the 1980s.[16] The mineral compounds resemble bone precursors and their inherent porous nature makes these materials good osteoconductive and osteointegrative agents. Although such agents as TCP may have initial structural strength, with remodeling and replacement the structural stability is finite before bony deposition. They lack inherent osteoinductive or osteogenic aptitude.

These highly porous compounds act as scaffolds and induce fibrovascular ingrowth, inward margination of bone-producing cells, and osteoid deposition onto their well-developed surface area. Mineralization and remodeling occur with eventual replacement by mature bone. These agents are available in paste, putty, solid matrix, or granule form.

Coralline HA

Coralline HA is derived from marine coral, which has an inherently highly porous and regular skeleton. The processing of the marine coral includes removal of organic matter and treatment of the calcium carbonate backbone. Naturally occurring coralline HA is sterilized calcium carbonate, which is very brittle and quick to resorb. Most coralline HA is now processed with ammonium phosphate and sterilized, thus converting the calcium carbonate skeleton to crystalline HA. This organized framework closely resembles that of trabecular bone. Coralline HA comes in granule or block form.

Uses of coralline HA have extended to distal radius and tibial plateau fractures, primarily for addressing metaphyseal defects. Coralline HA is often combined with autograft and more recently has been shown to be an effective carrier for BMPs. Boden and colleagues[24] studied the arthrodesis rate in the posterolateral lumbar spine in a rabbit model and found that coralline HA was an excellent carrier for osteoinductive growth proteins. In a series of 40 patients with displaced tibial plateau fractures with metaphyseal defects, Bucholz and colleagues[25] examined the use of cancellous autograft versus interporous HA. Follow-up clinical and radiologic assessment demonstrated no significant difference between the two groups. Resultant bone voids after benign bone tumor resections, located in the humerus, tibia, femur, calcaneus, ileum, fibula, and ulna, have been successfully managed with coralline HA.[26] Wolfe and colleagues[27] used coralline HA in 21 patients with distal radius fractures and found that it was an effective alternative to autograft for maintenance of articular congruity when used with external fixation and percutaneous Kirschner wires.

ProOsteon (Interpore International, Irvine, CA) is one example of available coralline HA. Despite its bonelike appearance, coralline HA has not been shown to have osteoclastic resorption, thus limiting the potential for true bony remodeling. This material has good compressive strength but low tensile strength, may be quite brittle, and may have delayed resorption. The implant is resorbed approximately 5% to 10% per year and remains visible on radiographs.[28] ProOsteon averages $200 to $600 for standard upper extremity use.[12]

Ceramics

The synthetic mineral salts, HA and β-TCP, are calcium phosphate–based ceramics. Ceramics are inorganic solids produced in a highly thermal process known as "sintering," where they are heated between 700°C and 1300°C to form their crystalline structure. This allows for improved strength but slower resorption.[2,28]

The chemical nature of HA ($Ca_{10}[PO_4]_6[OH]_2$,) is similar to the mineral phase of bone and is very osteoconductive and osteointegrative. HA-based products have been used in posterior lumbar fusions; coating of implants, such as femoral stems and cups; and external fixator pins to assist in osteointegration at the host–bone interface. Synthetic HA shows a delayed rate of resorption and is brittle in tensile strength.[19,29] Baer and colleagues[30] evaluated their results with Endobon (HA ceramic; Biomet, Warsaw, IN) for use in filling the defect after curettage of enchondromas or cysts in the upper extremity and showed excellent 5-year follow-up results. The authors' conclusion was that HA ceramic was a valid alternative to autogenous graft without donor morbidity. Werber and colleagues[31] used ceramic HA as a structural bone substitute to correct bone defects after distal radius fractures in 14 patients treated with internal or external fixation. Osseous integration and incorporation was demonstrated by magnetic resonance imaging and biopsy and the authors concluded that HA is a well-tolerated acceptable alternative to bone graft in distal radius fractures with bone defects. Some available HA products include Cerabone and Ostim (aap Implante AG, Berlin, Germany); Endobon (Biomet, Warsaw, IN); and ProOsteon 500 (Biomet, Warsaw, IN).

The composition of β-TCP ($Ca_3[PO_4]_2$) is also akin to the mineral phase of bone. This compound, like HA, is extremely porous and interconnected, helping to direct fibrovascular invasion and eventual bony replacement. A portion of TCP undergoes conversion to HA. These substances act as bioactive osteoconductive scaffolds and integrate well with host bone.[2] TCP is more porous, resorbs at a quicker rate than HA, and is mechanically weaker in compression than HA.[18,32] There are several potentially usable agents in the TCP category including ChronOS (Synthes, Paoli, PA); Vitoss (Orthovita, Malvern, PA); Cerasorb (Curasan-AG, Frankfurt, Germany); Conduit TCP and Orthograft (Depuy, Raynham, MA); and Osferion (Olympus, Tokyo, Japan).

HA and TCP are available in granule, block, powder, or putty forms. Both have compressive strength similar to cancellous bone graft and are brittle, with poor resistance to shear. HA notably seems to have delayed resorption, whereas resorption of TCP is by osteoclast and varies between 6 and 24 months. Both are beneficial materials to act as scaffolds in periarticular fractures treated with fixation, such as distal radius and tibial plateau fractures. TCP has been described for use in nonunion of the femur, tibia, calcaneus, humerus, and radius.[33] HA, in particular, has been described broadly for implant coating.[34,35] TCP and HA have been used as combination products and to combat the slower resorption of the HA. TCP has been described as void filler after curettage of benign bone tumors in the upper extremity. Vitoss (TCP; Orthovita, Malvern, PA) has also been shown in some studies to decrease short-term postoperative pain when used to fill iliac crest donor sites.[36–38]

Composites

These products are often used as expanders for bone autograft, combined with bone marrow, and as carriers for osteoinductive BMP.[28] Chapman and colleagues[9] showed the benefits of the composite Collagraft (collagen, HA, TCP, Zimmer, Warsaw, IN) with BMA over autograft in a multicenter randomized prospective clinical trial treating long bone fractures. In a rat model, Collagraft, Collagraft plus BMA, and BMA alone were compared for bone formation; Collagraft plus BMA showed significantly higher bone formation.[39] Kon and colleagues[40] studied bone marrow–derived cells seeded on a HA ceramic carrier in a sheep model to repair tibial gaps. In the cell-seeded HA carrier group, bone formation was found to occur within the porous HA carrier and around it as compared with being primarily limited to growth around the HA cylinder in the HA group. Stiffness was also improved in the cell-seeded carrier group. Their results suggest that use of autologous cells seeded on a HA carrier results in more expedient bone healing than HA alone.

There are many composite products available including Collagraft (bovine collagen/HA/TCP; Zimmer, IN); MBCP (HA and TCP; Citagenix, Quebec, Canada); OpteMx (HA and TCP; Exactech, Gainesville, FL); and Healos (HA-coated bovine collagen; Depuy, Raynham, MA). These are often mixed with BMA or as bone graft extenders. Eclipse (HA and TCP; Citagenix, Quebec, Canada) may be mixed with DBM, as can BoneSave (TCP and HA; Stryker, Hopkinton, MA). List prices range from $500 to $1500 per unit with varying size, with 1-mL aliquots around $200.[12]

Cements

Cements were developed to improve the profile of calcium phosphate bone substitutes with more moldability to custom-fill defects and withstand compressive loads. Calcium phosphate–based cements crystallize to dahllite, a carbonated HA that maintains a similar structure to most of the mineral phase of bone. Because bone cement is a paste before setting, it may be conveniently injected to fill a bone defect. Their innate strength lies in their osteoconductive capability, osteointegrative capability, malleability, and having increased compressive strength once set.

These compounds are available as injectable liquid or moldable putty and set with an isothermic reaction. They resorb by dissolution and osteoclast resorption.

Disadvantages include weakness in torsion and shear. One very significant concern is the potential extrusion of the cement into soft tissues or joints during injection, thus potentially damaging surrounding tissues.

Antibiotics and chemotherapeutic agents may be used to augment the cements. Calcium phosphate cements were initially approved for augmenting distal radius fractures and are now frequently used in cavitational metaphyseal defects of the distal radius, tibial plateau, and calcaneal fractures with concomitant internal-external fixation. Widespread use has been described for vertebroplasties and reinforcement of pedicle screw fixation in burst fractures of the vertebrae.[19] A meta-analysis by Bajammal and colleagues[41] reviewed available studies in the orthopedic literature with regards to the use of calcium phosphate–based cements in the management of intertrochanteric femoral, femoral neck, calcaneal, tibial plateau, and distal radius fractures. Compared with those patients who were treated with autograft, patients managed with calcium phosphate cement had significantly less loss of fracture reduction. Additional significant findings included less pain with the use of cement. In the upper extremity, Zimmermann and colleagues[42] used injectable calcium phosphate bone cement in their prospective study of 52 osteoporotic, menopausal women with unstable intra-articular distal radius fractures. The 2-year outcomes of percutaneous pinning with cast immobilization for 6 weeks versus the use of injectable calcium phosphate bone cement with pin and screw fixation and immobilization for 3 weeks were compared. The patients managed with bone cement to augment pin fixation showed better functional outcome, restoration of motion, and grip strength. These patients had significantly less loss of reduction compared with the control (nonbone cement) group. In a prospective randomized multicenter study, 323 patients with distal radius fractures were randomized to closed reduction and immobilization with Norian SRS cement for 6 weeks or closed reduction, immobilization, or external fixation for 6 to 8 weeks. Early results were better in the Norian group. However, at 1 year, no clinical differences were detected.[43,44]

Two examples of currently used products include BoneSource (Stryker, Hopkinton, MA) and Norian SRS (Synthes, Paoli, PA). Bone Source is tetracalcium phosphate and dicalcium phosphate dehydrate that when mixed forms a paste that hardens in situ forming a porous HA. One disadvantage of BoneSource is the requirement of a dry environment for setting. Norian SRS is monocalcium phosphate monohydrate, α-TCP, calcium carbonate, and sodium phosphate solution. This compound is an injectable liquid, radiopaque, and can be percutaneously injected under fluoroscopy to fill a bony void or fracture site. Additional products available include ChronOS Inject (Synthes, Paoli, PA); Callos (Acumed, Hillsboro, OR); Hydroset (Stryker, Hopkinton, MA); Alpha BSM (Etex, Cambridge, MA); Mimix and Calcibon (Biomet, Warsaw, IN). Calcium phosphate cements are costly, with 5 mL costing more than $1000.[12]

Calcium Sulfate

Calcium sulfate (Ca[SO_4]; plaster of Paris) has been available as a void filler for more than 100 years. Calcium sulfate is heated gypsym and made into powder form, with eventual crystalline structure described as alphahemihydrate. It is primarily osteoconductive in nature, with better compressive strength than cancellous bone, but poor tensile strength. The structural support of calcium sulfate seems to be less than the calcium phosphate formulations. Primary drawbacks include inconsistency in crystalline structure during setting and rapid resorption by dissolution of the product, which may create an imbalance between bony replacement and resorption. There is also an association with serous wound drainage after use.[11,45]

Available forms include pellets, blocks, and more recently injectable pastes. Calcium sulfate combination products have been described for similar indications to the previous bone cements and ceramics, including metaphyseal injuries, acetabular fractures, lumbar pedicle screws, tumor voids, and patellar and calcaneal fractures.[46] Available products include BonePlast (Interpore Cross International, Irvine, CA); MIIG X3 and Osteoset (Wright Medical Technology, Arlington, TN); Stimulan (Biocomposites, Wilmington, NC); and Calceon (Synthes, Paoli, PA).

The realm of calcium sulfate products has widened to include calcium sulfate mixed with other bone substitute products, DBM, and antibiotics. Calcium sulfate is also not infrequently used to augment and extend autograft for long bone injuries. Calcium sulfate products can be impregnated with antibiotics, such as the product Osteoset (Wright Medical Technology, Arlington, TN).

These products may be used to fill osteomyelitic bone voids with slowly eluting antibiotics. Allomatrix (DBM with osteoset calcium sulfate; Wright Medical Technology, TN) is another example of a composite bone substitute, taking advantage of the osteoconductive properties of Osteoset with the osteoinductive properties of DBM. Prodense (Wright Medical Technology, TN) is a composite calcium phosphate and calcium sulfate that has been described for treatment of subchondral bone loss. Pro-Stim (Wright Medical Technology, Arlington, TN) is Prodense calcium phosphate and calcium sulfate with added DBM. Calcium sulfate products can range from $400 for 5-mL products to more than $2000 depending on the composition with additional bone-augmentation products.[12]

Bioactive Glass

Bioactive glass is a solid material composed of sodium oxide, calcium oxide, silicone dioxide, and phosphorus. Bioactivity, the interaction between host bone and graft, depends on the silicone content of the glass, with ideal bonding with 45% to 52% silica in the agent. These agents demonstrate strong host–graft bonding as the silica breaks down after exposure to host fluids, forming a silica layer from which HA is then laid down. This results in a strong integrative response at the tissue–agent interface, creating an enriched osteoconductive environment. Advantages of bioactive glass include its strong and unique bonding capability, osteoconductive properties, ability to modify the composition, possible osteostimulation, and good resorption. However, bioactive glass offers little structural support.

The product is available as microspheres, fibers, paste, and porous implants. These agents may be injected into a defect or molded into putty. Bioactive glass has been described for use in screw augmentation especially for osteoporotic bone, vertebroplasty, distal radius fractures, and tibial plateau fractures.[28,47] A case report has described the use of bioactive glass in an intra-articular distal radius fracture in a female with osteoporosis.[48] Bioactive glass is currently available for use in trauma and orthopedic surgery but no evidence-based guidelines have been published for upper extremity surgery. Bioactive glass products available include Cortoss and Rhakoss (Orthovita, Malvern, PA) and NovaBone (NovaBone, Jacksonville, FL). Although the accurate industry average price of Cortoss was unable to be obtained, one estimate suggested a starting price of $800.[49]

Bone Morphogenetic Proteins

Bone formation requires growth factors, osteogenic cells, and extracellular matrix. A progenitor cell arises from a stem cell with eventual preosteoblast and subsequent osteoblast formation. Osteoblasts create the bony matrix. When osteoblasts become trapped within the matrix that has developed, they become osteocytes. These cells are an integral part of bone turnover. When fractures occur, a hematoma develops and cells within the hematoma secrete growth factors, which then stimulate bone formation. Growth factors are polypeptides that promote cell growth by binding to certain receptors. The TGF superfamily is a subset of these factors that has been shown to be influential in regulating development from the embryonic stage to bony healing. BMPs, a subset of the TGF family, are critical in instigating the mitogenesis of the multipotential mesenchymal cells to form osteoprogenitor cells. These specific factors are important in inducing migration of progenitor cells, differentiation, angiogenesis, and vascular ingrowth. They also help direct the mineralization and remodeling of formed bone. Growth factors are therefore primarily osteoinductive in nature, with no osteogenic, osteoconductive, or structural capability. This lack of osteoconductive ability is why BMPs require an osteoconductive carrier, such as collagen or bone mineral substitute. The osteoinductive capability of growth factors makes this a desirable product to exploit for fracture healing and nonunions and the popularity of BMPs has grown considerably.[11]

Although multiple BMPs have been identified, available recombinant factors include rhBMP-2, rhBMP-7, TGF-β, platelet-derived growth factor (PDGF), and fibroblast growth factor. Clinically available factors are Op-1 (recombinant growth factor rhBMP-7 and collagen carrier; Stryker Biotech, Hopkinton, MA); Infuse (rhBMP-2 and collagen carrier; Medtronic Sofamor Danek, Memphis, TN); Ossigel (basic fibroblast growth factor; DePuy, Warsaw, IN); and more recently Augment (rhPDGF-derived growth factor; BioMimetic, Franklin, TN). Numerous animal studies have shown the effectiveness of these products in long bone fractures, nonunions, spinal fusions, metaphyseal fractures, and hindfoot and ankle fusions.[45]

These agents are often delivered in powder form, which is reconstituted with saline to a paste and then implanted to the fracture site. In large prospective randomized controlled multicenter clinical trial, Friedlaender and colleagues[50] compared the use of Op-1 (rhBMP-7) delivered with type-1 collagen vehicle, with autograft in 124 tibial nonunions. Eighty-one percent of the Op-1 group versus 85% of the autograft group was clinically judged to have been treated successfully. Chronic donor site pain was found in greater than 20% of those patients managed with autograft. In the multicenter

prospective randomized clinical trial by the BMP-2 Evaluation in Surgery for Tibial Trauma-Allograft group, autogenous bone graft was compared with cancellous allograft with rhBMP-2 plus collagen carrier in the treatment of tibial fractures with significant diaphyseal cortical bone loss. At the 12-month follow-up, there was no significant difference in clinical healing outcome; however, more pain was noted in the autogenous group at the donor site.[51] In a multinational, prospective randomized controlled clinical trial, the effectiveness of rhBMP-2 on a collagen sponge (Infuse; Medtronic, TN) was evaluated for open tibial fractures in 450 patients. The group with higher-dose rhBMP-2 placement had faster time to union, improved wound healing, less infections, and fewer secondary interventions compared with the other two groups.[52] Augment (rhPDGF; Biomimetic, TN) was compared with autograft in a prospective randomized multicenter trial studying ankle and hindfoot fusion. Time to radiographic union, full weightbearing, and outcomes were similar between the two groups.[53] BMPs are not currently approved by the Food and Drug Administration (FDA) for use in the upper extremity and, as such, few published clinical studies are available. One small study by Ekrol and colleagues[54] compared autograft with rhBMP-7 in the treatment of osteotomy for malunion of distal radius fractures. Osteolysis was found in the rhBMP-7 group when used in conjunction with external fixation and slower healing rate than autograft when used with internal fixation.

Although the effectiveness of BMP makes a compelling clinical case for its use in a wide variety of indications, BMP products are exceedingly expensive and are often not reimbursed by insurance companies. Also, these factors are not currently FDA approved for use in the upper extremity. Institutional review board approval is often necessary for the use of Op-1. Current FDA indications for Infuse include anterior lumbar spinal fusion at a single level with a threaded interbody cage, open fracture of the tibia, and oral maxillofacial reconstruction with a collagen sponge. Current indications for Op-1 include revision posterolateral fusions and the management of tibial nonunion after internal fixation or Intramedullary nailing.[55] However, both are often used off-label. Recent studies suggest that these benefits may be especially attractive for older patients with osteoporosis who are more likely to have little harvestable bone and are less likely to be able to tolerate a second surgery. However, this use remains to be better elucidated.

Contraindications for the use of BMP include pregnancy, history of cancer, skeletal immaturity, and history of bone tumors. Antibodies to Op-1

		Osteogenesis	Osteoinduction	Osteoconduction	Structural strength	Forms available	Product examples	Comments
Autograft	Cancellous	+	+	+	-	cortical, corticocancellous, cancellous		Harvested from patient, many donor sites
	Cortical	+/-	+	+	+			
Allograft	Cancellous	-	+/-	+	-	powder, chips, wedges, pegs, or struts	Allopure (Wright Medical Technology, TN), Graftech (Osteotech, NJ)	Allograft carry risk of disease transmission and immune reaction. Preparation of allograft to reduce risk of disease transmission impairs osteoinductivity and mechanical strength.
	Cortical	-	-	+	+	whole allograft can be used, such as distal radius		
Bone Marrow Aspirate (BMA)		+	+	-	-	N/A	BMA + Collagraft(osteoconductive collagen/HA/TCP, Zimmer, IN); BMA +Healos (HA coated bovine collagen, Depuy, MA)	Often used to augment osteoconductive carriers by adding precursor cells and osteoinductive environment. Less invasive than autograft harvesting.
Demineralized Bone Matrix (DBM)		-	+	+	+/- if solid dbm	moldable paste, putty, strips, gel, powder, and granules	Grafton DBM (Osteotech, NJ)	DBM often used as composite with other bone substitutes to take advantage of its osteoinductive properties. Osteoconductivity is variable amongst donors and processing methods. Potential in vivo reaction to carrier, ie glycerol.
	Composite	+BMA/ Autograft	+	+	+corticocancellous allograft	granule, solid	Opteform (DBM with corticocancellous allograft, Exactech)	
Coralline Hydroxyapatite (coralline HA)		-	-	+	-	granule or block	ProOsteon (Interpore International, CA)	Can be brittle and slow to resorb. In an animal study, coralline HA plus BMP was superior to coralline HA+autograft in spinal fusion.
Mineral Derived Ceramic		-	-	+		granule, block, powder, or putty	Endobon (HA, Biomet, IN), Vitoss (TCP, Orthovita, PA)	HA has slower resorption, TCP resorbs by 6-24 months. HA well described for implant coating.
	Composite	+BMA	+BMP	+	-	solid, paste, strip, sponge	Healos (HA coated bovine collagen, Depuy, MA)	Autograft, BMA, DBM, and BMPs all described in combination with ceramics.
Calcium Phosphate Cement		-	-	+	+	injectable liquid or moldable putty	Norian SRS (Synthes, PA)	Increased compressive strength in early fracture healing. Can extrude into joint/soft tissue during injection.
Calcium Sulfate		-	-	+	-	pellets, blocks, injectable pastes	MIIG X3 (Wright Medical Technology, TN)	Quick resorption profile 6-12 weeks.
	Composite	+ autograft	+DBM	+	-	pellets, paste	Allomatrix (DBM + calcium sulfate, Wright Medical Technology, TN)	If composite with TCP - will delay resorption profile and increase strength
Bioactive Glass		-	-	+	+	microspheres, fibers, injectable paste, granules	Cortoss (Orthovita, PA), Novabone (NovaBone, FL)	Described for use in screw augmentation in osteoporotic bone. Strong osteointegration profile.
Bone Morphogenetic Proteins (BMP)		-	+	+carrier	-	powder, putty, sponge	Op-1 ((rhBMP-7 + collagen carrier, Stryker Biotech, MA)	Indication for use in fracture nonunion in place of autograft.

+=present -=absent +/-=variable

Fig. 1. Table of bone replacement agents. +, present; −, absent; ±, variable.

have been encountered, with no adverse events reported to date.[14] There has been recent evidence bringing to light clinical concerns about the safety and efficacy of BMPs. Carragee and colleagues[56] performed an investigation of available literature using rhBMP-2 in spinal fusion. In 13 industry-sponsored rhBMP-2 publications reviewed, methodologic bias was found. More recent evidence of unpublished adverse events was encountered, including life-threatening events, radiculitis, ectopic bone formation, osteolysis, and poorer global outcomes. Cost may also be a major obstacle to the use of BMPS, with costs ranging from $3500 to more than $5000.[12]

PRODUCT COMPARISONS: PROPERTIES AND COST

The profiles of the existing agents have many strengths and weaknesses and are illustrated in **Fig. 1**. Although clinical evidence should dictate use, few of the available products have clinical evidence above level V and further randomized prospective clinical trials will further elucidate the appropriate agent for individual problems.[3]

Relative cost is also an important consideration.[16] There seems to be a market shift toward nonallograft bone substitutes. In an analysis of multiple hospital purchasing databases in 2008, purchases of allograft bone and DBM products decreased with increasing clinical use of nonallograft bone substitutes in recent years (**Fig. 2**).[12] Analysis of cost further sheds light on the difficult decisions on clinical use: allograft prices for cancellous chips and 1-mL aliquots of DBM can start in the low hundreds of dollars but rise to thousands

of dollars. The cost of the newer products is significantly higher than their predecessors, such as osteoinductive BMPs currently costing in the $3500 to $5000 price range. These high costs, coupled with off-label use, and decreasing insurance reimbursement for BMPs should cause hesitation in current use for upper extremity surgery until better evidence demonstrates superior performance.[12,57] Mineral-based cements have some clinical evidence supporting their use in metaphyseal loss of distal radius fractures, but their use or the use of bioactive glass should be measured alongside their significant cost. Evidence-based guidelines need to be better established in most of the bone-replacement agents for this reason.

SUMMARY

Autogenous graft remains the gold standard bone replacement substance of choice. Clinical trials have revealed that bone graft substitutes have made substantial advances in comparative bone restoration. With the emergence of a multitude of bone replacement materials, it can be difficult to determine the optimal grafting material for each situation and not all bone replacement products behave the same. Of utmost importance for fracture or nonunion management is appropriate alignment and stabilization, along with maintenance of the soft tissue envelope. Consideration for bone replacement material should include critical examination of the healing environment and whether there is primarily a structural bony deficit, a large bone cavity, or difficulty with osteoinduction or osteogenesis in those cases with poor bone healing.

In the upper extremity, limited large clinical studies and market-driven analysis have made decisions related to bone grafts and substitutes challenging. Autogenously derived graft (ie, autogenous bone graft or BMA combinations) is the only option with significant osteogenic ability and continues to be the gold standard in cases with poor vascularity, such as scaphoid fractures or nonunions. For metaphyseal deficits, such as a distal radius fracture, osteoconductive grafts, such as allograft, mineral-based graft, calcium sulfate composite, or bioactive glass, can all be considered with fracture stabilization in a well-vascularized environment. For diaphyseal defects less than 5 to 6 cm, such as radial diaphysis, cortical or corticocancellous autograft or allograft plus or minus BMP may be considered. Vascularized bone graft should be used for larger diaphyseal defects. After curettage of enchondromas or large cysts DBM, cancellous allograft, coralline HA, TCP, HA, or calcium sulfate are all good options in addition to autograft.[18,28]

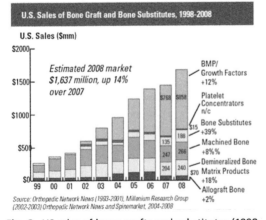

Fig. 2. US sales of bone grafts and substitutes (1998–2008). Market analysis of bone substitutes 1998–2008. Market shift away from allograft and DBM toward BMP and other bone substitutes in recent years. (*From* Mendenhall Associates Inc. Bone grafts and substitutes. Ortho Net News 2008;19(4):18–21; with permission.)

With current market competition, the upper extremity surgeon is confronted with a quandary of choice. Choice of autograft versus bone substitutes should be based on reasonable proof-based clinical evidence for the specific problem at hand. Expense and limited clinical evidence currently limit the use of the bone-replacement materials to situations in which there is inadequate healing potential, extreme comminution or bone loss, nonunion, or advanced age. In an environment of limited reimbursement, physicians need to justify the use of bone-replacement products to situations in which they have been proven to be clinically superior.

REFERENCES

1. Cypher TJ, Grossman JP. Biologic principles of bone graft healing. J Foot Ankle Surg 1996;35:413–7.
2. Moore WR, Graves SE, Bain GI. Synthetic bone graft substitutes. ANZ J Surg 2001;71:354–61.
3. Hartigan BJ, Cohen MS. Use of bone graft substitutes and bioactive materials in treatment of distal radius fractures. Hand Clin 2005;21:449–54.
4. Younger EM, Chapman MW. Morbidity at bone graft donor sites. J Orthop Trauma 1989;3:192–5.
5. Hill NM, Horne JG, Devane PA. Donor site morbidity in the iliac crest bone graft. Aust N Z J Surg 1999; 69(10):726–8.
6. Robertson PA, Wray AC. Natural history of posterior iliac crest bone graft donation for spinal surgery: a prospective analysis of morbidity. Spine 2001; 26(13):1473–6.
7. Burkus JC, Sandhu HS, Longley MG, et al. Use of rhBMP-2 in combination with structural cortical allografts: clinical and radiographic outcomes in anterior lumbar spinal surgery. J Bone Joint Surg 2005; 87:1205–12.
8. Connolly JL, Guse R, Lippiello L, et al. Development of an osteogenic bone marrow preparation. J Bone Joint Surg Am 1989;71:684–91.
9. Chapman MW, Bucholz R, Cornell C. Treatment of acute fractures with a collagen-calcium phosphate graft material: a randomized clinical trial. J Bone Joint Surg Am 1997;79:495–502.
10. Tiedeman JJ, Connolly JF, Strates BS, et al. Treatment of nonunion by percutaneous injection of bone marrow and demineralized bone matrix: an experimental study in dogs. Clin Orthop Relat Res 1991;268:294–302.
11. Ladd AL, Ilan DI. Bone graft substitutes. Operat Tech Plast Reconstr Surg 2003;9(4):151–60.
12. Mendenhall Associates Inc. Bone grafts and substitutes. Ortho Net News 2008;19(4):18–21.
13. Sandhu HS, Grewal HS, Parvataneni H. Bone grafting for spinal fusion. Orthop Clin North Am 1999; 30(4):685–98.
14. Jahangir AA, et al. Bone-graft substitutes in orthopaedic surgery. AAOS; 2008. Available at: http://www.aaos.org/news/aaosnow/jan08/reimbursement2.asp. Accessed January 1, 2012.
15. De Long WG, McKee M, Watson T, et al. Bone grafts and bone graft substitutes in orthopaedic trauma surgery. J Bone Joint Surg Am 2007;89(3):649–58.
16. Ladd AL, Pliam NB. Bone graft substitutes in the radius and upper limb. J Hand Surg 2003;3(4):227–45.
17. Giannoudis PV, Dinopoulos H, Tsirides E. Bone substitutes: an update. Injury 2005;36:S20–7.
18. Finkemeier CG. Current concepts review: bone-grafting and bone-graft substitutes. J Bone Joint Surg Am 2002;84(3):454–64.
19. Keating JF, Mcqueen MM. Substitutes for autologous bone graft in orthopaedic trauma. J Bone Joint Surg Br 2001;83(1):3–8.
20. Sassard WR, Eidman DK, Gray PM. Augmenting local bone with grafton demineralized bone matrix for posterolateral lumbar spine fusion: avoiding second site autologous bone harvest. Orthopedics 2000;23: 1059–65.
21. Hierholzer C, Sama D, Toro JB. Plate fixation of ununited humeral shaft fractures: effect of type of bone graft on healing. J Bone Joint Surg Am 2006;88:1442–7.
22. Segalman KA, Clarg GL. Un-united fractures of the distal radius: a report of 12 cases. J Hand Surg Am 1998;23:914–9.
23. Kelly CM, Watson JT, Kim PT, et al. The use of a surgical grade calcium sulfate as a bone graft substitute: results of a multicenter trial. Clin Orthop Relat Res 2001;382:42–50.
24. Boden SD, Ugbo JL, Hutton WC, et al. The use of coralline hydroxyapatite with bone marrow, autogenous bone graft, or osteoinductive bone protein extract for posterolateral lumbar spine fusion. Spine 1999;24(4): 320–7.
25. Bucholz RW, Carlton AR, Holmes R. Interporous hydroxyapatite as a bone graft substitute in tibial plateau fractures. Clin Orthop Relat Res 1989;240: 53–62.
26. Irwin RB, Bernhard M, Biddinger A. Coralline hydroxyapatite as bone substitute in orthopedic oncology. Am J Orthop 2001;30:544–50.
27. Wolfe SW, Sigart CR, Grauer J, et al. Augmented external fixation of distal radius fractures: a biomechanical analysis. J Hand Surg Am 1998;23: 127–34.
28. Van der Stok J, El-Massoudi Y, Patka P, et al. Bone substitutes in the Netherlands: a systematic literature review. Acta Biomater 2011;7:739–50.
29. Nandi SK, Mukherjee P, Basu D, et al. Orthopaedic applications of bone graft and graft substitutes: a review. Indian J Med Res 2010;132:15–30.
30. Baer W, Schaller P, Carl HD. Spongy hydroxyapatite in hand surgery: a five year follow-up. J Hand Surg Br 2002;27(1):101–3.

31. Werber KD, Brauer RB, Becker K, et al. Osseous integration of bovine hydroxyapatite ceramic in metaphyseal bone defects of the distal radius. J Hand Surg Am 2000;25:833–41.

32. Ogosea A, Hoshinoa M, Endoa N, et al. Histological assessment in grafts of highly purified beta-tricalcium phosphate (OSferion) in human bones. Biomaterials 2006;27(8):1542–9.

33. Galois L, Mainard D, Delagoutte JP. Beta-tricalcium phosphate ceramic as a bone substitute in orthopaedic surgery. Int Orthop 2002;26(2):109–15.

34. Cook SD, Thomas KA, Jarcho M, et al. Hydroxyapatite-coated implant applications. Clin Orthop Relat Res 1988;232:225–43.

35. Thanner J, Herberts P, Malchau H, et al. Hydroxyapatite and tricalcium phosphate-coated cups with and without screw fixation: a randomized study of 64 hips. J Arthroplasty 2000;15(4):405–12.

36. Hinz P, Wolfe E, Schwesinger G, et al. A new resorbable bone void filler in trauma: early clinical experience and histologic evaluation. Orthopedics 2005; 25:597–600.

37. Anker CJ, Holdridge SP, Baird B, et al. Ultraporous tricalcium phosphate is well incorporated in small cavitary defects. Clin Orthop Relat Res 2005;434:251–7.

38. Sakano H, Koshino T, Takeuchi R. Treatment of the unstable distal radius fracture with external fixation and hydroxyapatite spacer. J Hand Surg Am 2001; 26(5):923–30.

39. Alvis M, Hornby S, Reddi AH, et al. Osteoinduction by a collagen mineral composite combined with isologous bone marrow in a subcutaneous rat model. Orthopedics 2003;26(1):77–80.

40. Kon E, Cancedda R, Quarto R, et al. Autologous bone marrow stromal cells loaded onto porous hydroxyapatite ceramic accelerate bone repair in critical size defects of sheep long bones. J Biomed Mater Res 2000;49:328–37.

41. Bajammal SS, Einhorn TA, Bhandari M, et al. The use of calcium phosphate bone cement in fracture treatment: a meta-analysis of randomized trials. J Bone Joint Surg Am 2008;90:1186–96.

42. Zimmermann R, Gschwentner M, Pechlaner S, et al. Injectable calcium phosphate bone cement Norian SRS for the treatment of intra-articular compression fractures of the distal radius in osteoporotic women. Arch Orthop Trauma Surg 2003;123:22–7.

43. Cassidy C, Jupiter JB, Ladd A, et al. Norian SRS cement compared with conventional fixation in distal radius fractures. J Bone Joint Surg Am 2003;85(11):2127–37.

44. Russell TA, Leighton RK. Comparison of autogenous bone graft and endothermic calcium phosphate cement for defect augmentation in tibial plateau fractures: a multicenter prospective randomized study. J Bone Joint Surg Am 2008;90(10):2057–61.

45. Mauffrey C, Lichteb P, Al-Rayyan M, et al. Bone graft substitutes for articular support and metaphyseal comminution: what are the options? Injury 2011;42: S35–9.

46. Helgeson MD, Tucker CJ, Shawen SB, et al. Antibiotic-impregnated calcium sulfate use in combat-related open fractures. Orthopedics 2009; 32(5):323.

47. Heikkila JT, Kukkonen J, Mattila K, et al. Bioactive glass granules: a suitable bone substitute material in the operative treatment of depressed lateral tibial plateau fractures: a prospective, randomized 1 year follow-up study. J Mater Sci Mater Med 2011;22:1073–80.

48. Smit RS, van der Velde D, Hegeman JH. Augmented pin fixation with Cortoss for an unstable AO-A3 type distal radius fracture in a patient with a manifest osteoporosis. Arch Orthop Trauma Surg 2008; 128(9):989–93.

49. Datamonitor Research Store: Available at: http:// www.datamonitor.com/store/News/orthovita_cortoss_ could_generate_high_sales_in_the_spinal_fracture_ market?productid=1AE201D1-E6E5-4EAD-85F2-205968C4FA11. Accessed January 5, 2012.

50. Friedlaender GE, Laforte AJ, Yin S, et al. Osteogenic protein-1 (bone morphogenetic protein-7) in the treatment of tibial nonunions: a prospective, randomized clinical trial comparing rhop-1 with fresh bone autograft. J Bone Joint Surg Am 2001;83(Suppl 1 (Pt 2)): S151–8.

51. Jones AL, Bucholz RW, Valentin-Opran A, et al. Allograft compared with autogenous bone graft for reconstruction of diaphyseal tibial fractures with cortical defects: a randomized, controlled trial. J Bone Joint Surg Am 2006;88(7):1431–41.

52. Govender S, Courtenay B, Feibel R, et al. Recombinant human bone morphogenetic protein-2 for treatment of open tibial fractures: a prospective, controlled, randomized study of four hundred and fifty patients. J Bone Joint Surg Am 2002;84:2123–34.

53. Digiovanni CW, Baumhauer J, Lin SS, et al. Prospective, randomized, multi-center feasibility trial of rhpdgf-bb versus autologous bone graft in a foot and ankle fusion model. Foot Ankle Int 2011;32(4):344–54.

54. Ekrol I, Hajducka C, Mcqueen MM, et al. A comparison of RhBMP-7 (OP-1) and autogenous graft for metaphyseal defects after osteotomy of the distal radius. Injury 2008;39(2):S73–82.

55. Kraiwattanapong C, Ugbo JL, Hutton WC, et al. Comparison of healos/bone marrow to INFUSE(rhBMP-2/ACS) with a collagen-ceramic sponge bulking agent as graft substitutes for lumbar spine fusion. Spine 2005;30(9):1001–7.

56. Carragee EJ, Hurwitz EL, Weiner BK. A critical review of recombinant human bone morphogenetic protein-2 trials in spinal surgery: emerging safety concerns and lessons learned. Spine J 2011;11:479–91.

57. Greenwald AS, Boden SD, Goldberg VM, et al. Bone-graft substitutes: facts, fictions, applications. J Bone Joint Surg Am 2001;83(2):98–103.

Reverse Total Shoulder Arthroplasty
Early Results of Forty-One Cases and a Review of the Literature

Adam B. Shafritz, MD[a],*, Scott Flieger, MBA[b]

KEYWORDS

- Reverse total shoulder • Scapular notching • Acromion fracture • Base plate failure
- Pulmonary embolism • Instability

KEY POINTS

- Reverse total shoulder arthroplasty is proving to be one of the most exciting advances in upper extremity surgery in the past quarter-century.
- This article reviews the previous literature and the results of 41 reverse shoulder arthroplasties implanted in 39 patients by a single orthopedically trained hand and upper extremity surgeon at a single institution from November 2004 until July 2011.
- Complications occurred in 17.1% of shoulders replaced, which was consistent with other published studies, making this operation a high-risk, high-reward procedure.

INTRODUCTION
Background

In 2003, the US Food and Drug Administration approved reverse shoulder arthroplasty for use in patients with rotator cuff tears and glenohumeral arthritis, because no other good solutions existed to successfully improve shoulder function and eliminate pain. This operation has been one of the most significant advances in shoulder arthroplasty in the past 20 years. However, reversed, semiconstrained, or constrained shoulder prosthetic arthroplasty is not a new concept or design idea.[1] The first reported total shoulder arthroplasty, implanted by Pean in 1893, was a linked constrained shoulder arthroplasty. In the early 1970s, many shoulder prostheses were either linked or reversed to overcome soft tissue or bony loss. With the exception of the Kessel prosthesis,[2] reverse total shoulder implants had relatively short lives and high failure rates; therefore, they were largely abandoned.

In 1985, Dr Paul Grammont reintroduced reverse shoulder arthroplasty to treat patients with rotator cuff tears and anterior-superior instability of the glenohumeral joint. His prosthesis medialized the center of rotation of the glenohumeral joint and also lowered the center of rotation of the joint line. The rationale behind this design was to create a more stable fulcrum and longer moment arm for the deltoid muscle to act against. Medialization of the center of rotation was thought to reduce shear forces at the glenoid bone–prosthetic interface. During the 1980s and early 1990s, Grammont's prosthetic design was formally modified several times and ultimately, in the year 2003, the Food and Drug Administration approved the Delta III reverse total shoulder arthroplasty for use in patients with rotator cuff insufficiency, instability, and arthritis of the glenohumeral joint.

The authors have nothing to disclose.
[a] College of Medicine, University of Vermont, 95 Carrigan Drive, Stafford Hall, Burlington, VT 05405, USA;
[b] Fletcher Allen Healthcare, 192 Tilley Drive, South Burlington, VT 05401, USA
* Corresponding author.
E-mail address: adam.shafritz@uvm.edu

Hand Clin 28 (2012) 469–479
http://dx.doi.org/10.1016/j.hcl.2012.08.009
0749-0712/12/$ – see front matter © 2012 Elsevier Inc. All rights reserved.

Since the initial launch of this product in the United States, additional design modifications have been released by various manufacturers. Design updates were prompted by specific problems associated with the earlier device, including dissociation of the components, scapular notching, baseplate loosening, and instability. In 2004, 8% of total shoulders implanted in the United States were of reverse design. Over the past 3 years, reverse shoulder arthroplasty has been one of the fastest growing areas in shoulder arthroplasty. In 2010, approximately 25,600 reverse total shoulder arthroplasties were performed in the United States, which is 29% of all shoulder prostheses implanted in this country.[3]

Alternatives to Reverse Total Shoulder Arthroplasty

Before 2003, there was no solution for patients with the combination of rotator cuff tears, arthritis, and instability of the shoulder. Before the advent of reverse shoulder arthroplasty, the only option for patients with these conditions was hemiarthroplasty with either a standard or bipolar humeral component. Although early published studies suggested that hemiarthroplasty for patients with rotator cuff tears and arthritis was a good option to treat pain and dysfunction, a study performed by Sanchez-Sotelo and colleagues[4] confirmed what many physicians with vast experience performing hemiarthroplasty for rotator cuff tears and arthritis had seen in their own practices; namely, that approximately one-third of patients either were not significantly helped with this surgical procedure or had a poor outcome with reduced function and increased pain after hemiarthroplasty. A recent study by Leung and colleagues[5] compared the functional outcome of reverse total shoulder replacement with that of hemiarthroplasty for the treatment of rotator cuff tear arthropathy. They found that active forward elevation and the Shoulder Pain and Disability Index were significantly better in the patients treated with reverse shoulder arthroplasty; yet, a complication rate of 25% was the same for both cohorts of patients.

Biomechanics

Numerous published studies have demonstrated that the deltoid muscle is the prime mobilizer of the glenohumeral joint. The muscles and tendons of the rotator cuff serve as primary stabilizers of the humeral head in the glenoid during elevation and rotation and also act to internally and externally rotate the glenohumeral joint. In settings where the tendons or muscles of the rotator cuff are no longer functional, it may become impossible for the humeral head to remain centered in the glenoid on initiation of motion. This phenomenon tends to occur in patients in whom at least two of the four rotator cuff muscles are nonfunctional. Classically, with insufficiency of the supraspinatus and infraspinatus muscles and tendons, the humeral head tends to translate superiorly under the acromion. During forward elevation, the coracoacromial arch stabilizes the humeral head beneath the scapula. Over time, this arch may become insufficient from wear or, alternatively, was made insufficient as a result of a prior acromioplasty with release of the coracoacromial ligament during arthroscopic or open procedures. With loss of the coracoacromial arch and rotator cuff function, the humeral head tends to subluxate anteriorly and superiorly as the deltoid is activated to elevate the arm. This instability anteriorly and superiorly puts the deltoid at a significant mechanical disadvantage and it may become impossible for patients to abduct or forward elevate their arm, such that functional overhead activity becomes impossible. This syndrome, which has been termed "pseudoparalysis," is the primary indication for use of a reverse shoulder arthroplasty (**Fig. 1**). The reversed design of the implant allows the translational force of the deltoid on the humeral head to be converted to a rotational force, thereby allowing the humeral head to remain centered in the glenohumeral joint. As a result of this newly created stability, the arm is able once more to elevate overhead.[6]

Further indications for the use of reverse shoulder arthroplasty include (1) revision of failed total shoulder arthroplasties in the setting of rotator cuff insufficiency, (2) revisions of hemiarthroplasty for fracture with failed fixation of the tuberosities or resorption of the tuberosities leading to clinically apparent rotator cuff insufficiency and instability, and (3) primary fracture treatment when tuberosity repair is not possible. Because of relatively high complication rates, and an unknown life expectancy of the prothesis, it is generally recommended that patients maintain low activity levels, are at least 70 years old, and will place low demands on the prosthesis. Contraindications to reverse total shoulder arthroplasty include patients who cannot be compliant with postoperative rehabilitation or activity limitations; those with severe bone loss to the glenoid, such that the glenoid component cannot be supported; those with an active infection; and patients with neurologic conditions that result in a nonfunctioning deltoid muscle.

MATERIALS AND METHODS

A retrospective review of prospectively collected data was performed at the University of Vermont

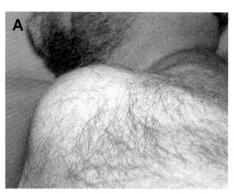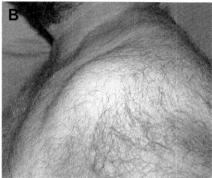

Fig. 1. Anterior-superior instability of the shoulder. (*A*) Humeral head escaping from under the deficient coracoacromial arch as the patient initiates forward elevation. (*B*) Return of the humeral head under the acromion when the patient relaxes his deltoid muscle.

College of Medicine on all patients undergoing reverse total shoulder arthroplasty from November 2004 until July 2011. This study was approved the Institutional Review Board of the University of Vermont. Medical records were compiled from the surgical schedule at the institution. Forty-two reverse total shoulder arthroplasties were identified. The first 12 patients were randomly assigned to receive either a Delta (DePuy International, Warsaw, IN) prosthesis or a Reverse Shoulder Prosthesis (RSP) (DJO Surgical, Austin, TX) in an alternating case-by-case fashion. All subsequent patients with one exception received a RSP because of concerns about scapular notching that was becoming apparent on follow-up radiographs in the Delta but was not noted in the RSP. One patient received a Zimmer Inverse (Zimmer, Warsaw, IN).

The indications for surgical intervention were patients with a failed shoulder arthroplasty in the setting of rotator cuff insufficiency, patients who had failed prior rotator cuff repair surgery and developed glenohumeral arthritis and their rotator cuff tear was determined to be irreparable, patients who had failed prior arthroscopic debridement procedures for massive irreparable rotator cuff tears and arthritis, and patients who had the diagnosis of a pseudoparalytic shoulder in the setting of a massive rotator cuff tear. A pseudoparalytic shoulder was defined as 60 degrees or less of forward elevation with associated anterior and superior shoulder instability.

Preoperatively, patients were assessed for forward elevation, external rotation, and internal rotation, measured in the standard planes. The infraspinatus function was tested as resistance to external rotation with the arm at the side. Patients with significant rotator cuff insufficiency or suprascapular nerve disfunction are not able to hold the arm in external rotation with the arm in adduction. The teres minor was assessed for its strength with the arm at 90 degrees of abduction and 90 degrees of external rotation. Loss of these two muscle functions is an indication for the addition of latissimus dorsi with or without teres major tendon transfer to a reverse total shoulder arthroplasty,[7] although no patients in this cohort required this procedure.

Patient-oriented outcomes were obtained using the Disabilities of the Arm, Shoulder and Hand (DASH) score and Simple Shoulder Test (SST)[8] preoperatively and postoperatively at a minimum of 6 months and at yearly intervals postoperatively. In addition, functional ranges of motion were measured in forward elevation and internal and external rotation. Preoperative and postoperative Visual Analog Scale (VAS) pain scores were recorded.

Radiographic evaluation at 6 months and then at yearly intervals was performed specifically looking for scapular notching based on the Sirveaux classification.[9] Grade 1 notching lesions are limited to the pillar of the scapula. Grade 2 lesions contact the inferior screw. Grade 3 lesions extend beyond the inferior screw. Grade 4 lesions approach the central peg of the baseplate and extend significantly under the baseplate (**Fig. 2**). Grade 3 and 4 lesions are associated with poor function.

All patients undergoing reverse total shoulder arthroplasty obtained a preoperative computed tomography scan to evaluate for glenoid bone stock and potential bone loss. In 2009, Frankle and colleagues[10] reported a new classification of glenoid morphology in patients undergoing reverse shoulder arthroplasty, comparing the computed tomography scan with observed pathology at surgery. They observed normal glenoid bony morphology in 63% of cases. The presence of abnormal morphology could be classified

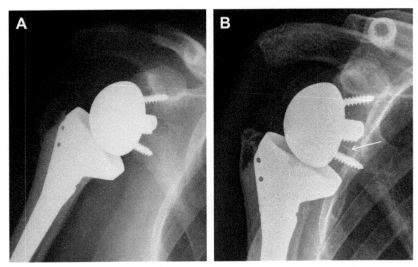

Fig. 2. Scapular notching in Grammont-based reverse total shoulder arthroplasty. (*A*) Immediate postoperative radiograph of the Delta prosthesis. (*B*) Sirveaux grade 3 scapular notching (*arrow*) 5 years postoperative.

into four subgroups based on location: (1) superior, (2) posterior, (3) anterior, and (4) global erosions. They cautioned surgeons that in the presence of abnormal morphology, the average centerline of the glenoid vault drops by 9 mm. Additionally, the area for peripheral screw placement drops by 42%, limiting it to the inferior and anterior quadrants. This result could lead to inadequate baseplate fixation or improper version of the glenoid component. In the current study, if glenoid bone depth was decreased to 15 mm or less, bone graft from the patient's humeral head or allograft femoral head was used to support the glenoid component.

Surgery was performed with patients in the beach-chair position with a deltopectoral approach under general anesthesia. Pneumatic compression devices were placed on the lower legs and used for deep venous thrombosis (DVT) prophylaxis. Routine anterior arthrotomy with release of the subscapularis off from bone and subsequent repair at the end of the procedure was performed in every case where subscapularis muscle, tendon, and anterior capsule were present. A Hemovac drain was used for 48 hours postoperatively and then removed. All patients were treated in a shoulder immobilizer and were discharged on postoperative Day 2. No formal physical therapy was used and patients were instructed to remain in their shoulder immobilizer for 6 weeks with the exception of free elbow, hand, and wrist range of motion, which was allowed beginning on postoperative Day 2. Follow-up evaluations were performed at 2 weeks, 6 weeks, 3 months, 6 months, and 1 year postoperatively, and subsequently at 6-month to 1-year

intervals. All clinical evaluations included examination of function, a visual analog pain scale, a DASH score, SST filed by the patient, and standard radiographs.

RESULTS

During the period of study, 42 reverse total shoulder arthroplasties were performed on 40 patients. Of these shoulders, one patient with one shoulder replacement was lost to follow-up at 2 months postoperatively, and although she did not experience any intraoperative or immediate postoperative complications, because she did not have 6 months minimum follow-up she was eliminated from the tabulation. In addition, during the 7.5-year study period, five patients with five shoulder arthroplasties died from causes unrelated to shoulder surgery. These patients were included using the data from their last follow-up visit.

The mean patient age was 73 years (range, 51–87 years). The mean follow-up was 2.5 years (range, 6 months–7.5 years). Of the procedures performed, 3 of the 40 shoulder replacements were done as revision shoulder arthroplasties. Two patients had undergone prior hemiarthroplasty for symptomatic rotator cuff tear arthropathy. They continued to have pain and instability and were subsequently converted from hemiarthroplasty to reverse total shoulder arthroplasty. The third case had an initial total shoulder arthroplasty that subsequently developed rotator cuff insufficiency, ultimately developing glenoid loosening. The glenoid component had been removed; the patient continued to have superior erosion wear, pain, instability, and poor function, and his shoulder hemiarthroplasty was subsequently converted to reverse total shoulder arthroplasty.

Twenty-one shoulders had at least one prior shoulder operation (mean, 1.5 surgeries; range, 1–4 surgeries). Twelve patients had a failed prior rotator cuff repair. Ten patients had prior arthroscopic debridement for either rotator cuff tears that were deemed irreparable or had prior rotator cuff repair surgery that had subsequently failed. Twenty shoulders had reverse total shoulder arthroplasty performed as a primary procedure. Preoperative anterior acromial insufficiency was noted in four shoulders. Three patients (7.1%)

had severe glenoid bone loss and required structural bone grafts, two autografts, one allograft (**Fig. 3**). At the most recent follow-up, all grafts appeared stable and incorporated.

The functional results and patient outcomes are summarized in **Table 1**. The average preoperative pain score was 7, with a range from 1 to 10. Preoperative DASH score averaged 54, with a range from 12 to 91. Preoperative SST score averaged 2, with a range from 0 to 8. Postoperatively, all scores improved with a mean pain score noted at 1, range 0 to 7; mean DASH score equaled 24, with a range 1 to 70; and mean SST was 8, with a range 0 to 12. Mean forward elevation was

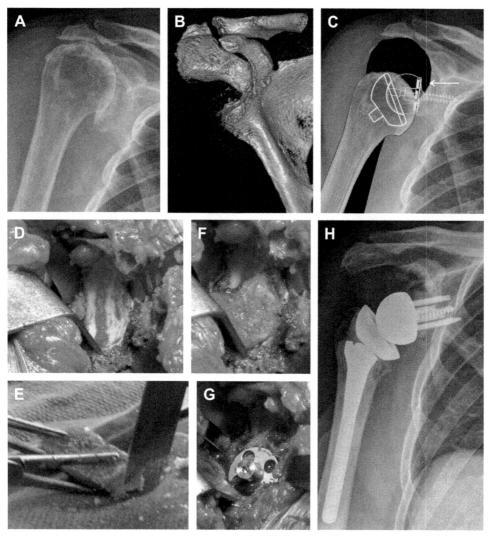

Fig. 3. Bone grafting for glenoid deficiency. The radiograph (*A*) and computed tomography scan (*B*) show severe superior bone loss to the glenoid. (*C*) Preoperative templating demonstrates the amount of bone necessary to place the glenoid component in an appropriate position. The glenoid is exposed (*D*) and the resected humeral head (*E*) is placed into the defect (*F*). It is provisionally fixed with k-wires, and definitively held with the screws of the baseplate (*G*). Follow-up radiographs (*H*) show the baseplate to be stable at 1 year.

Table 1
Results of reverse total shoulder arthroplasty

	Preoperative	Postoperative	Improvement factor
Pain	7 (1–10)	1 (0–7)	7
Forward elevation	74 degrees (0–140)	135 degrees (60–170)	1.8
External rotation	22 degrees (0–60)	35 degrees (15–60)	1.6
DASH score	54 (12–91)	24 (1–70)	2.25
Simple shoulder test	2 (0–8)	8 (0–12)	4

74 degrees (range, 0–140 degrees) preoperatively and improved to 135 degrees postoperatively (range, 60–170 degrees). External rotation improved from a mean of 22 degrees preoperatively (range, 0–60 degrees) to a mean of 35 degrees postoperatively (range, 15–60 degrees). Internal rotation spinal level did not change and averaged to the level of the sacrum. In evaluating collected data, the DASH score improved by a factor of 2.25; SST improved by a factor of 4; and forward elevation and external rotation improved by a factor of 1.8 and 1.6, respectively. The VAS pain score decreased by a factor of 7.

Five patients (five shoulders) experienced at least one major early complication. Two of these same patients also incurred an additional late major complication (acromion fractures). Two additional patients (two shoulders) had minor early complications but these problems did not require an intervention. The most common complication was instability (7.3%): three dislocations occurred in two patients and one patient exhibited subluxation of the glenohumeral joint. All dislocations occurred within the first 2 weeks postoperatively and required a closed reduction under general anesthesia. All dislocations and subluxations occurred as a result of noncompliance with postoperative immobilization and weight bearing on the arm. The one patient who experienced subluxation was reminded to keep his arm in the postoperative immobilizer for the recommended 6 weeks postoperatively. No patient developed recurrent instability.

Two patients had hematomas that required evacuation and drainage in the operating room (4.9%). Two patients had pulmonary embolisms (4.9%) within several days after surgery, but duplex Doppler evaluations failed to demonstrate DVT. One patient developed a nondisplaced acromial stress fracture at 4 months but this healed without intervention by 6 months. One patient had glenoid baseplate failure that occurred early at 10 months; her glenoid baseplate was subsequently revised. This baseplate also subsequently failed 14 months after the revision. However, she was salvaged by converting to a hemiarthroplasty with an Achilles allograft and humeral stabilization (**Fig. 4**).

During the initial phase of this study, five DePuy Delta prosthesis were implanted: four Delta-IIIs and one Delta-XTEND. Early scapular notching was noted in all patients receiving these prostheses. Progressive scapular notching was noted in four of the five prostheses. Additionally, one Zimmer Inverse was implanted and the baseplate failed at 10 months postoperative. During this time period, a similar number of RSPs were placed and no scapular notching was noted early. Because of the concerns associated with scapular notching and possible catastrophic failure from loosening, all subsequent patients received RSPs. With follow-up of 6 months to 5.25 years postoperatively, grade 1 scapular notching was detected in two patients with RSPs placed 4 years and 5.25 years prior. This is a rate of 5.7% in the RSP prosthesis versus 100% in patients receiving Delta prostheses. No patients' baseplates failed as a result of notching (**Fig. 5**).

DISCUSSION
Complications in Reverse Total Shoulder Arthroplasty

Several published studies have noted that reverse shoulder arthroplasty has the highest complication rate of all shoulder arthroplasty procedures performed.[11] In 2005, Werner and colleagues[12] reviewed 58 cases with a complication rate of 50% and an overall reoperation rate of 33%. Wierks and colleagues[13] reviewed the learning curve associated with single-surgeon experience comparing the first 10 cases with the second 10. The complication rate was higher for the first 10 cases and patients in the second group were only 10% as likely to have an intraoperative complication. The overall incidence was 11 cases with 22 intraoperative complications, and 8 patients with 11 postoperative complications. The conversion of a failed shoulder

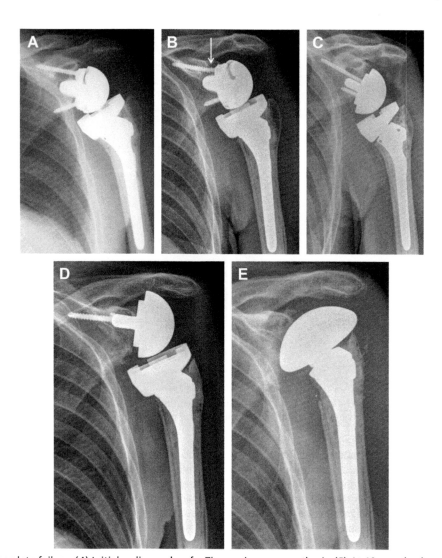

Fig. 4. Base plate failure. (*A*) Initial radiographs of a Zimmer inverse prosthesis. (*B*) At 10 months the patient had pain and radiographs revealed the superior screw had broken (*arrow*) indicating the base plate was loose. (*C*) The patient was revised using the Zimmer trabecular metal baseplate and glenosphere with impaction allografting to the glenoid. (*D*) At 14 months, this baseplate showed migration and the patient complained of continued pain with motion. The patient was revised to a hemiarthroplasty with Achilles tendon allograft stabilization and additional bone grafting of the glenoid. (*E*) At 1 year postoperatively, the shoulder is functional but there has been bone loss to the glenoid.

hemiarthroplasty or total shoulder arthroplasty to reverse total shoulder arthroplasty has an even higher complication rate. Levy and colleagues[14] reviewed 29 patients converted from failed hemiarthroplasty for fractures to reverse total shoulder arthroplasty. They had a total complication rate of 38% with only 55% of patients classified as having good to excellent results.

Scapular Notching

In the current study, scapular notching was noted in seven patients (17.1%). Publications that track

the function and longevity of reverse shoulder arthroplasties note that there is a major concern for inferior glenoid and scapular notching that occurs with designs based on the Grammont prosthesis.[15] Scapular notching is defined as bone loss under the most inferior and lateral portion of the baseplate. Melis and colleagues[16] recently reported an 88% rate of scapular notching in Grammont-designed shoulders at 8 to 12 years follow-up. The cause of inferior scapular notching has not been well established. Theories as to its origins involve the possibility of the

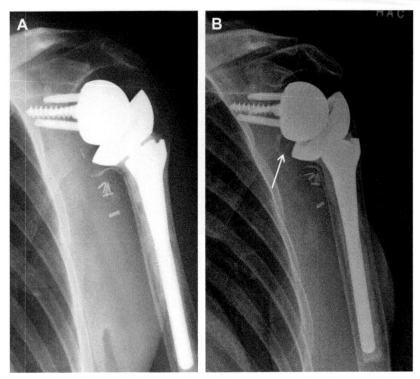

Fig. 5. Grade 1 scapular notching in the RSP prosthesis. (*A*) Postoperative Grashey view. (*B*) The radiograph is a 5.25-year postoperative Grashey view. The *arrow* points to the inferior notching.

humeral component contacting the inferior and lateral border of the scapula, and the possibility of polyethylene debris and osteolysis.[17] The concern about notching is that ultimately it leads to glenoid component failure by baseplate failure, because there is a progressive loss of bony architecture to support the glenoid components. However, there are not enough long-term data to support or refute this possibility. The release of a non-Grammont design–based reverse shoulder system has been shown to almost eliminate notching,[18] whereas technique changes in Grammont-based implant systems suggest inferior tilt of the baseplate and placing the baseplate as low as possible might help reduce the risk of scapular notching.[19]

Acromion Fractures

Postoperative acromion fractures occurred in three patients (**Fig. 6**); however, displaced fractures occurred in two (4.9%). Displaced fractures represent previously unseen complications in shoulder arthroplasty that have recently surfaced with the use of reverse shoulder implants. These acromial fractures are thought to be the result of increased forces associated with lengthening of the deltoid muscle, leading to increased stress

being placed across the acromion. Anterior and lateral fractures of the acromion are very difficult to treat and manage surgically, especially if there is minimal bone stock available for fixation. Fractures occurring at the base of the acromion or at the scapular spine are generally treated surgically with open reduction and internal fixation. Crosby and colleagues[20] suggests that the superior and posterior screw for glenoid baseplate fixation may create a stress riser at its tip, causing or predisposing patients to developing these acromial fractures. In a recent report on 457 reverse total shoulder procedures, 9% of patients had pre-existing acromial pathology and 0.9% developed an acromion fracture during the 9-year surveillance period.[21] They reported that the presence of acromial pathology preoperatively had no effect on outcome, but development of a fracture postoperative had a significant effect on pain and function and that treatment was uncertain.

Instability

Glenohumeral instability after reverse shoulder arthroplasty occurred in three patients (7.3%). Published rates range from 5% to 31%.[22] The surgical approach used may play a role in the development of instability postoperatively. Edwards and

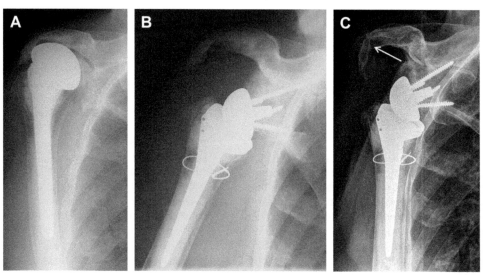

Fig. 6. Acromion fracture in reverse total shoulder arthroplasty. (*A*) Preoperative status of the shoulder. Note the original humeral component was placed high possibly contributing to rotator cuff failure. (*B*) Postoperative Grashey view. Note the acromion is thin but intact. (*C*) This patient sustained an atraumatic displaced acromion fracture (*arrow*) 2 years postoperative. The patient presented with pain, loss of forward elevation, and noted a deformity of his shoulder girdle contour.

colleagues[23] reviewed 138 consecutive reverse total shoulder arthroplasties performed through a deltopectoral approach. In 55% of patients the subscapularis was irreparable and seven of these cases developed postoperative instability (9% in this group and 5% of the total). They concluded that a deltopectoral approach without repair of the anterior structures was a significant risk factor for dislocation postoperatively. In contrast, Clark and colleagues[24] did not find that subscapularis repair reduced the rate of postoperative dislocations. Interestingly, in the current study, all three patients had deltopectoral approaches, but all of the events occurred because of patient noncompliance with postoperative instructions.

Baseplate Failure

One patient in this cohort had a failure of their baseplate twice. All designs of reverse shoulders rely on bony in-growth into a metal baseplate fixed to the glenoid. This baseplate supports the glenosphere. Published rates of failure range from 0.4% to 11.2%.[11] After the baseplate has failed, options are limited. Holcomb and colleagues[25] reviewed 14 cases of revision reverse total shoulder arthroplasty for baseplate failure. They followed these cases for 33 months on average after they reimplanted a new baseplate. Fourteen percent of patients required additional revision surgery, one for baseplate failure and one for instability. Other options for baseplate failure include conversion

to hemiarthroplasty; however, no published series exists concerning the outcome of this procedure. In this study, the one patient who was converted to hemiarthroplasty had good functional activity: 130 degrees forward elevation, 30 degrees of external rotation, DASH of 18, SST of 7, and was pain free at 1 year follow-up from the final procedure.

Hematoma

Two patients (4.9%) developed a postoperative hematoma despite use of a drain for 48 hours postoperatively. One patient developed the hematoma as the result of over anticoagulation to treat a pulmonary embolism, and the other patient had a huge preoperative synovial fluid effusion that resulted in a tremendous available "dead space" to reaccumulate fluid postoperatively. Both cases required surgical drainage. Published rates of hematoma formation range as high as 20%,[12] and it was one of the earliest reported complications of this operation.[26]

DVT and Pulmonary Embolism

There were two nonfatal pulmonary embolisms in this study (4.9%). In a study performed at the Hospital for Special Surgery of 100 consecutive total shoulder arthroplasties, the prevalence of DVT was 13%.[27] Six of the patients had an upper extremity DVT and seven had lower extremity DVTs. A prevalence of about 10% was noted at postoperative Day 2, a 6% incidence was noted at 3 months. The rate of pulmonary embolism was 3%; two patients had nonfatal pulmonary embolisms, and one patient had a fatal pulmonary embolism. Currently, no formal recommendations have been made regarding DVT prophylaxis in shoulder arthroplasty.

SUMMARY

It is clear that reverse shoulder arthroplasty is a rapidly expanding and changing field in upper extremity surgery. The early results are dramatic improvements in upper limb function and make this procedure an extremely attractive alternative for patients and surgeons. On average, the DASH score improved by a factor of 2.25; SST improved by a factor of 4; forward elevation and external rotation improved by a factor of 1.8 and 1.6, respectively; and the VAS pain score dropped by a factor of 7. Complications occurred in 17.1% of shoulders replaced, making reverse total shoulder arthroplasty a high-risk, high-reward procedure. This study demonstrates that orthopedic hand surgeons with an interest and additional training in shoulder surgery are capable of obtaining results that are equivalent to those published in the literature.

The technology is relatively new and major questions are yet to be answered. How can implant longevity be increased? Can the risk of complications be lowered? New developments in this field center on updated designs of the reversed prosthesis, attempting to address and correct existing problems, including baseplate loosening or failure, improving range of motion, reducing instability, reducing scapular notching, and improving instrumentation systems for surgeons to make the surgical procedure less demanding. It is clear that the success rates of these procedures are increasing and that initial predictions of short life span of these implants may not be justified. As shoulder arthroplasty technology continues to evolve, it is expected that results will continue to improve, approaching success rates similar to hip and knee replacement.

REFERENCES

1. Flatow EL, Harrison AK. A history of reverse total shoulder arthroplasty. Clin Orthop Relat Res 2011;469:2432–9.
2. Wretenberg PF, Wallensten R. The Kessel total shoulder arthroplasty. A 13- to 16-year retrospective followup. Clin Orthop Relat Res 1999;365:100–3.
3. A 2011 extremity update. Orthopedic Network News 2011;22(1):9–13.
4. Sanchez-Sotelo J, Cofield RH, Rowland CM. Shoulder hemiarthroplasty for glenohumeral arthritis associated with severe rotator cuff deficiency. J Bone Joint Surg Am 2001;83-A(12):1814–22.
5. Leung B, Horodyski M, Struk AM, et al. Functional outcome of hemiarthroplasty compared with reverse total shoulder arthroplasty in the treatment of rotator cuff tear arthroplasty. J Shoulder Elbow Surg 2012;21(3):319–23.
6. Walker M, Brooks J, Willis M, et al. How reverse shoulder arthroplasty works. Clin Orthop Relat Res 2011;469(9):2440–51.
7. Gerber C, Pennington SD, Lingenfelter EJ, et al. Reverse Delta-III total shoulder replacement combined with latissimus dorsi transfer. A preliminary report. J Bone Joint Surg Am 2007;89(5):940–7.
8. Lippitt SB, Harryman DT II, Matsen FA III. A practical tool for evaluation function: the simple shoulder test. In: Matsen FA III, Fu FH, Hawkins RJ, editors. The shoulder: a balance of mobility and stability. Rosemont (IL): American Academy of Orthopaedic Surgeons; 1993. p. 501–18.
9. Sirveaux F, Favard L, Oudet D, et al. Grammont inverted total shoulder arthroplasty in the treatment of glenohumeral osteoarthritis with massive rupture of the cuff. J Bone Joint Surg Br 2004;86-B:388–95.
10. Frankle MA, Teramoto A, Luo Z, et al. Glenoid morphology in reverse shoulder arthroplasty: classification and surgical implications. J Shoulder Elbow Surg 2009;18:874–85.
11. Cheung E, Willis M, Walker M, et al. Complications in reverse total shoulder arthroplasty. J Am Acad Orthop Surg 2011;19:439–44.
12. Werner CM, Steinmann PA, Gilbart M, et al. Treatment of painful pseudoparesis due to irreparable rotator cuff dysfunction with the Delta III reverse-ball-and-socket total shoulder prosthesis. J Bone Joint Surg Am 2005;87(7):1476–86.
13. Wierks C, Skolasky RL, Ji JH, et al. Reverse total shoulder replacement: intraoperative and early postoperative complications. Clin Orthop Relat Res 2009;467(1):225–34.
14. Levy J, Frankle M, Mighell M, et al. The use of the reverse shoulder prosthesis for the treatment of failed hemiarthroplasty for proximal humeral fracture. J Bone Joint Surg Am 2007;89(2):292–300.
15. Favard L, Levigne C, Nerot C, et al. Reverse prostheses in arthropathies with cuff tear: are survivorship and function maintained over time? Clin Orthop Relat Res 2011;469(9):2469–75.
16. Melis B, Defranco M, Ladermann A, et al. An evaluation of the radiological changes around the Grammont reverse geometry shoulder arthroplasty after eight to 12 years. J Bone Joint Surg Br 2011;93(9):1240–6.
17. Simovitch RW, Zumstein MA, Lohri E, et al. Predictors of scapular notching in patients managed with

the Delta III reverse total shoulder replacement. J Bone Joint Surg Am 2007;89(3):588–600.

18. Cuff D, Pupello D, Virani N, et al. Reverse shoulder arthroplasty for the treatment of rotator cuff deficiency. J Bone Joint Surg Am 2008;90(6):1244–51.

19. Levigne C, Boileau P, Favard L, et al. Scapular notching in reverse shoulder arthroplasty. J Shoulder Elbow Surg 2008;17(6):925–35.

20. Crosby LA, Hamilton A, Twiss T. Scapula fractures after reverse total shoulder arthroplasty: classification and treatment. Clin Orthop Relat Res 2011;469:2544–9.

21. Walch G, Mottier F, Wall B, et al. Acromial insufficiency in reverse shoulder arthroplasties. J Shoulder Elbow Surg 2009;18(3):495–502.

22. Zumstein MA, Pinedo M, Old J, et al. Problems, complications, reoperations, and revisions in reverse total shoulder arthroplasty: a systematic review. J Shoulder Elbow Surg 2011;20:146–57.

23. Edwards TB, Williams MD, Labriola JE, et al. Subscapularis insufficiency and the risk of shoulder dislocation after reverse shoulder arthroplasty. J Shoulder Elbow Surg 2009;18(6):892–6.

24. Clark JC, Ritchie J, Song FS, et al. Complication rates, dislocation, pain, and postoperative range of motion after reverse shoulder arthroplasty in patients with and without repair of the subscapularis. J Shoulder Elbow Surg 2012;21(1):36–41.

25. Holcomb JO, Cuff D, Petersen SA, et al. Revision reverse shoulder arthroplasty for glenoid baseplate failure after primary reverse shoulder arthroplasty. J Shoulder Elbow Surg 2009;18(5):717–23.

26. Baulot E, Chabernaud D, Grammont PM. Results of Grammont's inverted prosthesis in omarthritis associated with major cuff destruction: Apropos of 16 cases. Acta Orthop Belg 1995;61(Suppl 1):112–9 [in French].

27. Willis AA, Warren RF, Craig EV, et al. Deep vein thrombosis after reconstructive shoulder arthroplasty: a prospective observational study. J Shoulder Elbow Surg 2009;18(1):100–6.

Platelet-Rich Plasma and the Upper Extremity

Allan Mishra, MD[a],*, Pietro Randelli, MD[b],
Cameron Barr, MD[c], Tazio Talamonti, MD[b],
Vincenza Ragone, MEng[d], Paolo Cabitza, MD[b]

KEYWORDS

- Platelet-rich plasma • Tennis elbow • Lateral epicondylitis • Rotator cuff repair • Tendinopathy
- PRP

KEY POINTS

- Platelet-rich plasma (PRP) is a fraction of whole blood containing powerful growth factors and cytokines.
- Not all PRP has the same biologic characteristics.
- A PRP classification system exists is based on the presence or absence of white blood cells and whether the PRP is used in an activated or unactivated form.
- Studies support the use of PRP instead of cortisone for patients with chronic lateral epicondylar tendinopathy.
- Data suggest certain types of PRP enhance the healing of rotator cuff tears of less than 3 cm.
- Novel formulations and applications of PRP will continue to emerge.

INTRODUCTION

Orthopedic surgeons can count themselves among the pioneers in the use of biologic options to treat specific medical conditions. The use of bone grafting dates back to 1911 when a portion of a tibia was used to treat Pott disease.[1] The concept of platelet-rich plasma (PRP) emerged in the medical literature in 1954.[2] It was not until the late 1990s, however, that Marx and colleagues[3] published the seminal paper on the use of PRP to augment maxillofacial bone grafting. In 2006, Mishra and Pavelko[4] published a pilot study suggesting PRP may have value in the treatment of chronic lateral epicondylar tendinopathy. Two years later, Randelli and colleagues[5] published the first paper examining the use of PRP in rotator cuff repair.

It is important for researchers, clinicians, and patients to understand that not all PRP has the same biologic characteristics. Technically, PRP contains elevated concentrations of platelets when compared with whole blood. Within platelets are alpha granules that contain a cornucopia of cytokines, including, but not limited to, platelet-derived growth factor, transforming growth factor-beta, and vascular endothelial growth factor. Platelets also have dense granules that

Disclosures: Biomet Biologics provided research support for some of the articles discussed in this review.
Financial disclosure: Dr Mishra has license agreements with Biomet Biologics, BioParadox, and ThermoGenesis.
[a] Department of Orthopaedic Surgery, Menlo Medical Clinic, Stanford University Medical Center, 1300 Crane Street, Menlo Park, CA 94025, USA; [b] Università degli Studi di Milano, IRCCS Policlinico San Donato, Piazza Edmondo Malan, 2 20097 San Donato Milanese, Milano, Milan, Italy; [c] Department of Orthopaedic Surgery, Stanford University Medical Center, 450 Broadway Street, M/C 6342, Redwood City, CA 94063, USA; [d] Biomedical Engineer, IRCCS Policlinico San Donato, Piazza Edmondo Malan, 2 20097 San Donato Milanese, Milano, Milan, Italy
* Corresponding author.
E-mail address: am@totaltendon.com

hand.theclinics.com

house a variety of important bioactive molecules, such as serotonin, calcium, and adenosine.[6] More than 300 proteins have been identified in platelet releasate using a proteomics approach. These proteins function in an autocrine or paracrine fashion to modulate cell signaling and chemotaxis.[7] PRP may be prepared via centrifugation (**Fig. 1**) as a pure platelet concentrate suspended in plasma or as a mixture with white blood cells. These versions have been known as leukocyte-poor and leukocyte-rich, respectively.[8] White blood cells come in several varieties, including, but not limited to, neutrophils, lymphocytes, and monocytes. The interaction of platelets with these white blood cell subtypes in a small volume of plasma has not been studied extensively. Recent investigations have shown that there are clear differences in PRP formulations in terms of growth factor concentration and catabolic enzyme content.[9]

PRP application techniques are also variable. Platelets can be activated ex vivo with thrombin and/or calcium. A network of fibrin then forms, resulting in a membrane-like material that can be incorporated into a suture construct. This technique can result in immediate release of the growth factors. Use of PRP in an unactivated manner, without thrombin or calcium, allows for application via a syringe or catheter and relies on in-vivo activation via endogenous collagen. This methodology has been shown to result in up to 80% more growth factor release over time.[10]

To better understand and communicate about the value of PRP for sports medicine applications, Mishra and colleagues[6] devised a classification system. The system relies on the presence or absence of white blood cells and whether the PRP is used in an activated or unactivated form. Further delineation, based on platelet concentration, is also incorporated into the classification (**Table 1**). Most chronic lateral epicondylar tendinopathy studies have used type 1 PRP (unactivated with white blood cells). The rotator cuff literature has studied a variety of PRP formulations and techniques. Within this context, the application of PRP in the upper extremity will be explored. Emphasis is placed on published, peer review data. The future horizons for this novel biologic treatment will be outlined.

PRP AND LATERAL EPICONDYLAR TENDINOPATHY

Lateral epicondylar tendinopathy, also known as tennis elbow, commonly occurs in patients with overuse or overloading of the elbow and forearm. The cause of the disorder has been attributed to microscopic tearing of the extensor carpi radialis brevis tendon coupled with an angiofibroblastic reparative response.[11] Most patients respond to some combination of nonoperative interventions and time. For those who fail to respond to these treatments, surgery is often considered. Of the surgical patients, 80% to 90% can expect a good or excellent outcome with an open or arthroscopic operation. At 5 years after surgery, however, 9% of patients continue to report moderate to severe pain and up to 28% may complain of persistent low-grade symptoms.[12] Importantly, most surgical techniques recommend some form of local biologic stimulation such as drilling or abrasion of bone near the extensor carpi radialis brevis origin to augment healing.

PRP, as a stand-alone treatment of lateral epicondylar tendinopathy, was initially investigated in 140 subjects by Mishra and Pavelko[4] in 2006 (**Table 2**). It was postulated that a single injection of PRP, via its bioactive cytokines, could

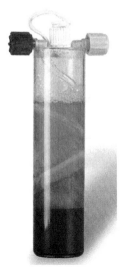

Fig. 1. PRP is prepared via a centrifugation process that separates blood into its components by density.

Table 1		
PRP classification		
	White Blood Cells (WBCs)	**Activated?**
Type 1	Increased over baseline	No
Type 2	Increased over baseline	Yes
Type 3	Minimal or no WBCs	No
Type 4	Minimal or no WBCs	Yes
—	A: >5x Platelets B: <5x Platelets	—

Data from Mishra A, Harmon K, Woodall J, et al. Sports medicine applications of platelet rich plasma. Curr Pharm Biotechnol 2012;13(7):1185–95.

Table 2
PRP and lateral epicondylar tendinopathy: controlled clinical studies

Study	Authors	Subjects	PRP Type	Comments
Level 1	Gosens et al,[14] 2011	100	1A Biomet GPS (Biomet Biologics, Warsaw, IN, USA)	PRP better than cortisone at 2 y. Success rate: PRP 77% vs cortisone 43%, P<.0001
Level 1	Peerbooms et al,[13] 2010	100	1A Biomet GPS (Biomet Biologics, Warsaw, IN, USA)	PRP better than cortisone at 1 y. Improvement in pain scores: PRP 64% vs cortisone 24%, P<.001
Level 1	Creaney et al,[15] 2011	150	1B manual centrifuge	Higher conversion to surgery with whole blood 20% vs PRP 10%; no differences in pain scores at 6 mo.
Level 1	Thanasas et al,[16] 2011	28	1A Biomet GPS (Biomet Biologics, Warsaw, IN, USA)	PRP better than whole blood at 6 wk. Improvement in pain scores: PRP 61% vs whole blood 42%, P<.05. No differences in pain scores at 6 mo.
Level 2	Mishra and Pavelko,[4] 2006	20	1A Biomet GPS (Biomet Biologics, Warsaw, IN, USA)	PRP better than bupivacaine at 8 wk. Improvement in pain scores PRP 60% vs bupivacaine 16%, P = .001. PRP subjects 93% better at 2 y.

significantly reduce pain in subjects with chronic lateral epicondylar tendinopathy. All of the subjects in this pilot trial initially underwent a standardized nonoperative protocol. Twenty subjects (14%) continued to have significant pain and disability. Of these subjects with continued pain, 15 were treated with PRP (type 1A) and 5 control subjects were given bupivacaine. The PRP was injected in an unactivated fashion using a peppering technique with five to seven penetrations of the extensor carpi radialis brevis tendon at or near its origin (**Figs. 2 and 3**). Initial pain scores were 8.0 for the PRP subjects and 8.6 for the bupivacaine subjects. At 8 weeks after treatment, the PRP subjects reported a 60% improvement in pain compared with a 16% improvement in the control subjects (P = .001). After this follow-up time, most of the control subjects elected to pursue other treatments, leaving only the PRP subjects for further evaluation. At a mean of 25.6 months of follow-up (range 12–38 months), the PRP subjects reported a 93% reduction in pain scores. Significant improvements in a modified Mayo elbow score were also reported in the PRP subjects. A lack of full randomization and the small

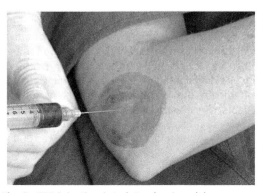

Fig. 2. PRP injection into lateral epicondyle.

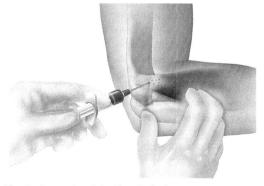

Fig. 3. Peppering injection technique.

number of subjects were limitations of this initial human investigation of PRP in the treatment of chronic lateral epicondylar tendinopathy.

Peerbooms and colleagues[13] evaluated a cohort of 100 subjects with lateral epicondylar tendinopathy who had failed physical therapy and other treatments in a double-blind prospective randomized trial. This study used the same type of PRP (1A) and injection techniques as the first pilot investigation by Mishra.[4] The study was specifically designed to evaluate the value of PRP versus cortisone. Initial pain scores were 6.9 for the PRP subjects and 6.6 for the cortisone subjects. At 6 months, the PRP subjects reported a 53% improvement in pain scores compared with 14% in the cortisone subjects (P<.001). When the subjects were reevaluated at 1 year, the PRP subjects noted a 63% improvement versus 24% for the cortisone subjects (P<.001). Gosens and colleagues[14] published a further evaluation of these subjects at 2 years. The PRP subjects reported a 69% improvement in pain score versus 36% for the cortisone subjects (P<.0001). Furthermore, there was a significant improvement in disabilities of the arm, shoulder, and hand (DASH) scores at the 2-year mark for the PRP group compared with the cortisone group (67.6% and 15.7% improvement, respectively; P<.0001).

The value of treating a patient with PRP versus whole blood has also been investigated in a prospective single-blind randomized trial of 150 subjects.[15] Subjects with lateral epicondylar tendinopathy were required to have had symptoms for 6 months and to have failed conservative measures. The patient-related tennis elbow evaluation (PRTEE) score was used as a single outcome measurement at 1 month, 3 months, and 6 months. A buffy coat PRP preparation with an average of 2.8 times baseline whole blood platelet concentration (type 1B) was used in the study. Two injections were given under ultrasonic guidance 1 month apart. A higher conversion rate to surgery was noted in the whole blood group (20%) compared with the PRP group (10%). After the first evaluation, the subjects who opted for surgical intervention were excluded, thus significantly altering the data set in favor of the whole blood group. The investigators specifically state that this caused "a false elevation in mean PRTEE scores for the remaining patients in the cohort." Despite this potentially significant design issue, the investigators go on to report that there was no difference in success rates between the two groups at 3 and 6 months. No data is reported about initial pain scores in these subjects, precluding direct analysis with other investigations.

Thanasas and colleagues[16] studied 28 subjects with lateral epicondylar symptoms of at least 3 months in a prospective fashion. Subjects were randomized to receive either PRP (type 1A) or whole blood injection under ultrasonic guidance using the same peppering technique and platelet concentration device as outlined in the initial human trial by Mishra and Pavelko.[4] They reported the platelet concentration to be 5.5 times baseline with white blood cells consistent with a type 1A PRP. Initial pain scores were 6.0 for the PRP subjects and 6.1 for the whole blood subjects. Subjects were evaluated at 6 weeks, 3 months, and 6 months. At 6 weeks, the PRP subjects reported a statistically significant 61% improvement in pain scores compared with a 42% improvement in the whole blood subjects. The pain score improvements continued to be larger at the 3- and 6-month follow-up appointments, but the data were not statistically significant. There were also no differences in the Liverpool elbow score.

Wolf and colleagues[17] evaluated blood, saline, and corticosteroid injections in a prospective randomized controlled trial. This study investigated subjects with symptoms of less than 6 months duration. The preinjection visual analog pain scores were 5.0 for the blood group, 4.9 for the saline group, and 4.7 for the steroid group. This represents a group of subjects with moderate symptoms who have not failed a specific set of treatments. At the final follow-up of 6 months postinjection, the pain scores were 2.8, 1.3, and 2.1, respectively. The differences were not significant between the groups in terms of pain or DASH scores. These data indicate that any of these injections in this type of patient will likely result in pain improvement but not complete elimination of reported discomfort.

PRP AND ROTATOR CUFF REPAIR

Rotator cuff tendon tears are a common source of shoulder pain and combine both traumatic and degenerative elements. The incidence of this condition is increasing along with an aging population.[18] The management of rotator cuff tears is complex and multifactorial. Partial thickness tears may heal with conservative management and avoidance of the predisposing factors. Operative treatment allows primary repair to be performed either as an open or arthroscopic procedure. Despite satisfactory results for primary rotator cuff repair, the incidence of persistent tendon defects, or re-tears, is still significant.[19–21]

Several studies have demonstrated that native tendon-bone insertions are not restored after tendon-to-bone repair.[22] Healing of repaired tendons occurs via fibrous scar tissue formation rather than via the regeneration of a histologically normal insertion and, thus, repaired tendons have inferior mechanical properties and are more susceptible to retearing.[23–25] Considering the relatively high percentage of repair failure, reported at 11% to 94%,[19–21,26–28] it is important to explore techniques of biologic augmentation to reduce the postsurgical recurrence rate and improve long-term shoulder function after rotator cuff repair. Autologous PRP added during surgery is an attractive biologic strategy to augment healing of rotator cuff tears.

Randelli and colleagues[5] published the first paper investigating the use of PRP in rotator cuff repair (**Table 3**). Fourteen subjects received an intraoperative injection of activated PRP (type 2) at the end of the surgical procedure (**Figs. 4** and **5**). The PRP was obtained by centrifugation of 54 mL of whole blood drawn preoperatively from the subjects. The PRP was mixed with concentrated plasma and activated with an autologous thrombin component. A single-row suture anchor technique was used to repair the rotator cuff tears. The PRP was delivered between the bone and the repaired rotator cuff in a dried subacromial space. Subjects started passive assisted exercises at 10 days after surgery and were prospectively followed for 24 months. A significant improvement in term of visual analog score; University of California, Los Angeles score; and Constant score was observed during the follow-up period compared with the

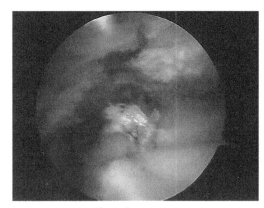

Fig. 4. Rotator cuff repair.

preoperative values. This pilot study concluded that their technique for PRP application in arthroscopic surgery was effective and safe with no reported complications. However, this investigation did not include a control group and no evaluation of the repair integrity was performed at last follow-up.

Using a similar PRP technique, Randelli and colleagues[29] published results of a randomized controlled study on the efficacy of intraoperative use of PRP in arthroscopic rotator cuff repair. The subjects were randomly divided into two groups. Subjects in the treatment group received a local injection of type 2 PRP at the end of the

Table 3
PRP and rotator cuff repair: controlled clinical studies

Study	Authors	Subjects	PRP Type	Comments
Level 4	Randelli et al,[5] 2008	14	Type 2 Biomet GPS (Biomet Biologics, Warsaw, IN, USA)	PRP safe to use, no complications at 24 mo follow-up.
Level 1	Castricini et al,[30] 2011	88	Type 4 Cascade (Musculoskeletal Transplant Foundation, Edison, NJ, USA)	No difference in Constant scores at 16 mo. PRP treated subjects had better restoration of footprint.
Level 1	Randelli et al,[29] 2011	53	Type 2 Biomet GPS (Biomet Biologics, Warsaw, IN, USA)	PRP subjects with better clinical outcomes at 3 mo. Smaller tears treated with PRP did better at medium and longer term follow-up.
Level 2	Jo et al,[33] 2011	42	Type 4 cell separator system	Trend for lower re-tearing in the PRP group. No accelerated recovery in the PRP group. 20 mo follow-up.
Level 2	Barber et al,[32] 2011	40	Type 4 Cascade (Musculoskeletal Transplant Foundation, Edison, NJ, USA)	Lower re-tear rates in the PRP group. Better healing rates in smaller tears with PRP.

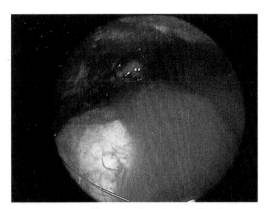

Fig. 5. Rotator cuff repair after PRP application.

surgical repair. The control group did not receive any additional treatment outside of the standard arthroscopic repair. All subjects had the same accelerated rehabilitation protocol. The pain score in the treatment group was lower than the control group at 3, 7, 14, and 30 days after surgery (P<.05). Clinical outcomes were significantly higher in the treatment group than the control group at 3 months after surgery (P<.05). There was no difference between the two groups after 6, 12, and 24 months. MRI studies at a minimum of 1-year follow-up showed no significant difference in the healing rate of the rotator cuff repair (PRP group, 40%; control group, 52%; P>.05). In the subgroup of subjects with smaller tears, strength in external rotation in the PRP group was significantly higher at 3, 6, 12, and 24 months postoperative (P<.05). The number of identified re-tears was two (14%) in the PRP subgroup and six (37%) in the control subgroup (P>.05).

Castricini and colleagues[30] performed a prospective randomized controlled double-blind study of 88 subjects undergoing arthroscopic rotator cuff repair with (43 subjects) and without (45 subjects) augmentation with autologous platelet-rich fibrin matrix. The membrane of autologous suturable fibrin was obtained by processing 9 mL of venous blood drawn from subjects before surgery. This PRP fibrin matrix construct did not have thrombin activation and the presence of white blood cells was minimal. A second spin of the PRP was done in the presence of calcium chloride for 25 minutes (type 4). This resulting membrane was incorporated into the suture construct and placed at the interface between the tendon and the greater tuberosity under continuous saline lavage. A double-row suture anchor technique was used in all cases. Passive and assisted active exercises were initiated after 3 weeks of immobilization. At the 16-month follow-up evaluation, there was no statistically significant difference in functional outcomes

as measured by Constant score or by MRI appearance. However, the re-tear rate was 10.5% in the control group compared with 2.5% in the treatment group, with a statistical trend approaching significance (P = .07). Arnoczky[31] reevaluated the MRI data from this paper using the binomial chi-squared test. He concluded that the PRP-augmented rotator cuff repairs result in a statistically significant return to normal footprint (P = .02) and signal intensity (P<.001).

Using the same PRP technique (type 4), Barber and colleagues[32] prospectively compared 40 subjects undergoing arthroscopic rotator cuff repair with and without PRP augmentation. The PRP group protocol consisted of drawing 18 mL of whole blood from subjects preoperatively to form two membranes of autologous suturable fibrin that were then inserted between the tendon and bone during the surgical repair. An arthroscopic single-row rotator cuff repair was performed in all cases and passive rehabilitation was allowed at 6 weeks. MRI studies obtained at 4 months after surgery showed persistent full-thickness tendon defects in 60% of the control group compared with 30% of the PRP augmented group (P = .03). In tears of less than 3 cm, the PRP group had an 86% healing rate compared with a 50% healing rate in the control group (P<.05). No difference was observed in clinical outcome scores at the unique final follow-up (average: 31 months).

Jo and colleagues[33] augmented his surgical treatment of 19 subjects with full-thickness rotator cuff tears using PRP activated with 10% calcium gluconate. He compared this treatment group to a control group of 23 subjects who underwent standard repair. PRP collection was performed 1 day before surgery and was prepared via plateletpheresis. A minimal amount of white blood cells were found in the PRP gel. An attempt was made to standardize the PRP at a target concentration of 3.5-fold increase above baseline. This technique resulted in a type 4B PRP. It was applied in the form of a gel threaded to a suture and placed at the interface between tendon and bone. The rotator cuff repair was performed using a transosseous equivalent technique in all cases. Passive range of motion and active-assisted exercises were allowed at 4 to 6 weeks after surgery depending on the size of the tear. Higher functional scores were observed in the control group at 3 months postoperatively; however, bias existed in this data set. The PRP group contained a larger proportion of subjects with massive tears that began rehabilitation 6 weeks after surgery, whereas the control group favored those with small-to-large tears that began rehabilitation at 4 weeks. No significant difference was seen at

6, 12, and at final follow-up. Despite the greater proportion of large-to-massive tears in the PRP group, MRI showed a re-tear rate of 26.7% in the PRP group compared with 41.2% in control group at a minimum of 9 months after surgery (P>.05). In tears less than 3 cm, the re-tear rate was 12.5% (1 of 8) for subjects in the PRP group and 35.7% (5 of 14) for subjects in the control group (P>.05).

Bergeson and colleagues[34] recently prospectively evaluated subjects with rotator cuff tears at risk for repair failure. These subjects had a combination of larger tear size, fatty atrophy, and older age. Single-row or double-row techniques were used to repair the tendon in combination with two suturable fibrin clots prepared from whole blood via a centrifugation process. This is consistent with type 4 PRP. These subjects were then compared with historical controls. The investigators reported higher re-tear rates in the PRP group (65.2% vs 38.1% P = .024) when compared with controls. There were no differences in functional outcomes between the two groups (P>.55). The small number of subjects in this highly variable subject population and the variability in repair techniques in addition to the use of retrospective controls limit the value of this investigation. The data do, however, suggest that type 4 PRP rotator repair constructs are not helpful for large or massive tears with fatty atrophy in an older patient population.

DISCUSSION

PRP research is rapidly evolving. A search of PubMed reveals approximately 6,000 references with several hundred additions within the last year. This explosion of data has led to a better understanding of the various types and potential applications of PRP. Presently, PRP exists in two primary versions. One contains concentrated platelets and white blood cells and the other contains concentrated platelets without white blood cells. These versions can be used clinically in an unactivated or activated manner. A new classification system (see **Table 1**) arose from these four basic versions of PRP. This system allows for better comparison of studies and outcomes.

PRP has been proposed as a primary or adjuvant treatment of a variety of orthopedic conditions and disorders. The most studied tissue type to date, however, is tendon. Significant preclinical data support the use of PRP for tendon repair and regeneration.[35–38] Kajikawa and colleagues[39] studied the effects of PRP on migration of bone marrow–derived cells. They demonstrated how a PRP injection into a tendon enhanced migration and incorporation of these reparative cells.

Preclinical data have also shown improved biomechanical structure of tendons when treated with PRP.[40] Finally, PRP protects human tenocytes against cell death and senescence induced by ciprofloxacin and dexamethasone.[41]

In the upper extremity, PRP has been used clinically for more than a decade—mainly for tendon-related injuries and disorders. Published, controlled studies have investigated the use of unactivated PRP with white blood cells (type 1) in approximately 300 subjects with lateral epicondylar tendinopathy.[4,13–16] No controlled investigations have been published using activated PRP (type 2) or PRP without white blood cells (types 3 and 4). It is, therefore, not possible to extrapolate the published findings outlined below to these types of PRP. There are also differences between the studies, including the initial level of pain reported by the subjects and the tools used to evaluate the subjects. Level-one data, however, now clearly support the use of type 1 PRP instead of cortisone for subjects with chronic lateral epicondylar tendinopathy.[13,14] Data also suggest PRP may prevent progression to surgery compared with whole blood and reduce pain in the short term (6 weeks).[15] At 3 and 6 months, no significant differences in pain scores are noted in subjects with moderate (6 out of 10) pain initially when whole blood is compared with PRP.[15,16] Longer term follow-up at 1 year and 2 years for PRP versus whole blood has not been published. The differences in subjects who report moderate pain (6 out of 10) versus subjects with significant pain initially (8 out of 10) are also not clear and this may affect outcomes. In subjects with mild to moderate symptoms (pain less than or equal to 5 out of 10) of less than 6 months duration, the literature supports using autologous blood, saline, or cortisone injections.[17] None of these studies reported any significant complications associated with the use of PRP in the treatment of lateral epicondylar tendinopathy. Further prospective, randomized trials of PRP versus saline and surgical treatment as controls have been initiated. Overall, the efficacy rate of PRP for subjects with chronic lateral epicondylar tendinopathy that has failed standard treatments is about 75% to 93%. This has important implications for the cost of treating these patients. No detailed data are available. However, the total cost of treating a patient with PRP is lower than the total cost of treating a patient with surgery—especially when the outpatient facility and anesthesia fees are included. Further prospective trials that include complete cost data would help specify these potential savings. Finally, private and government payers are presently evaluating the cost-effectiveness of

PRP as a treatment of patients with chronic lateral epicondylar tendinopathy.

Although clinical studies have produced conflicting results, PRP data suggest a beneficial effect on the healing process when applied during a rotator cuff repair. Importantly, no complications have been reported from its use for this application. Definitive conclusions on the efficacy of PRP in rotator cuff repair presently are difficult to draw. Clinical studies published so far have had different experimental design and the strength of evidence has ranged from one to four. These trials used several PRP strategies, including application of activated PRP (type 2) or incorporation of platelet rich fibrin matrix (type 4) into the repair, implantation of PRP membrane during the continuously saline irrigation, and PRP injection in a dried subacromial space. Also, the surgical techniques (transosseous equivalent, single-row or double-row technique) and rehabilitation protocols (standard or accelerated) were not the same across the trials.

In this review, a trend toward a lower rotator cuff re-tear rate as measured by MRI was found. This trend was most prominent when a stratified analysis was made to analyze the results of small and medium tears. The re-tear rate ranged from to 2.5% to 14% in subjects with tears less than 3 cm treated with type 4 PRP. Subjects receiving conventional surgical repair alone had a higher re-tear rate ranging from 36% to 50%.[30,32,33] Although pooling data were not possible given variation in the surgical techniques and PRP formulation, it was observed that the re-tear rate was more than 2.5 times higher in the control group. Using a type 2 PRP injected in a dried subacromial space, Randelli and colleagues[29] found a similar risk ratio in subjects with less extensive tears (grade 1 or 2). Furthermore, these investigators reported accelerated recovery in subjects who received the PRP treatment compared with the control group.

One other study investigating healing time in PRP-augmented rotator cuff repairs showed conflicting results; however, the study had some inherent weaknesses.[33] It was a nonrandomized design and the PRP group had a larger proportion of massive tears that affected the time to start the rehabilitation after surgery. These findings support the use of PRP in small rotator cuff tears that may be more prone to the biologic enhancement by PRP. A continuous saline lavage, level of platelet concentration, and the timing of a postoperative rehabilitation protocol can all affect the efficacy of applying PRP in conjunction with a rotator cuff repair. More precise prospective randomized controlled studies are needed to determine the role of PRP in improving healing when compared with standard treatment especially in small-to-medium sized tears. To show a significant difference in recurrence rate of 25% with an alpha level of 5% and power of 80%, 50 subjects for each group are needed. A prospective randomized controlled study of 100 subjects using the same PRP type and surgical technique would clarify the role of this biologic tool in conjunction with rotator cuff repair.

As outlined above, published clinical studies using PRP have focused on lateral epicondylar tendinopathy and rotator cuff tears. Some of the data within these papers also support the use of PRP for medial epicondylar tendinopathy. Anecdotal reports of PRP being used to treat partial rotator cuff tears, biceps tendinopathy, and partial tears of the medial collateral ligament (MCL) of the elbow do exist but not in any peer reviewed published reports. Recently presented data, however, suggest type 1 PRP may help athletes return to sport after partial elbow MCL injuries. Crow and colleagues[42] reported that 16 of 17 athletes who had failed nonoperative treatment of partial elbow MCL injuries were able to return to their sport an average of 10 weeks after an ultrasonic-guided injection of type 1 PRP. DASH scores also improved significantly compared with baseline ($P = .003$). This study supports further investigation of PRP for this specific indication. Other potential applications in the upper extremity that have been proposed but not studied include de Quervain tenosynovitis, carpal tunnel syndrome, and shoulder arthritis. No data, however, on these applications have been published to date. In the lower extremity, PRP in various formulations has been studied in Achilles tendinopathy, patellar tendinopathy, and knee osteoarthritis.[43–47] Preclinical data also suggest certain types of PRP may be useful in the treatment of degenerative disc disease.[48] Any attempt to generalize about the value of PRP based on a meta-analysis of the literature would be difficult. There are simply too many different application techniques and poor documentation of what was actually given to the subjects.

As PRP continues to evolve, more research is needed to understand its mechanism of action in addition to clinical data. It is possible that the soup of cytokines within PRP modifies neural pain receptors and the extracellular matrix while stimulating cellular proliferation. Data already exist demonstrating how PRP modulates IL-1 production from macrophages.[49,50] It is also clear that large clinical trials are needed to define the best type of PRP to be used and for what specific clinical application. This is simple to call for but difficult to execute. Prospective randomized trials that are designed and powered appropriately are expensive and take years to complete. Who will pay for such trials? Institutions or industry may be motivated to do so but only with better clarity about potential regulatory and payment approvals. For now, it is clear that type 1 (See **Table 1**) PRP is a safe and effective option for patients with chronic lateral epicondylar tendinopathy when compared with cortisone and may be better at helping patients avoid surgery when compared with whole blood. The data are less clear with regard to the rotator cuff, but a trend toward improved healing rates and faster clinical recovery for smaller and medium sized tears is emerging.

SUMMARY

Novel formulations of PRP will continue to emerge. Fractionation of the white blood cell population within PRP, specifically depleting neutrophils, may be of significant value for certain clinical conditions. PRP may, in the future, be used in combination with cellular or gene therapies such as adipose-derived stem cells. A better point-of-care measurement of PRP potency is also needed. It is clear that some patients respond dramatically to PRP and others do not. Understanding the reasons why this occurs and then treating only those patients that are likely to respond would be of significant value. Finally, it may soon be possible to sample a patient's blood or connective tissue and predict via genetic markers if that person could be successfully treated with PRP. In some respects, PRP in its present state is similar to arthroscopy in its early stages in the 1970s. The data supporting its use are immature but this biologic technology has the potential to transform the practice of musculoskeletal medicine and orthopedic surgery.

REFERENCES

1. Albee FH. Transplantation of a portion of the tibia into the spine for Pott's disease: a preliminary report 1911. Clin Orthop Relat Res 2007;460:14–6.
2. Kingsley CS. Blood coagulation; evidence of an antagonist to factor VI in platelet-rich human plasma. Nature 1954;173:723–4.
3. Marx RE, Carlson ER, Eichstaedt RM, et al. Platelet-rich plasma: growth factor enhancement for bone grafts. Oral Surg Oral Med Oral Pathol Oral Radiol Endod 1998;85:638–46.
4. Mishra A, Pavelko T. Treatment of chronic elbow tendinosis with buffered platelet-rich plasma. Am J Sports Med 2006;34:1774–8.
5. Randelli PS, Arrigoni P, Cabitza P, et al. Autologous platelet rich plasma for arthroscopic rotator cuff repair. A pilot study. Disabil Rehabil 2008;30:1584–9.
6. Mishra A, Harmon K, Woodall J, et al. Sports medicine applications of platelet rich plasma. Curr Pharm Biotechnol 2012;13(7):1185–95.
7. Coppinger JA, Cagney G, Toomey S, et al. Characterization of the proteins released from activated platelets leads to localization of novel platelet proteins in human atherosclerotic lesions. Blood 2004;103:2096–104.
8. Dohan Ehrenfest DM, Bielecki T, Mishra A, et al. In search of a consensus terminology in the field of platelet concentrates for surgical use: platelet-rich plasma (PRP), platelet-rich fibrin (PRF), fibrin gel polymerization and leukocytes. Curr Pharm Biotechnol 2011;13(7):1131–7.
9. Sundman EA, Cole BJ, Fortier LA. Growth factor and catabolic cytokine concentrations are influenced by the cellular composition of platelet-rich plasma. Am J Sports Med 2011;39:2135–40.
10. Harrison S, Vavken P, Kevy S, et al. Platelet activation by collagen provides sustained release of anabolic cytokines. Am J Sports Med 2011;39:729–34.
11. Nirschl RP, Pettrone FA. Tennis elbow. The surgical treatment of lateral epicondylitis. J Bone Joint Surg Am 1979;61:832–9.
12. Cohen MS, Romeo AA. Open and arthroscopic management of lateral epicondylitis in the athlete. Hand Clin 2009;25:331–8.
13. Peerbooms JC, Sluimer J, Bruijn DJ, et al. Positive effect of an autologous platelet concentrate in lateral epicondylitis in a double-blind randomized controlled trial: platelet-rich plasma versus corticosteroid injection with a 1-year follow-up. Am J Sports Med 2010;38:255–62.
14. Gosens T, Peerbooms JC, van Laar W, et al. Ongoing positive effect of platelet-rich plasma versus corticosteroid injection in lateral epicondylitis: a double-blind randomized controlled trial with 2-year follow-up. Am J Sports Med 2011;39:1200–8.
15. Creaney L, Wallace A, Curtis M, et al. Growth factor-based therapies provide additional benefit beyond physical therapy in resistant elbow tendinopathy: a prospective, single-blind, randomised trial of autologous blood injections versus platelet-rich plasma injections. Br J Sports Med 2011;45:966–71.
16. Thanasas C, Papadimitriou G, Charalambidis C, et al. Platelet-rich plasma versus autologous whole blood for the treatment of chronic lateral elbow epicondylitis: a randomized controlled clinical trial. Am J Sports Med 2011;39:2130–4.
17. Wolf J, Ozer K, Scott F, et al. Comparison of autologous blood, corticosteroid and saline injection in the treatment of lateral epicondylitis: a prospective,

randomized, controlled multicenter study. J Hand Surg 2011;36:1269–72.

18. Sher JS, Uribe JW, Posada A, et al. Abnormal findings on magnetic resonance images of asymptomatic shoulders. J Bone Joint Surg Am 1995;77: 10–5.

19. Boileau P, Brassart N, Watkinson DJ, et al. Arthroscopic repair of full-thickness tears of the supraspinatus: does the tendon really heal? J Bone Joint Surg Am 2005;87:1229–40.

20. Galatz LM, Ball CM, Teefey SA, et al. The outcome and repair integrity of completely arthroscopically repaired large and massive rotator cuff tears. J Bone Joint Surg Am 2004;86-A:219–24.

21. Gerber C, Fuchs B, Hodler J. The results of repair of massive tears of the rotator cuff. J Bone Joint Surg Am 2000;82:505–15.

22. Burkhart SS, Danaceau SM, Pearce CE Jr. Arthroscopic rotator cuff repair: Analysis of results by tear size and by repair technique-margin convergence versus direct tendon-to-bone repair. Arthroscopy 2001;17:905–12.

23. Cheung EV, Silverio L, Sperling JW. Strategies in biologic augmentation of rotator cuff repair: a review. Clin Orthop Relat Res 2010;468:1476–84.

24. Galatz LM, Sandell LJ, Rothermich SY, et al. Characteristics of the rat supraspinatus tendon during tendon-to-bone healing after acute injury. J Orthop Res 2006;24:541–50.

25. Rodeo SA, Arnoczky SP, Torzilli PA, et al. Tendon-healing in a bone tunnel. A biomechanical and histological study in the dog. J Bone Joint Surg Am 1993; 75:1795–803.

26. Levy O, Venkateswaran B, Even T, et al. Mid-term clinical and sonographic outcome of arthroscopic repair of the rotator cuff. J Bone Joint Surg Br 2008;90:1341–7.

27. Lafosse L, Brzoska R, Toussaint B, et al. The outcome and structural integrity of arthroscopic rotator cuff repair with use of the double-row suture anchor technique. Surgical technique. J Bone Joint Surg Am 2008;90(Suppl 2 Pt 2):275–86.

28. Bishop J, Klepps S, Lo IK, et al. Cuff integrity after arthroscopic versus open rotator cuff repair: a prospective study. J Shoulder Elbow Surg 2006; 15:290–9.

29. Randelli P, Arrigoni P, Ragone V, et al. Platelet rich plasma in arthroscopic rotator cuff repair: a prospective RCT study, 2-year follow-up. J Shoulder Elbow Surg 2011;20:518–28.

30. Castricini R, Longo UG, De Benedetto M, et al. Platelet-rich plasma augmentation for arthroscopic rotator cuff repair: a randomized controlled trial. Am J Sports Med 2011;39:258–65.

31. Arnoczky SP. Platelet-rich plasma augmentation of rotator cuff repair: letter. Am J Sports Med 2011; 39:NP8–9 [author reply: NP-11].

32. Barber FA, Hrnack SA, Snyder SJ, et al. Rotator cuff repair healing influenced by platelet-rich plasma construct augmentation. Arthroscopy 2011;27: 1029–35.

33. Jo CH, Kim JE, Yoon KS, et al. Does platelet-rich plasma accelerate recovery after rotator cuff repair? A prospective cohort study. Am J Sports Med 2011; 39:2082–90.

34. Bergeson AG, Tashjian RZ, Greis PE, et al. Effects of platelet-rich fibrin matrix on repair integrity of at-risk rotator cuff tears. Am J Sports Med 2012; 40:286–93.

35. Anitua E, Andia I, Sanchez M, et al. Autologous preparations rich in growth factors promote proliferation and induce VEGF and HGF production by human tendon cells in culture. J Orthop Res 2005; 23:281–6.

36. de Mos M, van der Windt AE, Jahr H, et al. Can platelet-rich plasma enhance tendon repair? A cell culture study. Am J Sports Med 2008;36:1171–8.

37. Visser LC, Arnoczky SP, Caballero O, et al. Growth factor-rich plasma increases tendon cell proliferation and matrix synthesis on a synthetic scaffold: an in vitro study. Tissue Eng Part A 2010;16:1021–9.

38. Wang X, Qiu Y, Triffitt J, et al. Proliferation and differentiation of human tenocytes in response to platelet rich plasma: an in vitro and in vivo study. J Orthop Res 2012;30(6):982–90.

39. Kajikawa Y, Morihara T, Sakamoto H, et al. Platelet-rich plasma enhances the initial mobilization of circulation-derived cells for tendon healing. J Cell Physiol 2008;215:837–45.

40. Virchenko O, Aspenberg P. How can one platelet injection after tendon injury lead to a stronger tendon after 4 weeks? Interplay between early regeneration and mechanical stimulation. Acta Orthop 2006;77:806–12.

41. Zargar Baboldashti N, Poulsen RC, Franklin SL, et al. Platelet-rich plasma protects tenocytes from adverse side effects of dexamethasone and ciprofloxacin. Am J Sports Med 2011;39:1929–35.

42. Crow S, Podesta L, Yocum L. Treatment of the elbow partial ulnar collateral ligament tears with platelet rich plasma. Presented at the American Academy of Orthopaedic Surgery Annual Meeting. San Francico (CA); Feb. 7–11, 2012.

43. de Vos RJ, Weir A, van Schie HT, et al. Platelet-rich plasma injection for chronic Achilles tendinopathy: a randomized controlled trial. JAMA 2010;303: 144–9.

44. Monto RR. Platelet-rich plasma (PRP) effectively treats chronic Achilles tendonosis. Presented at the American Academy of Orthopedic Surgery Annual Meeting. New Orleans (LA); March 9–13, 2010.

45. Kon E, Filardo G, Delcogliano M, et al. Platelet-rich plasma: new clinical application: a pilot study for treatment of jumper's knee. Injury 2009;40:598–603.

46. Kon E, Buda R, Filardo G, et al. Platelet-rich plasma: intra-articular knee injections produced favorable results on degenerative cartilage lesions. Knee Surg Sports Traumatol Arthrosc 2010;18:472–9.

47. Filardo G, Kon E, Della Villa S, et al. Use of platelet-rich plasma for the treatment of refractory jumper's knee. Int Orthop 2010;34:909–15.

48. Gullung G, Woodall J Jr, Tucci M, et al. Platelet-rich plasma effects on degenerative disc disease: analysis of histology and imaging in an animal model. Evid Based Spine Care J 2011;2(4):13–8.

49. Woodall J Jr, Tucci M, Mishra A, et al. Cellular effects of platelet rich plasmainterleukin1 release from PRP treated macrophages. Biomed Sci Instrum 2008;44: 489–94.

50. Mishra A, Woodall J Jr, Vieira A. Treatment of tendon and muscle using platelet-rich plasma. Clin Sports Med 2009;28:113–25.

Free Vascularized Medial Femoral Condyle Autograft for Challenging Upper Extremity Nonunions

David B. Jones Jr, MD, Peter C. Rhee, DO,
Alan T. Bishop, MD, Alexander Y. Shin, MD*

KEYWORDS

- Medial femoral condyle • Vascularized autograft • Nonunion

KEY POINTS

- The medial femoral condyle has a consistent, robust vascular supply based on the descending genicular artery and the superiomedial genicular artery.
- Free vascular corticocancellous grafts from the medial femoral condyle have proven valuable in treating nonunions of the scaphoid, metacarpals, and phalanges.
- Thin, flexible corticoperiosteal grafts from the medial femoral condyle have successfully been used in the treatment of long bone nonunions in the upper extremity.

INTRODUCTION

Vascularized bone grafts (VBG) have been used for over a century to address fracture nonunions, bony defects, and avascular necrosis (AVN). In 1905, Huntington[1] reported using a pedicled fibula graft to reconstruct a tibial bone defect. Then with the advancement of microvascular surgical techniques in the 1970s, the use of free vascularized bone grafts to treat remote nonunions became feasible and further expanded the potential and role of vascularized bone grafting.[2] Since that time, numerous other pedicled and free vascularized bone grafts have been described and have proven effective in promoting the healing of chronic nonunions; restoring vascularity to osteonecrotic bone; and reconstituting segmental bone defects resulting from trauma, infection, or tumor resection.

Vascularized grafts offer several advantages over nonvascularized autografts or allografts in the treatment of these challenging problems. Although nonvascularized grafts have limited osteogenic capacity and require creeping substitution of the graft bone, vascularized grafts preserve viable osteocytes and blood supply resulting in faster incorporation and healing, particularly in the biologically unfavorable setting.[3,4]

The medial femoral condyle (MFC) has been described as a valuable source of vascularized bone grafts. Grafts from this region were initially described by Hertel and Masquelet[5] as pedicled, reverse-flow periosteal and corticoperiosteal grafts based on branches of the descending genicular artery. They reported that these grafts could extend to the proximal and middle third of the tibia to address nonunions, segmental bone defects, or AVN about the knee. Sakai and colleagues[6] subsequently described free vascularized thin, corticoperiosteal flaps based on the articular branch of

---

The authors have nothing relevant to disclose.
Division of Hand Surgery, Department of Orthopedic Surgery, Mayo Clinic, 200 1st Street Southwest, Rochester, MN 55905, USA
* Corresponding author.
E-mail address: shin.alexander@mayo.edu

Hand Clin 28 (2012) 493–501
http://dx.doi.org/10.1016/j.hcl.2012.08.005
0749-0712/12/$ – see front matter © 2012 Elsevier Inc. All rights reserved.

the descending genicular artery (DGA) and vein or the superomedial genicular vessels that were used in the treatment of persistent nonunions of the humerus, ulna, and metacarpals. Then in 2000, Doi and colleagues[7] described harvesting corticocancellous grafts based on the same vascular pedicle, which they used as free vascularized grafts to treat scaphoid nonunions. Since that time, MFC grafts have been used most commonly to treat scaphoid nonunions[8–10] but have also been used in the successful salvage of tubular bone defects of the hand[11,12] and recalcitrant long bone nonunions.[13–18]

ANATOMY

The clinical success of free vascularized MFC grafts is evidence of the robust and consistent vascularity of this region. The highly vascular nature of the distal femur was recognized by Rogers and Gladstone[19] in 1950 when they labeled this the "area cribrosa vasorum condyloidae medialis and lateralis" given the observation of numerous foramina evenly distributed over the medial and lateral condylar surfaces. They studied the vascular foramina of the distal femora of 200 adults, 4 juveniles, and 16 infants. They also described an anastomosis between "the deep branch of the highest genicular artery and the medial genicular artery" supplying multiple nutrient vessels to the medial femoral condyle.[19]

Scapinelli[20] subsequently described 3 branches of the supreme or highest DGA: the saphenous, deep oblique, and musculo-articular branch, which was noted to form an anastomotic arch parallel to the articular surface over the medial condyle with the medial superior genicular artery.[20] In their evaluation of the blood supply to the knee for allogenic transplantation, Kirschner and colleagues[21] also described this combined contribution to the MFC from the DGA and the superior medial genicular artery (SMGA). They described the DGA as originating from the femoral artery approximately 12 cm above the condyle and the SMGA originating from the popliteal artery approximately 4 cm above the condyle. Reddy and Frederick[22] studied the intraosseous and extraosseous blood supply of the distal femur as it relates to structures at risk during posterior cruciate ligament reconstruction and also noted this dual arterial supply to the medial femoral condyle.

This vascular anatomy has been further evaluated and defined in a cadaveric study at the authors' institution.[23] Nineteen specimens were studied, with the DGA present in 89% and the SMGA present in 100% of specimens with average distances proximal to the articular surface of 13.7 cm and 5.2 cm, respectively (**Fig. 1**). The DGA originates from the superficial femoral artery just proximal to the adductor hiatus and travels deep to the adductor magnus and sartorius tendons along the posterior aspect of the medial intermuscular septum before branching and becoming intimately invested with the periosteum an average of 6.0 cm (range 4.5–7.0 cm) from the articular surface. The SMGA originates from the popliteal artery and travels from behind the adductor magnus tendon to anastomose with the osteoarticular branch of the DGA supplying multiple perforating vessels to the periosteum and medial femoral condyle. The average number of

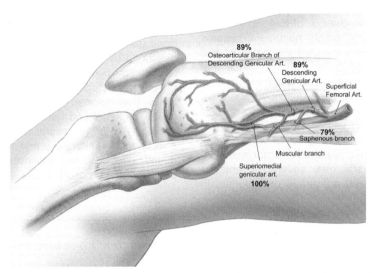

Fig. 1. The extraosseous arterial anatomy supplying the medial femoral condyle. (*Reprinted from* Larson AN, Bishop AT, Shin AY. Tech Hand Up Extrem Surg. Philadelphia: Lippincott Williams & Wilkins; 2007. p. 247; with permission from the Mayo Foundation.)

perforating vessels was greatest in the posterior distal quadrant of the condyle (**Fig. 2**). These vessels supplying the MFC were consistently noted to be of sufficient diameter and length to facilitate microvascular anastomosis (>1 mm).

Given the expanding indications for MFC grafts and the use of larger intercalary grafts from this region, Iorio and colleagues[24] recently reported on the proximal limits of these flaps supplied by the DGA. In their series of 18 cadaveric femora, the DGA branched from the superficial femoral artery 14.2 ± 2.4 cm from the articular surface and communicated with a proximally directed, previously unnamed arcuate branch they labeled the medial metaphyseal periosteal artery (MMPA). The medial distal femoral periosteum supplied by the DGA and MMPA averaged 13.7 ± 1.3 cm proximal to the articular surface. Therefore, based on this consistent and robust vascular anatomy, a variety of corticoperiosteal or corticocancellous flaps can be harvested.

INDICATIONS
Scaphoid Nonunion

Among the various applications of MFC grafts, the treatment of scaphoid nonunions has become one of the most common. Doi and Sakai[25] initially described the use of an onlay corticocancellous MFC vascularized bone grafts in the treatment of scaphoid nonunions with associated AVN as an alternative to the various pedicled bone grafts that had been used for scaphoid nonunion and

AVN. All 10 patients went on to union at an average of 12 weeks, with good or excellent results in 8 patients and fair results in 2 at an average of 3.5 years postoperatively. The investigators noted that the abundant vascularity of the graft and the relative ease of shaping the graft to fit the defect in the scaphoid made this a desirable alternative to the pedicled distal radius grafts.

The indications for the use of this graft were further clarified in a retrospective comparison of the MFC vascularized graft with the 1,2 intercompartmental supraretinacular (1,2 ICSRA) pedicled distal radius graft in the treatment of scaphoid nonunions complicated by AVN *and* carpal collapse or humpback deformity.[8] The technique had been modified slightly to use the graft as a structural, volar interposition graft to restore scaphoid geometry and carpal alignment.[10] Only 4 of the 10 patients treated with the 1,2 ICSRA at a median time to union of 19 weeks with no significant changes noted in the radiographic carpal angles, whereas all 12 nonunions treated with the MFC graft healed at a median time to union of 13 weeks with significantly improved carpal parameters. Given the poor results of the 1,2 ICSRA graft in achieving union in scaphoid nonunions with both AVN and humpback deformity, attributed at least in part to the failure in correcting the humpback deformity, the MFC graft was recommended as a better alternative in this challenging subset of scaphoid nonunions. Therefore, this graft is currently indicated in the treatment of scaphoid nonunions associated with

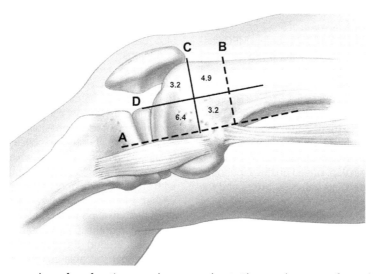

Fig. 2. The average number of perforating vessels per quadrant. The quadrants are formed by drawing lines along the insertions of the hamstring and medial collateral ligament (A dashed line), from the insertion of the adductor magnus (B dashed line) and then from the proximal pole of the patella (C solid line) and the anterior margin of the medial meniscus (D solid line). (*Reprinted from* with permission from the Mayo Foundation.)

both scaphoid foreshortening and proximal segment AVN.

Scaphoid foreshortening or humpback deformity is defined as a lateral intrascaphoid angle more than 45° (normal <35°). It is associated with dorsal intercalary segment instability deformity defined as a revised carpal height ratio less than 1.52 (normal = 1.57 ± 0.05) or radiolunate angle more than 15° (normal <10°). Proximal pole avascularity is evidenced by the preoperative radiographic finding of increased bone density or sclerosis, occasionally associated with the loss of trabecular structure, collapse of subchondral bone, and formation of bone cysts. Magnetic resonance imaging (MRI) is more helpful in assessing scaphoid vascularity, with low signal intensity on both T1 and T2 and diminished contrast uptake on gadolinium-enhanced MRI.[26] Ultimate confirmation of avascularity occurs at surgery by observation of white, sclerotic bone with absent punctate bleeding on tourniquet release.[27]

In the setting of prolonged AVN, the articular cartilage of the proximal pole of the scaphoid may begin to deteriorate. Although this has traditionally been a contraindication for vascularized bone grafting and an indication for a salvage procedure, a graft from the MFC, including the articular cartilage, has been described recently.[28]

Phalanx and Metacarpal Nonunions

The free corticoperiosteal MFC vascularized bone graft may be effective in the treatment of nonunions within the hand. The pliable nature of this graft allows for excellent conformation around the tubular bones of the hand up to an area of 5 × 7 cm.[29] Sakai and colleagues[6] used a corticoperiosteal MFC vascularized graft and cancellous bone graft to treat a second metacarpal shaft infected nonunion at 4 months postinjury (graft size: 4 × 3 cm, recipient vessel: dorsal branch of the radial artery).[6] Because of the excision of a sinus tract, simultaneous skin flap transfer was performed. Bone union was noted at 7 weeks postoperatively without any wound healing issues. The investigators concluded that a simultaneous sensory skin flap, based on the saphenous branch of the descending genicular artery and the saphenous nerve, was feasible in cases of bone and soft tissue loss about the hand. However, Giessler and Schmidt[11] cautioned against the use of the MFC graft as an osteocutaneous flap when applied to the finger because of the mismatch in thickness of the donor skin flap to the thin subcutaneous tissues over the phalanges. Instead, the investigators advocated soft tissue coverage with a full-thickness skin graft placed directly over the periosteum of the MFC graft, based on their successful results.

A free structural corticocancellous MFC vascularized bone graft can be useful for the reconstruction of small osseous defects within the hand. Sammer and colleagues[12] reported successful thumb metacarpophalangeal joint arthrodesis with a corticocancellous MFC graft (graft size: 3 × 1 × 1 cm, recipient vessel: end to side into the radial artery in the distal forearm) in a 44-year-old man with an infected nonunion, despite previous iliac crest corticocancellous bone grafting. Computed tomography confirmed graft consolidation at 6.5 months postoperatively. Similarly, Geissler and Schmidt[11] noted successful revision thumb interphalangeal joint arthrodesis with a corticocancellous MFC vascularized graft (graft size: ~2 cm, recipient vessel: dorsal branch of the radial artery) in a 22-year-old man with an open crush injury to the thumb proximal phalanx with a persistent pseudarthrosis, despite 3 previous attempts at fracture union with nonvascularized iliac crest bone grafting. Union was noted at 3 months, and the patient returned to full work duties. Additionally, Grant and colleagues[30] achieved successful index finger distal interphalangeal joint arthrodesis with a corticocancellous MFC graft (graft size: 1.0 × 1.5 cm², recipient vessel: end-to-end anastomosis to the radial digital artery) despite previous failed attempts at arthrodesis, including arteriovenous bundle implantation, in a 61-year-old woman treated initially for osteoarthritis. Union was observed at 3 months with full return to work as a typist.

Clavicle Nonunions

A free vascularized corticoperiosteal MFC graft can also be very useful in the treatment of clavicle nonunions.[14,15,25] The pliable graft can be easily conformed around the tubular clavicle without excessive bulk. Popularized by Doi and Sakai[25] in the treatment of many nonunions of the upper extremity, their initial report included one clavicle nonunion treated successfully with a corticoperiosteal MFC graft. Fuchs and colleagues[15] reported on 3 clavicle nonunions (2 of which were radiation-induced pathologic fractures) successfully treated with an onlay corticoperiosteal MFC graft (recipient vessel: thoracoacromial trunk) and rigid stainless steel plate fixation with bony union noted between 3 and 7 months postoperatively. The graft was wrapped around the clavicle and secured with heavy nonabsorbable sutures around the fracture site. The shoulder was immobilized postoperatively for 6 to 8 weeks at which point passive range of motion was initiated. Similarly, Choudry and colleagues[14] observed successful union with the corticoperiosteal MFC graft in 2 clavicle fractures after a failed open reduction and internal fixation.

Humerus Nonunions

Atrophic nonunions of the humerus can be successfully treated with a free vascularized corticoperiosteal MFC graft. Although free vascularized fibula grafts can provide both structural and osteogenic properties, especially in cases of large bone defects (>3 cm) with poor intrinsic stability at the nonunion site, Sakai and colleagues[6] and Doi and colleagues[25,31] recommended the free vascularized corticoperiosteal MFC graft for atrophic nonunions of the humerus at the time of revision fixation. Union after corticoperiosteal MFC grafting for humeral nonunion has been reported to be between 90% and 100%.[7,14,17,18,31–33] Choudry and colleagues[14] noted successful union in 3 out of 3 humerus nonunions with a free corticoperiosteal MFC graft (recipient vessel: end to side into the brachial artery) at a mean of 3 months (range: 2–4 months) with return to full, regular activities. Similarly, Yajima and colleagues[18] successfully treated 6 of 6 humerus nonunions with revision open reduction, internal fixation, and a free corticoperiosteal MFC graft (graft size: 4.0 × 2.5 cm to 5 × 3 cm, recipient vessel: brachial artery) with union noted at a mean of 3.3 months with 1 case of graft-site transient saphenous nerve paresthesia. Muramatsu and colleagues[31] reported the largest series of recalcitrant posttraumatic nonunions of the humerus treated with a variety of VBGs (fibula: n = 10, MFC: n = 10, and scapula: n = 3). Of these, 9 corticoperiosteal MFC grafts resulted in successful union at a mean of 4 months (range: 2–6 months) when used throughout the length of the humerus (distal: n = 4, middle: n = 4, proximal: n = 1) for bone defects of less than 1 cm. Complications included paresthesias near the graft donor site (n = 3), nonunion (n = 1), and venous thrombosis successfully revascularized with thrombectomy and reanastomosis (n = 1). Kakar and colleagues[17] stressed the importance of bony apposition at the nonunion site (up to 2 cm of shortening accepted), reestablishment of the intramedullary canal, stabilization of the inset graft (Kirschner wires, screws, or suture anchors), and judicious use of nonvascularized fibular strut allografts if significant bone loss was present.

Forearm Nonunions

Nonunions of the forearm bones with small osseous defects (<5 cm) can be effectively treated with rigid fixation and corticoperiosteal MFC vascularized grafts. Successful union rates in the treatment of nonunions involving the radius and ulna with use of the corticoperiosteal MFC graft has been reported to be 100%.[6,14,32–34] De Smet reported successful union in 6 out of 6 nonunions of the forearm (ulna n = 4 and radius n = 2) with a corticoperiosteal MFC graft (recipient vessel: end to side into the ulnar or radial artery) in addition to nonunion resection and fracture stabilization.[34] In this series, 1 patient sustained an insufficiency fracture through the supracondylar region of the femur at the graft donor site. Del Piñal and colleagues[32] noted successful union in 3 out of 3 nonunions of the forearm (ulna: n = 2, radius: n = 1) with revision rigid fixation, free corticoperiosteal MFC graft (graft size: 3 × 3 cm to 4 × 4 cm, recipient vessel: end-to-side into the radial, ulnar or brachial) wrapped around the nonunion site, with or without additional cancellous bone grafting, at 6 to 8 weeks postoperatively. In cases of segmental bone loss, Rodriguez-Vegas and Delgado-Serrano[33,35] recommended onlay of the corticoperiosteal MFC graft with cancellous bone graft placement into the resulting tubular structure, as described by Masquelet. They noted consolidation of the segmental osseous defect (3 cm) in one patient treated in this manner.

SURGICAL TECHNIQUE

The procedure is performed under general anesthesia. Patients are supine with the affected upper extremity prepped and positioned appropriately depending on the site to be bone grafted. A pneumatic tourniquet is placed on the ipsilateral lower extremity, which is then prepped free from the proximal thigh distally. A sandbag beneath the drapes is used to maintain knee flexion. The ipsilateral leg is selected for medial femoral condylar graft harvest because it facilitates simultaneous work on both surgical sites and allows use of an ambulatory aid in the contralateral hand postoperatively if necessary.

Under tourniquet control, a longitudinal incision is made over the posterior border of the vastus medialis, extending from the palpable joint line proximally for 18 to 20 cm (**Fig. 3**). The dissection is carried down to the fascia overlying the vastus medialis, which is incised along its posteromedial border. The vastus medialis is then elevated and retracted exposing the vessels supplying the MFC traveling along the floor of the muscle compartment to the periosteum overlying the medial femoral condylar and supracondylar region (**Fig. 4**). As described earlier, the MFC is supplied by the DGA, which originates from the superficial femoral artery just proximal to the adductor hiatus, and the SMGA, which arises from the popliteal artery. These vessels join to form an anastomotic

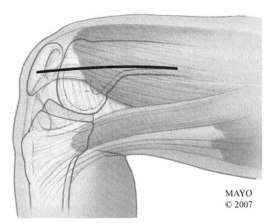

Fig. 3. The incision (*dark line*) for harvesting the free vascularized bone graft from the MFC is made over the posterior aspect of the vastus medialis extending from the joint line proximally 18 to 20 cm. (*Reprinted from* Larson AN, Bishop AT, Shin AY. Tech Hand Up Extrem Surg. Philadelphia: Lippincott Williams & Wilkins; 2007. p. 252; with permission from the Mayo Foundation.)

ring or whorl overlying and supplying the medial femoral condyle. The larger of the two arteries, most commonly the DGA, with its venae comitantes is selected as the vascular pedicle and mobilized taking care to ligate or cauterize any small muscular branches with bipolar cautery. The length of the vascular pedicle is determined by the recipient site anatomy. The DGA, if present, provides a longer pedicle.

Next, the extra-articular surface of the MFC is inspected and the graft site is selected. If the graft is to be harvested as a structural, corticocancellous graft, the site is selected based on the region of highest concentration of perforating vessels. As described earlier, this is most commonly in the posterior, distal quadrant. The medial collateral

ligament must be identified and protected. A rectangular area of sufficient size to reconstruct the bony defect is outlined and the periosteum is sharply incised. The bone is then cut with a small osteotome or microsagittal saw taking great care to protect the vascular pedicle. An additional cut is made angled 45° just distal to the graft to facilitate removal of the graft with less risk of fracturing or shearing the underlying cancellous bone from the corticoperiosteal layer (**Fig. 5**).

If the graft is to be harvested as a thin, corticoperiosteal flap, a broader area is outlined (**Fig. 6**). The proximal extent is limited to the region supplied by the DGA, which has been demonstrated to extend approximately 13 cm from the joint line if the MMPA is included in the graft.[24] The distal extent is limited by the articular surface and the medial collateral ligament. The width is limited by the posterior border of the femur and the medial patellar facet anteriorly (usually approximately 6 cm). The periosteum overlying the region to be harvested is sharply incised. The graft is then elevated using a curved osteotome working from the periphery toward the center of the graft (**Fig. 7**). Advancing a few millimeters at a time, the cortex is elevated from the underlying cancellous bone resulting in a thin potato chip–like corticoperiosteal flap. The thinner the cortical layer harvested,

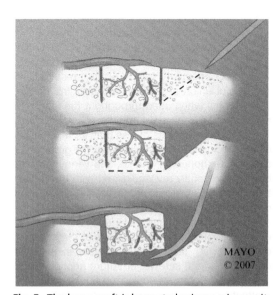

Fig. 5. The bone graft is harvested using a microsagittal saw and osteotomes, making an additional cut distal to the bone block angled toward the base of the graft to facilitate removing the graft without shearing the cortical bone from the underlying cancellous bone. (*Reprinted from* Larson AN, Bishop AT, Shin AY. Tech Hand Up Extrem Surg. Philadelphia: Lippincott Williams & Wilkins; 2007. p. 254; with permission from the Mayo Foundation.)

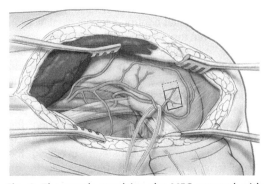

Fig. 4. The vessels supplying the MFC exposed with the vastus medialis retracted anteriorly. The area to be harvested as a vascularized corticocancellous graft is outlined. (*Reprinted from* with permission from the Mayo Foundation.)

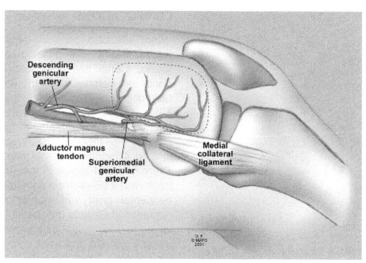

Fig. 6. The outlined area to be harvested as a thin, corticoperiosteal graft limited by the articular surface distally, the medial patellar facet anteriorly, and the posterior border of the femur posteriorly. (*Reprinted from* Choudry UH, Bakri K, Moran SL, et al. The vascularized medial femoral condyle periosteal bone flap for the treatment of recalcitrant bony nonunions. Ann Plast Surg 2008;60:174–80; with permission from the Mayo Foundation.)

the more flexible the graft will be. But care must be taken to preserve the cambium layer by avoiding shearing the periosteum from the cortical bone.

Once the graft is elevated, the tourniquet is released to evaluate bleeding from the periosteum and underlying bone. The vascular pedicle is then clamped, ligated, and divided at least 6 cm proximally. An additional cancellous bone graft can be harvested as necessary to fill any additional bony defects at the nonunion site. The defect in the MFC is then filled with a bone substitute, and the wound is then closed in layers with absorbable suture over a drain. A knee immobilizer is typically used in the immediate perioperative period for patient comfort.

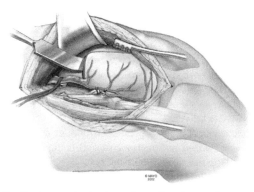

Fig. 7. A curved osteotome is used to elevate the cortex with overlying periosteum from the underlying cancellous bone. (*Reprinted from* Fuchs B, Steinmann SP, Bishop AT. The Journal of Shoulder and Elbow Surgery board of trustees. J Shoulder Elbow Surg; 2005. p. 266; with permission from the Mayo Foundation.)

Insetting and fixation of the graft depends on the bony defect and recipient site anatomy. If addressing scaphoid nonunion, the scaphoid is approached via an extended volar Russe-type incision. The dorsal intercalated segment instability deformity is corrected by flexing the wrist under fluoroscopic imaging until the radiolunate angle is neutral and then maintained with a temporary radiolunate Kirschner wire.[36] The wrist is then extended, gapping open the scaphoid nonunion site. Fibrous and necrotic tissue is debrided from the nonunion site and a sagittal saw is used to prepare flat edges to accept the graft. The size of the bony defect is measured after gentle distraction of the fragments with a small lamina spreader. The graft is then trimmed appropriately and inset with the periosteal surface facing volarly to preserve the vascular pedicle and allow its cortical bone to correct the humpback deformity (**Fig. 8**). The midcarpal and radioscaphoid joints are then carefully inspected for evidence of graft impingement, which is corrected by carefully removing small amounts of the graft in situ with a burr. The graft is fixed with a cannulated screw if the fragments are of sufficient size or with Kirschner wires if necessary. Microvascular anastomosis is performed in an end-to-side fashion to the radial artery and an end-to-end fashion to a vena comitans under an operating microscope.

If addressing a long-bone nonunion, the fracture site is freshened and fixed with rigid, internal fixation. If adequate bony apposition cannot be achieved, cancellous bone harvested from the MFC can be packed into the nonunion site. The

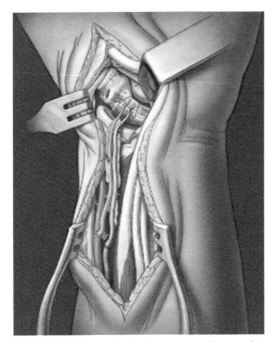

Fig. 8. The free vascularized corticocancellous graft is placed volarly to correct the scaphoid humpback deformity, and the arterial anastomosis is performed end to side to the radial artery and the venous anastomosis end to end to the vena comitans. (*Reprinted from Jones Jr DB, Burger H, Bishop AT, et al. The Journal of Bone and Joint Surgery Incorporated. J Bone Joint Surg Am; 2008. p. 2621; with permission from the Mayo Foundation.*)

thin corticoperiosteal flap is then conformed to and/or wrapped around the nonunion site and held in place with a heavy, nonabsorbable suture or suture anchors (**Fig. 9**). Microvascular anastomosis is then performed to the appropriate adjacent vessels (clavicle: thoracoacromial trunk, humerus: brachial artery, radius/ulna: radial or ulnar artery).

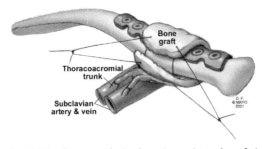

Fig. 9. The free vascularized corticoperiosteal graft is wrapped around the nonunion site and fixed with wire or nonabsorbable suture, and microvascular anastomosis is performed to the adjacent vessels. (*Reprinted from Fuchs B, Steinmann SP, Bishop AT. The Journal of Shoulder and Elbow Surgery board of trustees. J Shoulder Elbow Surg; 2005. p. 267; with permission from the Mayo Foundation.*)

COMPLICATIONS

Donor site pain generally resolves over 3 to 6 weeks. Rarely is a gait aid required beyond 3 weeks. Donor site complications are rare, with donor site seroma being the most commonly reported in 8% (2 out of 25[33]) to 25% (3 out of 12[14]) of patients, with several of those requiring irrigation and debridement. Saphenous nerve paresthesias have also been reported and resolve in 3 to 4 months with no long-term sequelae.[33] There is only 1 report in the literature of a femur fracture in a 58-year-old patient in which a corticoperiosteal graft was harvested for a forearm nonunion.[34] Despite this, patients are generally allowed to bear weight as tolerated postoperatively using a gait aid and knee immobilizer as needed for comfort. There have been no cases of knee instability reported.

SUMMARY

Free vascularized grafts from the MFC have demonstrated clinical success in achieving union in the treatment of persistent upper extremity nonunions. The graft is based on a consistent, robust vascular supply and can be harvested as either a structural corticocancellous graft or a flexible corticoperiosteal graft, making it a valuable and versatile option for addressing challenging recalcitrant nonunions.

REFERENCES

1. Huntington TW. VI. Case of bone transference: use of a segment of fibula to supply a defect in the tibia. Ann Surg 1905;41(2):249–51.
2. Ostrup LT, Fredrickson JM. Distant transfer of a free, living bone graft by microvascular anastomoses. An experimental study. Plast Reconstr Surg 1974;54(3):274–85.
3. Dell PC, Burchardt H, Glowczewskie FP. A roentgenographic, biomechanical and histologic evaluation of vascularized and non-vascularized segmental fibular canine autografts. J Bone Joint Surg Am 1985;67A(1):105–12.
4. Shaffer JW, Field GA, Goldberg VM, et al. Fate of vascularized and nonvascularized autografts. Clin Orthop Relat Res 1985;197:32–43.
5. Hertel R, Masquelet AC. The reverse flow medial knee osteoperiosteal flap for skeletal reconstruction of the leg. Description and anatomical basis. Surg Radiol Anat 1989;11(4):257–62.
6. Sakai K, Doi K, Kawai S. Free vascularized thin corticoperiosteal graft. Plast Reconstr Surg 1991;87(2):290–8.

7. Doi K, Oda T, Soo-Heong T, et al. Free vascularized bone graft for nonunion of the scaphoid. J Hand Surg Am 2000;25(3):507–19.

8. Jones DB Jr, Burger H, Bishop AT, et al. Treatment of scaphoid waist nonunions with an avascular proximal pole and carpal collapse. A comparison of two vascularized bone grafts. J Bone Joint Surg Am 2008;90(12):2616–25.

9. Jones DB Jr, Moran SL, Bishop AT, et al. Free-vascularized medial femoral condyle bone transfer in the treatment of scaphoid nonunions. Plast Reconstr Surg 2010;125(4):1176–84.

10. Larson AN, Bishop AT, Shin AY. Free medial femoral condyle bone grafting for scaphoid nonunions with humpback deformity and proximal pole avascular necrosis. Tech Hand Up Extrem Surg 2007;11(4): 246–58.

11. Giessler GA, Schmidt AB. Thumb salvage with skin grafted medial femoral corticoperiosteal free flap. J Plast Reconstr Aesthet Surg 2011;64(12):1693–6.

12. Sammer DM, Bishop AT, Shin AY. Vascularized medial femoral condyle graft for thumb metacarpal reconstruction: case report. J Hand Surg Am 2009; 34(4):715–8.

13. Bakri K, Shin AY, Moran SL. The vascularized medial femoral corticoperiosteal flap for reconstruction of bony defects within the upper and lower extremities. Semin Plast Surg 2008;22(3):228–33.

14. Choudry UH, Bakri K, Moran SL, et al. The vascularized medial femoral condyle periosteal bone flap for the treatment of recalcitrant bony nonunions. Ann Plast Surg 2008;60(2):174–80.

15. Fuchs B, Steinmann SP, Bishop AT. Free vascularized corticoperiosteal bone graft for the treatment of persistent nonunion of the clavicle. J Shoulder Elbow Surg 2005;14(3):264–8.

16. Cavadas PC, Landin L. Treatment of recalcitrant distal tibial nonunion using the descending genicular corticoperiosteal free flap. J Trauma 2008;64(1):144–50.

17. Kakar S, Duymaz A, Steinmann S, et al. Vascularized medial femoral condyle corticoperiosteal flaps for the treatment of recalcitrant humeral nonunions. Microsurgery 2011;31(2):85–92.

18. Yajima H, Maegawa N, Ota H, et al. Treatment of persistent non-union of the humerus using a vascularized bone graft from the supracondylar region of the femur. J Reconstr Microsurg 2007;23(2):107–13.

19. Rogers WM, Gladstone H. Vascular foramina and arterial supply of the distal end of the femur. J Bone Joint Surg Am 1950;32(A:4):867–74.

20. Scapinelli R. Studies on the vasculature of the human knee joint. Acta Anat (Basel) 1968;70(3):305–31.

21. Kirschner MH, Menck J, Hennerbichler A, et al. Importance of arterial blood supply to the femur and tibia for transplantation of vascularized femoral diaphyses and knee joints. World J Surg 1998; 22(8):845–51 [discussion: 852].

22. Reddy AS, Frederick RW. Evaluation of the intraosseous and extraosseous blood supply to the distal femoral condyles. Am J Sports Med 1998;26(3):415–9.

23. Yamamoto H, Jones DB Jr, Moran SL, et al. The arterial anatomy of the medial femoral condyle and its clinical implications. J Hand Surg Eur Vol 2010; 35(7):569–74.

24. Iorio ML, Masden DL, Higgins JP. The limits of medial femoral condyle corticoperiosteal flaps. J Hand Surg 2011;36(10):1592–6.

25. Doi K, Sakai K. Vascularized periosteal bone graft from the supracondylar region of the femur. Microsurgery 1994;15(5):305–15.

26. Anderson SE, Steinbach LS, Tschering-Vogel D, et al. MR imaging of avascular scaphoid nonunion before and after vascularized bone grafting. Skeletal Radiol 2005;34(6):314–20.

27. Green DP. The effect of avascular necrosis on Russe bone grafting for scaphoid nonunion. J Hand Surg 1985;10A:579–605.

28. Kalicke T, Burger H, Muller EJ. A new vascularized cartilague-bone-graft for scaphoid nonunion with avascular necrosis of the proximal pole. Description of a new type of surgical procedure. Unfallchirurg 2008;111(3):201–5 [in German].

29. Bishop AT. Vascularized bone grafting. In: Green DP, Hotchkiss RN, Pederson WC, et al, editors. Green's operative hand surgery. 5th edition. New York: Churchill Livingstone; 2005. p. 1777–811.

30. Grant I, Berger AC, Ireland DC. A vascularised bone graft from the medial femoral condyle for recurrent failed arthrodesis of the distal interphalangeal joint. Br J Plast Surg 2005;58(7):1011–3.

31. Muramatsu K, Doi K, Ihara K, et al. Recalcitrant posttraumatic nonunion of the humerus: 23 patients reconstructed with vascularized bone graft. Acta Orthop Scand 2003;74(1):95–7.

32. Del Pinal F, Garcia-Bernal FJ, Regalado J, et al. Vascularised corticoperiosteal grafts from the medial femoral condyle for difficult non-unions of the upper limb. J Hand Surg Eur Vol 2007;32(2):135–42.

33. Rodriguez-Vegas JM, Delgado-Serrano PJ. Corticoperiosteal flap in the treatment of nonunions and small bone gaps: technical details and expanding possibilities. J Plast Reconstr Aesthet Surg 2011; 64(4):515–27.

34. De Smet L. Treatment of non-union of forearm bones with a free vascularised corticoperiosteal flap from the medial femoral condyle. Acta Orthop Belg 2009;75(5):611–5.

35. Romana MC, Masquelet AC. Vascularized periosteum associated with cancellous bone graft: an experimental study. Plast Reconstr Surg 1990;85(4):587–92.

36. Tomaino MM, King J, Pizillo M. Correction of lunate malalignment when bone grafting scaphoid nonunion with humpback deformity: rationale and results of a technique revisited. J Hand Surg Am 2000;25(2):322–9.

Allograft Tendon for Second-Stage Tendon Reconstruction

Ren Guo Xie, MD, Jin Bo Tang, MD*

KEYWORDS

- Flexor and extensor tendons • Allograft • Deep-freeze-dried preservation
- Secondary reconstruction • Indications • Fate of grafted tendons

KEY POINTS

- We used allogenic tendons in 22 patients (30 flexor or extensor tendons) for second-stage reconstruction in the hand with the longest follow-up being 4.5 years.
- No particular problems have been found thus far, and the patients are generally satisfied with this procedure.
- Tendon allograft is encouraged in selected academic institutes to fully assess its merits and problems and to standardize the preservation process of allogenic tendons.

Lengthy defects of flexor or extensor tendons in the upper extremity may present after extensive or severe trauma that prohibit primary tendon repair and require secondary tendon graft reconstruction. The tendon defects are conventionally repaired by grafting functionally less important tendons harvested from the forearm (eg, palmaris longus) or the lower extremity (eg, toe extensors). Tendon autograft is currently a standard and popular means to reconstruct defective tendons. However, 2 clinical conditions may preclude such autogenous tendon grafting: (1) patients do not want to sacrifice their own normally functioning tendons; and (2) multiple tendon defects require more donor tendons than a patient can offer.

Over the past few decades, allograft tendon has been investigated in experimental settings, and several methods have been tested for preservation of tendon allograft for clinical use.[1–4] In theory, tendon has sparse cellularity and lower immunogenicity than other tissue types, and preservation of the tendon allograft is technically possible. Both of these factors allow exploratory clinical use to proceed carefully. To assess patients' attitude toward the use of an autograft versus an allograft, we sampled 35 patients who presented with defects requiring tendon grafting in the past 5 years. The patients were fully informed of the merits, potential problems, and cosmetic or functional aspects of both procedures if their tendon defect warranted a grafting procedure. Two-thirds of the patients thought that the loss of healthy tendons outweighs potential problems associated with a tendon allograft; they requested the allograft. We subsequently performed tendon allograft reconstruction of flexor or extensor tendons in 22 patients.

CLINICAL TENDON ALLOGRAFTS: INDICATIONS

Current indications for tendon allografts in our unit are as follows:

1. The patient has a clear and strong wish to use allogenic tendons instead of autogenic tendons for functional reconstruction after the surgeon has carefully explained to the patient the merits and potential problems of both sources of graft.

This work was supported by the Health Bureau of Jiangsu Province and the Natural Science Foundation. The authors have nothing to disclose.

Department of Hand Surgery, The Hand Surgery Research Center, Affiliated Hospital of Nantong University, 20 West Temple Road, Nantong 226001, Jiangsu, China
* Corresponding author.
E-mail address: jinbotang@yahoo.com

Hand Clin 28 (2012) 503–509
http://dx.doi.org/10.1016/j.hcl.2012.08.011

2. Need for reconstruction of multiple tendons in a patient, requiring multiple donor sites if autografts are used, as seen in the cases of multiple tendon loss on the dorsum of the hand and wrist or secondary reconstruction of multiple lacerated flexor tendons in the palm.
3. Reconstruction of a minor function, in which the patient does not wish to donate his or her own tendons. An example is a defect in a single extensor digitorum communis tendon, which only partly affects extension of a finger.

In the hand, allograft may also be used in ligament reconstruction, such as in the distal radioulnar, carpometacarpal, and metacarpophalangeal (MP) joints, and bridging gaps during tendon transfer to restore thumb opposition, abduction, and so forth.

PATIENTS AND OPERATIONS
Patients

Between August 2007 and June 2011, we performed tendon allografts in 22 patients (30 grafts). Patient ages ranged from 21 to 59 years, with an average of 38 years. There were 13 men and 9 women. Five patients with extensive crush injuries or replantation surgery at the wrist or palm had defects in multiple tendons and required grafts of 2 to 4 tendons. In the other 17 patients, the defects were in a single tendon, requiring graft reconstruction. The graft lengths ranged from 6 to 15 cm. The tendon graft reconstruction procedure was performed typically 4 to 12 months after injury or the initial surgery. At the time of surgery, the patients were confirmed to have pliable skin and soft tissues, mobile joints of the hand, and well-healed wounds.

The allografts were used to reconstruct 8 flexor digitorum profundus, 8 extensor digitorum communis, 5 extensor pollicis longus, 3 flexor pollicis longus, 2 extensor carpi ulnaris, and 4 other tendons in the hand. In 6 patients, tendon allograft was performed along with 1 or 2 other surgeries: removal of internal fixation (4 cases), flap defatting (2), and skin grafting (1). In the patients with multiple tendon lacerations, the little finger flexor or extensors were not reconstructed, because the little finger is less critical functionally, and functional return is less optimal.[5,6]

The Institutional Review Board approved the use of allograft in these patients, and patients were fully consented regarding the potential (unknown) problems associated with the allograft tendon. The allogenic tendons were harvested and transferred to deep-freeze preservation by a commercial company under strict working guidelines with the tissue bank of the Orthopedic Institute of the People's Liberation Army in Beijing. The fresh tendons were washed, immersed for a short time in nutritional fluid, separately sealed in sterile bags, and preserved at $-80°$. They were fully tested to exclude infectious diseases and sterilized to prevent risk of infection of grafts. The tendons were subjected to γ-irradiation before preservation. They were thawed the day before surgery and preserved at $0°$ overnight for use. The allograft tendons were flexor digitorum profundus, superficialis tendons, or digital extensor tendons.

Surgical Procedures

The surgical procedures for tendon allograft are the same as for conventional autogenous tendon grafting. Twelve of our patients receiving an allograft had injuries in digital extensor tendons presenting with defects between the MP joint and wrist level, or had secondary reconstruction of the zone 2 flexor tendon lacerations, which constitutes the bulk of our past experience with allografts. For the extensor pollicis longus, extensor digitorum communis, and extensor carpi ulnaris, the allografted tendons were woven into the residual stumps of the extensors. For the flexor pollicis longus and flexor digitorum profundus, the distal tendon-to-bone junction was achieved with strong direct suture to the distal stump of the tendon, or with tendon-to-bone junction with minianchors and the proximal tendon-to-tendon junction with woven sutures in the palm.

For secondary reconstruction of lacerated tendons in zone 2, we used the allograft in the cases that had indications of 1-stage graft reconstruction. These cases did not have extensive scar in the tendon bed and no destruction of major pulleys, and they had intact synovial sheath systems or fine tendon gliding bed when the sheath and tendon were exposed. These cases did not require staged tendon reconstruction. The surgical procedure for 1-stage reconstruction of the digitorum profundus tendon lacerated in zone 2 (**Figs. 1–5**) is as follows:

1. Surgical exposure: the digital flexor tendons are approached through a Bruner zigzag incision extending from the fingertip to the midpalm area (see **Figs. 1** and **2**). The flexor pulleys are carefully preserved; at least the A2, A3, and A4 pulleys should be preserved. If the synovial sheath is intact around these pulleys, the sheath is preserved as well. The lacerated flexor digitorum profundus and superficialis tendons are resected, but the distal tendon stump of about 1.5 cm attached to the distal phalanx is preserved. The proximal stump of

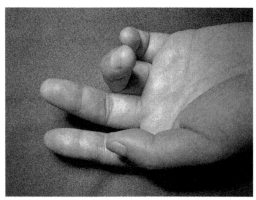

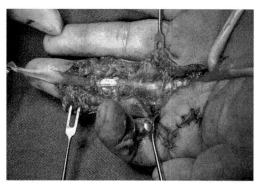

Fig. 1. A 45-year-old man had his left index and middle fingers lacerated and subsequently had no active flexion of the fingers for 5 months before referring to the author (JBT).

Fig. 3. The allogenic tendon was guided into the digital fibro-osseous tunnel, the size of which fits the sheath and pulleys well. Note that the synovial sheath and multiple pulleys were preserved for optimal function of the grafted tendon.

the flexor tendon is usually found retracted into the palm or even more proximally. The proximal stump is retrieved to the middle of the palm. At this time, the graft is taken out of the sealed bag, washed with saline, and placed in saline with antibiotics for 30 minutes before use. Particular attention is paid to ensuring that the graft should look solid and appear fresh, without any sign of softening. A few cycles of tension-relaxation confirms its elasticity. The graft is introduced into the digital sheath gliding tunnel, which consists of a series of preserved annular pulleys and synovial sheath (see Fig. 3). The test gliding of the grafted tendon should confirm that the tendon glides smoothly under the pulleys and is free from impingement at the pulley edges.

2. Distal tendon junction: we use either a strong direct suture (ie, a reinforced overlapping suture; see Fig. 4), or minianchors to achieve a distal tendon-to-bone junction. When inserting a mini-anchor, we first anchor the screws into the mid-portion of the distal phalanx; the screw is tagged with 4 suture threads. The distal stump of the allograft tendon is placed over the screw, and the 2 groups of sutures are tied over the tendon. The knots are secured and the tendon is lightly pulled to test the safety of the junction.

3. Proximal tendon junction: we place the proximal tendon-to-tendon junction into the midpalm level, and the grafted tendon is connected to the proximal stump of the injured flexor profundus tendon by means of Pulvertaft weave sutures using 4-0 Ethibon or 4-0 Prolene. The tendon is appropriately tensioned before tying the suture. We set the fingers into semiflexion to tension the tendon junction site when delivering the stitches.

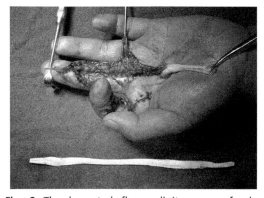

Fig. 2. The lacerated flexor digitorum profundus tendon was reconstructed with an allograft tendon (performed by JBT). Through a Bruner incision, the profundus tendon ends were identified. A silicone tube was placed into the preserved sheath and pulleys to introduce the donor tendon. The allogenic tendon (at bottom of picture) was taken out of the sealed bag and was ready to use.

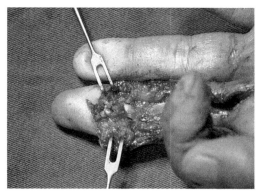

Fig. 4. Completion of the reinforced suture of the allograft tendon end to the distal residual stumps of the profundus tendon.

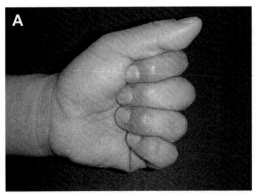
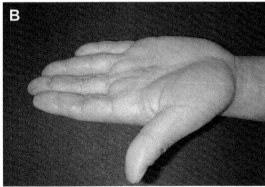

Fig. 5. The active flexion (*A*) and extension (*B*) of the operated left middle finger 8 months after tendon allograft. The patient was satisfied with the surgery and achieved excellent recovery of the finger flexion, without extension lag.

Postoperative care

For the flexor tendon reconstruction in the fingers, we now commonly use a passive-active motion regime commencing 3 to 5 days after surgery. The finger is protected with a dorsal thermoplastic splint, with the wrist in slight flexion and the MP joint in flexion of about 30°. The postsurgical finger is passively flexed over the full motion range for 20 to 30 times in each exercise session, followed by active finger flexion over a limited range to the extent to which patients are comfortable (ie, no resistance to active flexion). The number of daily exercise sessions prescribed to the patient varies from 3 to 6, depending on both the willingness and the needs of the patient. Patients with, or inclined to have, significant stiffness of the hand are prescribed more exercise sessions. Moderate to full range of active finger flexion starts at the end of 3 weeks. The dorsal wrist flexion splint is changed to a dorsal extension splint at week 3. The full range of hand motion exercise starts at week 6. Stretching, traction, ultrasound, and electrical stimulation are used to help improve the finger joint stiffness and reduce scar formation over the fingers when necessary. The normal use of the hand starts at week 8 or later. The timing to commence motion and the protocols we use after second-stage tendon grafting have some similarities with those we use after primary flexor tendon repair.[7–10] However, we generally are more conservative for second-stage reconstruction, because the incision is usually longer, and conditions of the hand vary greatly among patients. We have to individualize the amplitude of finger motion and rigor of exercise according to the severity of the injury of each patient. Full active extension of the finger joint is usually hard to achieve in the initial weeks, because the tension on the flexors is greater after grafting.

For the reconstruction of extensor tendons, we do not usually implement early tendon motion. Instead, we immobilize the hand at 30° of wrist extension to ease the tension for 3 weeks, followed by full range of passive motion and limited range of active motion of the involved fingers.

OUTCOMES

The tendon allograft procedure should be assessed with long-term follow-up, which is not yet available in our patient group with this operation. Our patients have been regularly followed thus far, with the longest follow-up being 4 years and 6 months (range 7 months to 4.5 years) as of January 2012. The major emphasis of the follow-up is to identify any abnormal tissue reactions of the hand and to detect particularly unfavorable functional results, which are likely to be caused by using allogenic tendons.

In the most recent follow-up conducted in December 2011 and January 2012, we asked the patients (1) whether they have any particular discomfort in the hand that may potentially be related to the allograft; (2) to grade the satisfaction levels (satisfied, rather satisfied, fairly satisfied, less satisfied, or not satisfied); (3) whether they would choose this type of graft again and whether their opinions have changed about the use of allograft or autograft; and (4) to rate the overall function of the hand. Four patients failed to return for follow-up, and those results are not included here. Sixteen patients who came to the latest follow-up are reported.

The follow-up results are as follows: (1) all patients reported no particular discomfort in the hand. (2) Eight were satisfied, 2 rather satisfied, 6 fairly satisfied, and none less satisfied or not at all satisfied. (3) All except 2 responded that they would choose tendon allograft again, given a similar injury. (4) Patients' overall rating of the hand function was 4 excellent, 7 good, 5 fair, and none poor (**Figs. 5** and **6**).

CONSIDERATION OF CURRENT INDICATIONS
Evidence from Basic Science Investigations

The basic investigations of preservation and clinical use of allogenic tendon grafts took place during the 1970s and 1980s.[1–3] Clinical use of tendon allografts in surgical treatment of hand problems has been sporadic.[11–15] Past investigations revealed that deep fresh or freeze-dried preservation can preserve the mechanical properties of the tendon, and that these preserved tendons are a good material for grafting.[1–4,13,14] Nevertheless, no long-term follow-up studies have been completed and potential problems associated with the allograft have been a concern. Our decision to use such allografts in a small series of clinical cases was based on evidence from basic scientific investigations accumulated over decades[1–3,13,14] and, in particular, the evidence of favorable clinical outcomes in a group of patients treated by Zhang and colleagues,[15] who started to use tendon allografts to reconstruct zone 2 tendon injuries in 1990. We explained to our patients the possibility of unforeseen problems with the graft and consequent functional and cosmetic drawbacks. These patients had full rights to accept or reject the procedure. We considered the current allograft protocol a clinical exploratory study, rather than a currently popular method, and thus have proceeded with care to regularly review the postoperative status of these patients.

Merits of Tendon as Allografts

Compared with many other tissues, an obvious advantage of the tendon as an allograft is its low cellularity and expected lower immunogenicity. Densely packed collagen constitutes the bulk of tendon substance, within which tenocytes are sparsely located. An allogenic tendon should elicit limited or minimal reactions from the body and is an ideal candidate for such grafting. Preliminary clinical reports have not documented any significant adverse reactions by the body after grafting of allogenic tendons.[11–13] Adhesions formed around the allogenic tendons, indicating no rejection.[15] Nevertheless, no information is available regarding long-term follow-up. These allografts should be given careful long-term follow-up, and this surgery should not be popularized until more data become available. Drawbacks of tendon allografts include limited sources, possibility of disease transmission, uncertain long-term problems, and high costs (and charges to patients) because of the rarity of the tendons and the necessary sterilization and preservation processes.

Fate of the Allogenic Tendon Graft

The fate of cells in tendon allografts remains unknown. There are a few possibilities regarding the changes of these cells. Most likely, cells lose some of their viability after harvest and deep-freeze preservation. It is unknown whether or when cells migrate from peritendinous sources into allogenic tendons after grafting. We assume that the cells from the surrounding tissues would

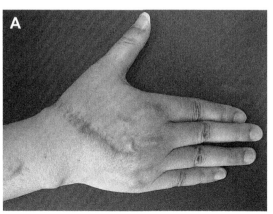
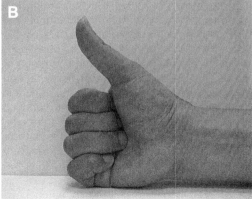

Fig. 6. A 49-year-old man had allogenic tendon grafting to reconstruct the extensor pollicis longus tendon 5 months after open trauma causing a fracture at the middle of the thumb metacarpus. Seven months after tendon allograft (*A*), and full active extension of the thumb (*B*).

seed into the grafted tendon and the grafted tendons may ultimately be repopulated with the patient's own cells. It remains undetermined whether the reseeding of the patients' cells into allogenic tendons is important for the function of the grafted tendons and whether these seeded cells can penetrate the tendon surface to reach the center. It has also not been established whether specific cellular apoptosis occurs in these grafts, something we have observed in healing tendons.[16,17] A series of laboratory studies conducted by Chang and colleagues[18–22] highlighted the possibility and merits of decellularization of the allogenic tendons and then reseeding them with autogenous cells before placing the allogenic tendons into the recipient. Chang and colleagues showed that seeded cells can repopulate the allogenic tendons.[19–21] In patients with tendon allograft in the hand who required tenolysis 4 to 15 months later, Sun and colleagues[23] found solid healing of the allograft tendon with the tendons of the patients, and that the grafted tendons were viable, forming adhesions with peritendinous tissues. It remains unclear which is more beneficial for allogenic tendon grafting: taking special measures to reseed the cells before grafting procedures, or allowing for gradual and natural reseeding of the cells after tendon grafting. These questions await future answers as the use of tissue engineered or preserved natural allogenic tendons undergoes further and more focused study. Nevertheless, the 2 types of allogenic grafts share common features, in that the collagen components in these tendons demand no particular modification, they cause minimal immunogenicity, and they seem to preserve mechanical properties such as elasticity and tensile strength, which are the fundamental requirements of a graft.[24–28]

FUTURE PERSPECTIVES

It is too early to comment on the ultimate clinical merits and problems associated with allogenic tendon grafts. Nevertheless, based on our experience of the use of this type of graft in a group of patients who needed extensor or flexor tendon reconstruction and their follow-up thus far, this type of allogenic graft does not seem to produce serious concern as a foreign tissue in the body, at least in the short term. Although it is not our intention to present data on functional recovery after this type of grafting, the information we have obtained thus far seems to support that this type of graft behaves similarly to autogenous tendons, and ultimately functional recovery is likely to be comparable with that achieved with autograft.

The considerations of the use of allografts discussed in this article are based on the assumption that this type of graft will have no major adverse reactions in the long term. Therefore, currently we cannot suggest the routine use of this procedure, but we do encourage application of tendon allografts in well-selected patients in some academic institutes where long-term follow-up and objective assessment are streamlined. That application will allow the potential merits and problems associated with this procedure to be fully evaluated and commented on, and the preservation process to become more standard and widely available.

SUMMARY

Tendons are made of compact dense collagen fibers with only sparse cellularity and naturally low immunogenicity. Over the past few decades, basic investigations indicated that allogenic tendons may be preserved through deep freezing methods, while retaining excellent mechanical properties after revitalization. Between 2007 and 2011, we used allogenic tendons in 22 patients (30 tendons) for second-stage tendon reconstruction in the hand. Preliminary results indicate no observable adverse tissue reactions, and functional recovery after tendon grafting does not seem different from reconstruction using tendon autografts. This type of allogenic graft does not seem to produce serious concern as a foreign tissue in the body, at least in the short term. Nevertheless, long-term follow-up information is not yet available. Routine use of this procedure cannot currently be recommended, but we encourage application of tendon allografts in well-selected patients in some academic institutes where objective assessment and long-term follow-up are streamlined, so that the merits and problems associated with this procedure can be fully evaluated and the preservation process of the donor tendon perfected.

ACKNOWLEDGMENTS

Dr Guheng Wang reviewed the patient data and outcomes for inclusion in this paper.

REFERENCES

1. Potenza AD, Melone C. Evaluation of freeze-dried flexor tendon grafts in the dog. J Hand Surg Am 1978;3:157–62.
2. Minami A, Ishii S, Ogino T, et al. Effect of the immunological antigenicity of the allogeneic tendons on tendon grafting. Hand 1982;14:111–9.

3. Webster DA, Werner FW. Mechanical and functional properties of implanted freeze-dried flexor tendons. Clin Orthop Relat Res 1983;180:301–9.

4. Zhao C, Sun YL, Ikeda J, et al. Improvement of flexor tendon reconstruction with carbodiimide-derivatized hyaluronic acid and gelatin-modified intrasynovial allografts: study of a primary repair failure model. J Bone Joint Surg Am 2010;92:2817–28.

5. Orkar KS, Watts C, Iwuagwu FC. A comparative analysis of the outcome of flexor tendon repair in the index and little fingers: does the little finger fare worse? J Hand Surg Eur 2012;37:20–6.

6. Dowd MB, Figus A, Harris SB, et al. The results of immediate re-repair of zone 1 and 2 primary flexor tendon repairs which rupture. J Hand Surg Br 2006;31:507–13.

7. Tang JB. Indications, methods, postoperative motion and outcome evaluation of primary flexor tendon repairs in zone 2. J Hand Surg Eur 2007;32:118–29.

8. Cao Y, Chen CH, Wu YF, et al. Digital oedema, adhesion formation and resistance to digital motion after primary flexor tendon repair. J Hand Surg Eur 2008;33:745–52.

9. Tang JB. Clinical outcomes associated with flexor tendon repair. Hand Clin 2005;21:199–210.

10. Tang JB. Tendon injuries across the world: treatment. Injury 2006;37:1036–42.

11. Asencio G, Abihaidar G, Leonardi C. Human composite flexor tendon allografts. A report of two cases. J Hand Surg Br 1996;21:84–8.

12. Krocker D, Matziolis G, Pruss A, et al. Reconstruction of the extensor mechanism using a free, allogenic, freeze-dried patellar graft. Unfallchirurg 2007;110:563–6.

13. Zhang Y, Yang K, Zhu W. Experimental research and clinical application of allogenic tendon grafting. Chin J Surg 1995;33:539–41.

14. Zhang YL, Yang KF, Gao XS, et al. An experimental study and clinical application of allogenic freeze-dried tendon grafting. Chin J Orthop 1997;17:59–62.

15. Zhang YL, Zhu W, Sun YK, et al. Comparative study of synovial tendon allograft and nonsynovial tendon autograft in digital flexor sheath area. Chin J Hand Surg 2006;22:131–2.

16. Wu YF, Chen CH, Cao Y, et al. Molecular events of cellular apoptosis and proliferation in the early tendon healing period. J Hand Surg Am 2010;35:2–10.

17. Wu YF, Zhou YL, Mao WF, et al. Cellular apoptosis and proliferation in the middle and late intrasynovial tendon healing periods. J Hand Surg Am 2012;37:209–16.

18. Chong AK, Riboh J, Smith RL, et al. Flexor tendon tissue engineering: acellularized and reseeded tendon constructs. Plast Reconstr Surg 2009;123:1759–66.

19. Woon CY, Pridgen BC, Kraus A, et al. Optimization of human tendon tissue engineering: peracetic acid oxidation for enhanced reseeding of acellularized intrasynovial tendon. Plast Reconstr Surg 2011;127:1107–17.

20. Angelidis IK, Thorfinn J, Connolly ID, et al. Tissue engineering of flexor tendons: the effect of a tissue bioreactor on adipoderived stem cell-seeded and fibroblast-seeded tendon constructs. J Hand Surg Am 2010;35:1466–72.

21. Thorfinn J, Angelidis IK, Gigliello L, et al. Bioreactor optimization of tissue engineered rabbit flexor tendons in vivo. J Hand Surg Eur 2011;37:109–14.

22. Momeni A, Grauel E, Chang J. Complications after flexor tendon injuries. Hand Clin 2010;26:179–89.

23. Sun Y, Zhang Y, Li X, et al. Analysis of reasons of tendon adhesions after tendon allograft. Chin J Reparative Reconstr Surg 2008;22:346–8.

24. Huang H, Zhang J, Sun K, et al. Effects of repetitive multiple freeze-thaw cycles on the biomechanical properties of human flexor digitorum superficialis and flexor pollicis longus tendons. Clin Biomech (Bristol, Avon) 2011;26:419–23.

25. Jung HJ, Vangipuram G, Fisher MB, et al. The effects of multiple freeze-thaw cycles on the biomechanical properties of the human bone-patellar tendon-bone allograft. J Orthop Res 2011;29:1193–8.

26. Nicholas SJ, Lee SJ, Mullaney MJ, et al. Clinical outcomes of coracoclavicular ligament reconstructions using tendon grafts. Am J Sports Med 2007;35:1912–7.

27. Carey JL, Dunn WR, Dahm DL, et al. A systematic review of anterior cruciate ligament reconstruction with autograft compared with allograft. J Bone Joint Surg Am 2009;91:2242–50.

28. McGuire DA, Hendricks SD. Allograft tissue in ACL reconstruction. Sports Med Arthrosc 2009;17:224–33.

Use of Suture Anchors and New Suture Materials in the Upper Extremity

Min Jung Park, MD, MMSc[a], Steven S. Shin, MD, MMSc[b,*]

KEYWORDS

- Suture • Anchor • Bio-absorbable

KEY POINTS

- Suture anchors have mostly obviated the need for multiple drill holes when striving for secure fixation of soft tissue to bone.
- As with most other orthopedic products, the designs of these anchors and the materials used to fabricate them have evolved as their use increased and their applications became more widespread. It is ultimately the surgeon's responsibility to be familiar with these rapidly evolving technologies and to use the most appropriate anchor for any given surgery.
- Besides the shoulder, the elbow is another joint in which the use of suture anchors has become popular for various surgical procedures.

INTRODUCTION

Suture anchors have revolutionized the way orthopedic surgeons perform upper limb surgery. They are designed to help surgeons achieve soft tissue–to-bone healing in cases where inadequate soft tissue stock on bone makes it impossible to perform a direct soft tissue–to–soft tissue repair.[1] Previously open surgical procedures may now be performed arthroscopically, thanks to the advent of suture anchors. This is particularly notable in the shoulder, where glenoid labrum repairs and rotator cuff repairs are now routinely performed arthroscopically.[2–9] Arthroscopic stabilization has become the gold standard treatment of shoulder instability, largely because of the introduction of suture anchors. Suture anchor tenodesis of the proximal biceps tendon is performed for the treatment of proximal biceps tendonitis and rupture,[10] although other techniques are also available for this condition.[11–13]

Besides the shoulder, the elbow is another joint in which the use of suture anchors has become popular for various surgical procedures. Although different techniques exist for ulnar collateral ligament reconstruction, suture anchors have been used for this procedure (**Fig. 1**).[14,15] They are also used in the repair of distal biceps tendon ruptures, conditions in which transosseous suture repair used to be the only surgical option. Some investigators have also described the use of the Corkscrew anchor (Arthrex, Naples, FL) in distal biceps tendon ruptures: implants that were originally designed for rotator cuff tendon fixation (**Fig. 2**).[16–20]

In the wrist and hand, smaller-sized suture anchors are used for various surgical procedures (**Fig. 3**). In the wrist, suture anchors are used for scapholunate or lunotriquetral ligament repair, capsulodesis procedures, and triangular fibrocartilage repair.[21,22] Suture anchors are also used in

The authors have nothing to disclose.

[a] Department of Orthopaedic Surgery, Perelman School of Medicine, University of Pennsylvania, 2501 Christian Street 103, Philadelphia, PA 19146, USA; [b] Kerlan-Jobe Orthopedic Clinic, 6801 Park Terrace, Los Angeles, CA 90045, USA
* Corresponding author.
E-mail address: orthohand@gmail.com

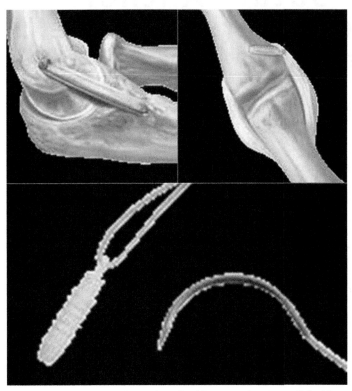

Fig. 1. Ulnar collateral ligament reconstruction using the biocomposite SutureTak. (*Courtesy of* Arthrex, Inc, Naples, FL; with permission.)

the repair of ulnar collateral ligament injuries of the thumb, as well as collateral ligament injuries of the finger metacarpophalangeal and interphalangeal joints.[23–25] Ruptures of the flexor digitorum profundus tendon are commonly repaired using suture anchors as well.[26–30]

HISTORY OF SUTURE ANCHOR MATERIALS AND COMPOSITION

Like many present-day suture anchors, the first suture anchors were made exclusively of metal and, for the most part, did quite well in facilitating soft tissue–to-bone healing. Over time, both product-related and surgeon-related complications of these implants were reported, such as fracture at the site of anchor placement, anchor pull-out, infection around the metal implant, and errant anchor placement (extraosseous or even intra-articular, causing chondral injury and foreign body reactions).[31–36] The presence of a metal anchor around a joint also impaired satisfactory visualization of the joint on magnetic resonance imaging (MRI), not to mention making revision

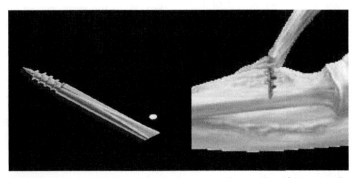

Fig. 2. (*Left*) A 3.5 x 10 mm Corkscrew FT. (*Right*) The Corkscrew anchor in distal biceps tendon repair. (*Courtesy of* Arthrex Inc, Naples, FL; with permission.)

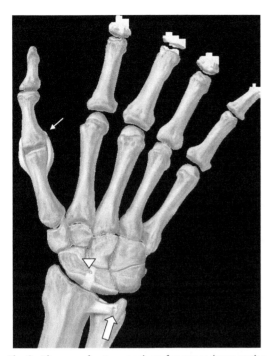

Fig. 3. The use of suture anchors for procedures at the hand and wrist: (*thin arrow*) repair of thumb ulnar collateral ligament, (*arrowhead*) repair of scapholunate interosseous ligament, (*thick arrow*) repair of triangular fibrocartilage complex. (*Courtesy of* Arthrex, Inc, Naples, FL; with permission.)

surgery even more difficult when anchor removal was necessary. The idea of a bioabsorbable, radiolucent device that lasts only as long as necessary for soft tissue healing to bone to occur and then was hydrolyzed was attractive to many surgeons. Just as bioabsorbable suture materials were developed as suture material technology advanced, so too were bioabsorbable suture anchors. The Suretac bioabsorbable device (Smith and Nephew, Andover, MA) was one of the first such implants; since its introduction, its tack design was replaced by a suture anchor design, as was its nonscrew-to-screw design.[37] Early clinical and animal data of bioabsorbable implants were promising[38]; however, as with the earlier metal implants, reports of complications, such as exuberant inflammatory reaction leading to

osteolysis and implant breakage surfaced as long-term follow-up data became available and the indications for these devices increased.[38–47] Although the material that was used to manufacture these initial bioabsorbable anchors was usually some variant of poly-lactic acid (PLA) or co-polymer of PLA and polyglycolic acid, it is unclear as to which factors (eg, material composition, isomer configuration, or implant design) contributed to the reported complications.[48,49] Surgeon technical error may also have played a role in some of the reports of bioabsorbable anchor failure.[50] Some suture anchors are now made of "biocomposite" materials (ie, a combination of tricalcium phosphate [TCP] and PLA derivatives), with the goals of decreasing inflammatory reaction in bone and faster implant-to-bone consolidation (**Fig. 4**).[31–36] Although some surgeons have advocated a move away from bioabsorbable suture anchors and back to traditional metal anchors, bioabsorbable anchors are still widely used.[44,51]

The mechanical properties and material compositions of suture anchors may contribute to the differences in potential clinical and/or mechanical failure, owing to premature anchor breakdown, loss of fixation, or osteolysis.[52,53] In a study by Park and colleagues,[54] a highly significant relationship was observed between failure of a superior labrum repair and the use of bioabsorbable poly-L/D-lactic acid (PLDLA) suture anchors as compared with nonabsorbable metallic or polyetherether ketone (PEEK) anchors. Although patient factors, such as workers compensation claim and smoking status, contributed to the reoperation rate, the strongest association was made with the use of bioabsorbable suture anchors. Even subtle differences in the manufacturing processes of PLDLA, oxidative degradation after or during manufacturing, and varying isomer compositions between anchors from different manufacturers may contribute to the different chemical properties of the final products.

With the development of new anchor materials and designs, Barber and colleagues[37,55–62] have been periodically reporting in vitro as well as anatomic site-specific biomechanical data on the performance of various suture anchors. Although

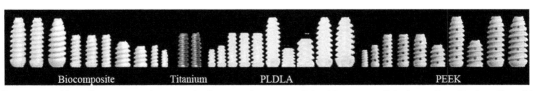

Fig. 4. Examples of suture anchors made from various materials. (*Courtesy of* Arthrex, Inc, Naples, FL; with permission.)

the data are an important guide for potential clinical performance, literature is scarce in terms of actual clinical performance of the individual anchor materials, design, and their modes of failure in vivo.

EVOLVING ANCHOR TECHNOLOGIES AND TECHNIQUES

Owing to some of the complications mentioned previously, many device manufacturers have been introducing new materials and designs for suture anchors. PEEK is a material that has gained popularity in recent years as an alternative to previously available suture anchor materials. Although not bioabsorbable, PEEK is a highly specialized plastic that currently has wide industrial applications because of its high material strength.

For osteoporotic bone, some investigators advocate the augmentation of suture anchors with either polymethylmethacrylate cement or bioabsorbable TCP cement, based on cadaveric study data.[63] It is unclear, however, whether this technique is clinically relevant. The recent development of biocomposite materials in the manufacture of suture anchors is a technically simpler and therefore more attractive option. As stated previously, biocomposite materials are made of some combination of TCP and PLA derivatives and were introduced to theoretically minimize the host reaction and enhance bony integration of the suture anchors. BioComposite SutureTak (Arthrex) and Biocryl Rapide (Depuy Mitek, Raynham, MA) are 2 examples of such products. Although

internal manufacturer data exist showing various levels of material resorption and bony integration, as of the time of this review, no peer-reviewed publication is available regarding the use of biocomposite materials in a clinical setting.

With regard to suture anchor design, knotless anchor designs have become an attractive alternative to the traditional suture anchor design, where knots are tied down close to the anchor and may be prominent and potentially impinge or cause intra-articular cartilage damage. Recently, an all-suture anchor concept was introduced in the JuggerKnot implant (Biomet, Warsaw, IN; **Fig. 5**), in which the "anchor" is made of a suture material instead of the typical metal or bioabsorbable material of traditional anchors. The suture is secured into the bone using a 1-cm strand of suture that encases the regular suture material; as the surgeon pulls on the suture strands, the central portion of the all-suture anchor bunches up as it contacts the cortical rim, thereby "anchoring" it within the bone. The JuggerKnot design allows for smaller drill holes compared with the designs of more traditional suture anchors that have comparable pullout strength. More data are needed to determine the long-term clinical benefits of this unique implant.

Of note, metal anchors have been widely used in hand surgery, with relatively few reported hardware complications. This is likely because of the generally open nature of the surgeries that allows for direct visualization of anchor placement and the relatively smaller size of the anchors used in hand and wrist procedures; however, errant

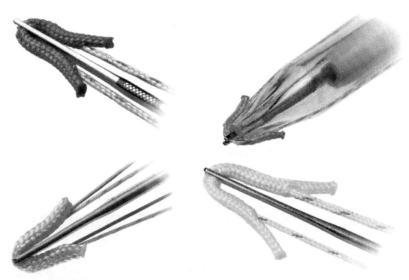

Fig. 5. (*Top left*) JuggerKnot soft anchor 1.4; (*top right*) JuggerKnot soft anchor 1.0 mini; (*bottom left*) JuggerKnot soft anchor 2.9; (*bottom right*) JuggerKnot soft anchor 1.5. (*Courtesy of* Biomet, Warsaw, IN; with permission.)

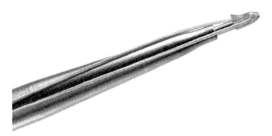

Fig. 6. The Microfix bio-absorbable suture anchor with Orthocord suture. (*Courtesy of* Depuy Mitek, Raynham, MA; with permission.)

anchor placement or preloaded suture breakage can prevent surgeons from achieving satisfactory anchor fixation and/or repair. Although relatively uncommon, preloaded suture breakage may be salvaged by putting an additional PDS suture through the anchor eyelet.[64] As the materials used for sutures and anchors evolve, the incidence of suture breakage after anchor insertion is unlikely. With the help of small Mitek anchors (Depuy Mitek), surgeons have reported successful collateral ligament reconstruction at the metacarpophalangeal joint and proximal interphalangeal joint with return to activities of daily living in 5 weeks and preinjury activities in 12 weeks (**Fig. 6**).[65,66]

Promising cadaveric study data exist for stainless steel anchors used for flexor digitorum profundus tendon repair.[27] Although bioabsorbable suture anchors are also widely used in hand and wrist procedures, they have not been shown to have a significant advantage over the well-tolerated metal anchors.

NEW SUTURE MATERIAL

Braided polyester sutures (Ethibond, Ethicon, Sommerville, NJ) were widely used in the past,

but improved, stronger suture materials, such as Fiberwire (Arthrex), made of ultra–high molecular weight polyethylene (UHMWPE), are now available. The Orthocord suture (Depuy Mitek) is made of a UHMWPE sleeve and a polydioxanone (PDS) core with polyglactin 910 coating. The introduction of the stronger suture material changed the mode of failure of the anchor/suture construct. Instead of suture breakage, the metal anchor failed by pulling out of bone, whereas the bioabsorbable anchor failed at the level of the anchor eyelet.[67,68] Suture knot configuration has been studied as well, as it is an essential part of the fixation construct. Although a static surgeon's knot provides the best balance of loop and knot security, a sliding knot with the addition of 3 reversing half-hitches on alternating posts can also provide adequate fixation for clinical use.[69] Sliding knots without reversing half-hitches on alternating posts should not be used.

Monofilament stainless steel sutures have been advocated in the past for flexor tendon repairs, but difficulties in handling the material (eg, kinking and plastic deformation) caused interest to fade quickly in this suture material. There have been recent developments in the manufacture of multifilament stainless steel sutures, however, with promising data reflecting its nonviscoelastic properties as compared with polymer sutures. The elimination of the previously described handling problems of the monofilament stainless steel suture, along with overcoming the shortcomings of stress relaxation and creep, as seen with polymer sutures, could make stainless steel suture material relevant again in flexor tendon repair.[70] Another theoretical advantage of the multifilament stainless steel suture is the option of using a crimp mechanism instead of suture knots during the tendon repair, thereby ensuring simultaneous and equal tensioning of the suture limbs (**Fig. 7**). Clinical

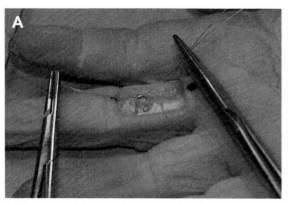
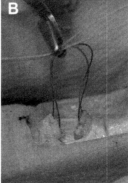

Fig. 7. (*A*) Multifilament stainless steel suture used in flexor tendon repair. (*B*) Multifilament stainless steel suture with crimp mechanism for securing the sutures and pretensioning. (*Courtesy of* Dr Leonard Gordon.)

data are still lacking, however, with regard to whether or not the use of this suture material leads to improved functional outcome.

SUMMARY

Suture anchors have been available since the early 1990s and are now an essential tool in the orthopedic surgeon's armamentarium. As with any other implant, the surgeon should be thoroughly educated on the characteristics of the anchor being used and the technique necessary for correct insertion of the anchor. With so many different types of new anchors and sutures available, the surgeon must take care in choosing the device that is most appropriate for the procedure and body part in question. Upper extremity surgical techniques will continue to be revisited, revised, and perhaps even reinvented, in no small part because of the introduction of new technologies, such as suture anchors and new suture materials.

REFERENCES

1. Barber FA, Cawley P, Prudich JF. Suture anchor failure strength—an in vivo study. Arthroscopy 1993;9(6):647–52.
2. Ahmad CS, Stewart AM, Izquierdo R, et al. Tendon-bone interface motion in transosseous suture and suture anchor rotator cuff repair techniques. Am J Sports Med 2005;33(11):1667–71.
3. Gartsman GM. Arthroscopic assessment of rotator cuff tear reparability. Arthroscopy 1996;12(5): 546–9.
4. Nebelung W, Ropke M, Urbach D, et al. A new technique of arthroscopic capsular shift in anterior shoulder instability. Arthroscopy 2001;17(4): 426–9.
5. Paulos LE, Evans IK, Pinkowski JL. Anterior labrum reconstruction with mini-capsular shift procedure. Iowa Orthop J 1994;14:53–64.
6. Paulos LE, Kody MH. Arthroscopically enhanced "miniapproach" to rotator cuff repair. Am J Sports Med 1994;22(1):19–25.
7. Richmond JC, Donaldson WR, Fu F, et al. Modification of the Bankart reconstruction with a suture anchor. Report of a new technique. Am J Sports Med 1991;19(4):343–6.
8. Snyder SJ. Technique of arthroscopic rotator cuff repair using implantable 4-mm Revo suture anchors, suture Shuttle Relays, and no. 2 nonabsorbable mattress sutures. Orthop Clin North Am 1997; 28(2):267–75.
9. Tauro JC. Arthroscopic rotator cuff repair: analysis of technique and results at 2- and 3-year follow-up. Arthroscopy 1998;14(1):45–51.

10. Ozalay M, Akpinar S, Karaeminogullari O, et al. Mechanical strength of four different biceps tenodesis techniques. Arthroscopy 2005;21(8):992–8.
11. Lafosse L, Shah AA, Butler RB, et al. Arthroscopic biceps tenodesis to supraspinatus tendon: technical note. Am J Orthop (Belle Mead NJ) 2011; 40(7):345–7.
12. Patzer T, Rundic JM, Bobrowitsch E, et al. Biomechanical comparison of arthroscopically performable techniques for suprapectoral biceps tenodesis. Arthroscopy 2011;27(8):1036–47.
13. Patzer T, Santo G, Olender GD, et al. Suprapectoral or subpectoral position for biceps tenodesis: biomechanical comparison of four different techniques in both positions. J Shoulder Elbow Surg 2012;21(1):116–25.
14. Hechtman KS, Tjin AT, Zvijac JE, et al. Biomechanics of a less invasive procedure for reconstruction of the ulnar collateral ligament of the elbow. Am J Sports Med 1998;26(5):620–4.
15. Hechtman KS, Zvijac JE, Wells ME, et al. Long-term results of ulnar collateral ligament reconstruction in throwing athletes based on a hybrid technique. Am J Sports Med 2011;39(2):342–7.
16. Citak M, Backhaus M, Seybold D, et al. Surgical repair of the distal biceps brachii tendon: a comparative study of three surgical fixation techniques. Knee Surg Sports Traumatol Arthrosc 2011;19(11):1936–41.
17. El-Hawary R, Macdermid JC, Faber KJ, et al. Distal biceps tendon repair: comparison of surgical techniques. J Hand Surg 2003;28(3):496–502.
18. Khan AD, Penna S, Yin Q, et al. Repair of distal biceps tendon ruptures using suture anchors through a single anterior incision. Arthroscopy 2008;24(1):39–45.
19. Khan W, Agarwal M, Funk L. Repair of distal biceps tendon rupture with the Biotenodesis screw. Arch Orthop Trauma Surg 2004;124(3):206–8.
20. Barnes SJ, Coleman SG, Gilpin D. Repair of avulsed insertion of biceps. A new technique in four cases. J Bone Joint Surg Br 1993;75(6):938–9.
21. Chou KH, Sarris IK, Sotereanos DG. Suture anchor repair of ulnar-sided triangular fibrocartilage complex tears. J Hand Surg Br 2003;28(6):546–50.
22. Moritomo H. Advantages of open repair of a foveal tear of the triangular fibrocartilage complex via a palmar surgical approach. Tech Hand Up Extrem Surg 2009;13(4):176–81.
23. Bovard RS, Derkash RS, Freeman JR. Grade III avulsion fracture repair on the UCL of the proximal joint of the thumb. Orthop Rev 1994;23(2):167–9.
24. Fairhurst M, Hansen L. Treatment of "Gamekeeper's Thumb" by reconstruction of the ulnar collateral ligament. J Hand Surg Br 2002;27(6):542–5.
25. Jarrett CD, McGillivary GR, Hutton WC. The 2.5 mm PushLock suture anchor system versus a traditional suture anchor for ulnar collateral ligament injuries of the thumb: a biomechanical study. J Hand Surg Eur Vol 2010;35(2):139–43.

26. Brustein M, Pellegrini J, Choueka J, et al. Bone suture anchors versus the pullout button for repair of distal profundus tendon injuries: a comparison of strength in human cadaveric hands. J Hand Surg 2001;26(3):489–96.

27. Gordon L, Tolar M, Rao KT, et al. Flexor tendon repair using a stainless steel internal anchor. Biomechanical study on human cadaver tendons. J Hand Surg Br 1998;23(1):37–40.

28. Lee SK, Fajardo M, Kardashian G, et al. Repair of flexor digitorum profundus to distal phalanx: a biomechanical evaluation of four techniques. J Hand Surg 2011;36(10):1604–9.

29. Ruchelsman DE, Christoforou D, Wasserman B, et al. Avulsion injuries of the flexor digitorum profundus tendon. J Am Acad Orthop Surg 2011;19(3): 152–62.

30. Schreuder FB, Scougall PJ, Puchert E, et al. The effect of mitek anchor insertion angle to attachment of FDP avulsion injuries. J Hand Surg Br 2006;31(3): 292–5.

31. Kaar TK, Schenck RC Jr, Wirth MA, et al. Complications of metallic suture anchors in shoulder surgery: a report of 8 cases. Arthroscopy 2001;17(1):31–7.

32. Benson EC, MacDermid JC, Drosdowech DS, et al. The incidence of early metallic suture anchor pullout after arthroscopic rotator cuff repair. Arthroscopy 2010;26(3):310–5.

33. Goeminne S, Debeer P. Delayed migration of a metal suture anchor into the glenohumeral joint. Acta Orthop Belg 2010;76(6):834–7.

34. Ticker JB, Lippe RJ, Barkin DE, et al. Infected suture anchors in the shoulder. Arthroscopy 1996;12(5): 613–5.

35. Gaenslen ES, Satterlee CC, Hinson GW. Magnetic resonance imaging for evaluation of failed repairs of the rotator cuff. J Bone Joint Surg Am 1996; 78(9):1391–6.

36. Wright PB, Budoff JE, Yeh ML, et al. The properties of damaged and undamaged suture used in metal and bioabsorbable anchors: an in vitro study. Arthroscopy 2007;23(6):655–61.

37. Barber FA, Herbert MA, Richards DP. Sutures and suture anchors: update 2003. Arthroscopy 2003; 19(9):985–90.

38. Matsusue Y, Hanafusa S, Yamamuro T, et al. Tissue reaction of bioabsorbable ultra high strength poly (L-lactide) rod. A long-term study in rabbits. Clin Orthop Relat Res 1995;317:246–53.

39. Athwal GS, Shridharani SM, O'Driscoll SW. Osteolysis and arthropathy of the shoulder after use of bioabsorbable knotless suture anchors. A report of four cases. J Bone Joint Surg Am 2006;88(8):1840–5.

40. Bos RR, Rozema FR, Boering G, et al. Degradation of and tissue reaction to biodegradable poly(L-lactide) for use as internal fixation of fractures: a study in rats. Biomaterials 1991;12(1):32–6.

41. Bostman OM, Pihlajamaki HK. Late foreign-body reaction to an intraosseous bioabsorbable polylactic acid screw. A case report. J Bone Joint Surg Am 1998;80(12):1791–4.

42. Burkart A, Imhoff AB, Roscher E. Foreign-body reaction to the bioabsorbable suretac device. Arthroscopy 2000;16(1):91–5.

43. Freehill MQ, Harms DJ, Huber SM, et al. Poly-L-lactic acid tack synovitis after arthroscopic stabilization of the shoulder. Am J Sports Med 2003;31(5): 643–7.

44. Nho SJ, Provencher MT, Seroyer ST, et al. Bioabsorbable anchors in glenohumeral shoulder surgery. Arthroscopy 2009;25(7):788–93.

45. Sassmannshausen G, Sukay M, Mair SD. Broken or dislodged poly-L-lactic acid bioabsorbable tacks in patients after SLAP lesion surgery. Arthroscopy 2006;22(6):615–9.

46. Park AY, Hatch JD. Proximal humerus osteolysis after revision rotator cuff repair with bioabsorbable suture anchors. Am J Orthop (Belle Mead NJ) 2011;40(3):139–41.

47. Galano GJ, Jiang KN, Strauch RJ, et al. Inflammatory response with osteolysis related to a bioabsorbable anchor in the finger: a case report. Hand (N Y) 2010;5(3):307–12.

48. Yao J, Dantuluri P, Osterman AL. A novel technique of all-inside arthroscopic triangular fibrocartilage complex repair. Arthroscopy 2007;23(12): 1357.e1–4.

49. Yao J. All-arthroscopic triangular fibrocartilage complex repair: safety and biomechanical comparison with a traditional outside-in technique in cadavers. J Hand Surg 2009;34(4):671–6.

50. Cole BJ, Provencher MT. Safety profile of bioabsorbable shoulder anchors. Arthroscopy 2007; 23(8):912–3 [author reply: 913–4].

51. Cummins CA, Strickland S, Appleyard RC, et al. Rotator cuff repair with bioabsorbable screws: an in vivo and ex vivo investigation. Arthroscopy 2003;19(3):239–48.

52. Glueck D, Wilson TC, Johnson DL. Extensive osteolysis after rotator cuff repair with a bioabsorbable suture anchor: a case report. Am J Sports Med 2005;33(5):742–4.

53. Burkhart SS. Case report by Drs. Glueck, Wilson, and Johnson entitled "Extensive osteolysis after rotator cuff repair with a bioabsorbable suture anchor" (May 2005, pages 742-744). Am J Sports Med 2005;33(11):1768.

54. Park MJ, Hsu JE, Harper C, et al. Poly-L/D-lactic acid anchors are associated with reoperation and failure of slap repairs. Arthroscopy 2011;27(10): 1335–40.

55. Barber FA, Coons DA, Ruiz-Suarez M. Cyclic load testing and ultimate failure strength of biodegradable glenoid anchors. Arthroscopy 2008;24(2):224–8.

56. Barber FA, Hapa O, Bynum JA. Comparative testing by cyclic loading of rotator cuff suture anchors containing multiple high-strength sutures. Arthroscopy 2010;26(Suppl 9):S134–41.

57. Barber FA, Herbert MA, Beavis RC. Cyclic load and failure behavior of arthroscopic knots and high strength sutures. Arthroscopy 2009;25(2):192–9.

58. Barber FA, Herbert MA, Beavis RC, et al. Suture anchor materials, eyelets, and designs: update 2008. Arthroscopy 2008;24(8):859–67.

59. Barber FA, Herbert MA, Coons DA, et al. Sutures and suture anchors—update 2006. Arthroscopy 2006;22(10):1063.e1–9.

60. Barber FA, Herbert MA, Hapa O, et al. Biomechanical analysis of pullout strengths of rotator cuff and glenoid anchors: 2011 update. Arthroscopy 2011; 27(7):895–905.

61. Barber FA, Herbert MA, Schroeder FA, et al. Biomechanical advantages of triple-loaded suture anchors compared with double-row rotator cuff repairs. Arthroscopy 2010;26(3):316–23.

62. Ruiz-Suarez M, Aziz-Jacobo J, Barber FA. Cyclic load testing and ultimate failure strength of suture anchors in the acetabular rim. Arthroscopy 2010; 26(6):762–8.

63. Oshtory R, Lindsey DP, Giori NJ, et al. Bioabsorbable tricalcium phosphate bone cement strengthens fixation of suture anchors. Clin Orthop Relat Res 2010;468(12):3406–12.

64. Othman D, Cocq HL, Majumder S. A safety technique for mitek anchor suture rupture: a new trick. J Hand Surg 2011;36(9):1532–3.

65. Kato H, Minami A, Takahara M, et al. Surgical repair of acute collateral ligament injuries in digits with the Mitek bone suture anchor. J Hand Surg Br 1999; 24(1):70–5.

66. Beauperthuy GD, Burke EF. Alternative method of repairing collateral ligament injuries at the metacarpophalangeal joints of the thumb and fingers. Use of the Mitek anchor. J Hand Surg Br 1997;22(6): 736–8.

67. De Carli A, Vadala A, Monaco E, et al. Effect of cyclic loading on new polyblend suture coupled with different anchors. Am J Sports Med 2005;33(2):214–9.

68. Lo IK, Burkhart SS, Athanasiou K. Abrasion resistance of two types of nonabsorbable braided suture. Arthroscopy 2004;20(4):407–13.

69. Lo IK, Burkhart SS, Chan KC, et al. Arthroscopic knots: determining the optimal balance of loop security and knot security. Arthroscopy 2004;20(5):489–502.

70. McDonald E, Gordon JA, Buckley JM, et al. Comparison of a new multifilament stainless steel suture with frequently used sutures for flexor tendon repair. J Hand Surg 2011;36(6):1028–34.

Advances in Treating Skin Defects of the Hand
Skin Substitutes and Negative-Pressure Wound Therapy

Andrew J. Watt, MD[a,e,*], Jeffrey B. Friedrich, MD[b,c,d], Jerry I. Huang, MD[a,e]

KEYWORDS

- Hand reconstruction • Skin substitute • Dermal substitute • V.A.C. • Integra

KEY POINTS

- By virtue of its position in space and function as the primary mode of physical interaction with the surrounding environment, the hand is notoriously prone to injury, infection, and, less commonly, carcinogenesis.
- The skin of the hand and its accessory structures, including the perionychium and nail, are highly specialized, reflecting their specific function.
- Soft tissue reconstruction of the hand has primarily adhered to the same reconstructive hierarchy applied by surgeons to other soft tissue defects throughout the body.
- The widespread availability of skin substitutes and the advent of negative pressure wound therapy provide adjunctive and alternative options to traditional reconstructive techniques for treating soft tissue defects of the hand.

INTRODUCTION

The distinctly specialized structure and function of the hand have remained a focus of interest and a source of surgical innovation for hand and reconstructive surgeons. By virtue of its position in space and function as the primary mode of physical interaction with the surrounding environment, the hand is notoriously prone to injury, infection, and, less commonly, carcinogenesis. These processes result not only in injury to the underlying osseous, ligamentous, and tendinous structures but also to the investing soft tissue cover of the hand. Adequate skin cover is a prerequisite for any complex osseous, ligamentous, or tendinous reconstruction within the hand. To view this investing skin envelope as simply a cover belies its complexity.

The skin of the hand and its accessory structures including the perionychium and nail are highly specialized, reflecting their specific function. The thick glabrous skin of the palm allows for fine, discriminate sensation and provides a durable cover for the working surface of the hand. In contrast, the dorsum of the hand is characterized by thin, supple skin that allows for nearly

Conflict of interest and financial disclosure: the authors have no financial disclosures or conflicts of interest. No external funding was used in the preparation of this article.
[a] Department of Orthopedic Surgery & Sports Medicine, University of Washington, WA, USA; [b] Division of Plastic Surgery, Department of Surgery, University of Washington, WA, USA; [c] Department of Orthopaedics, University of Washington, WA, USA; [d] Harborview Medical Center, 325 9th Avenue, Box 359796, Seattle, WA 98104, USA; [e] University of Washington Hand Center, 4245 Roosevelt Avenue Northeast, Box 354740, Seattle, WA 98105, USA
* Corresponding author. University of Washington Hand Center, 4245 Roosevelt Avenue Northeast, Box 354740, Seattle, WA 98105.
E-mail address: ajwatt50@gmail.com

Hand Clin 28 (2012) 519–528
http://dx.doi.org/10.1016/j.hcl.2012.08.010

unrestricted mobility. No other tissues throughout the body perfectly reproduce these functions when transplanted to the hand.

Soft tissue reconstruction of the hand has primarily adhered to the same reconstructive hierarchy applied by surgeons to other soft tissue defects throughout the body. In general, soft tissue reconstruction has ranged from healing via secondary intention to complex, microsurgical tissue transfers in an effort to recapitulate the structure and function of lost tissues. Each stage in this reconstructive algorithm has applicability to particular soft tissue defects of the hand. However, this hierarchy of reconstruction has notable limitations that are unique to the hand. The first unique characteristic relates to mobility. Mobility remains paramount in any reconstructive endeavor involving the hand and is often in direct opposition to some degree of immobility required to obtain tissue healing. The necessity of minimizing immobility favors reconstructive techniques that afford expeditious healing or allow for mobility while healing occurs. The second unique challenge relates to the number of critical, avascular structures that afford a poor, if not frankly hostile, wound bed for simpler reconstructive techniques, including skin grafting. These structures are close to the overlying skin and require motion independent of the skin envelope to allow for full function.

Local tissue reconstruction of the hand, which maintains the advantages of providing analogous, often sensate, tissue, has distinct limitations, including a relative shortage of skin with limited mobility. Local tissue reconstruction is therefore limited to the treatment of smaller wounds of the hand, and consideration must be afforded to the potential donor site morbidity. Larger wounds of the hand have traditionally required regional or free tissue transfer. Pedicled groin and abdominal flaps can provide for reliable and often functional reconstruction; however, they require a period of significant immobility as well as a second surgical procedure to divide the flap pedicle. Reverse radial forearm fascial and fasciocutaneous flaps provide a facile alternative to staged reconstruction; however, sacrifice of the radial artery and the presence of a complete palmar arch are necessities that may not be tenable in the setting of a traumatized extremity. Free tissue transfer provides the most versatile option for soft tissue reconstruction of the hand; however, this skill-set is not universally available and not all patients are potential candidates for these extensive operations.

These challenges have inspired surgeons and scientists to pursue alternative methods of reconstruction that may play an adjunctive role to, or completely supplant, these more traditional reconstructive modalities. This article provides an overview of these emerging techniques, with an emphasis on skin substitutes and negative-pressure wound therapy as they apply to the treatment of soft tissue defects of the hand. The indications, contraindications, and relative advantages and disadvantages of these techniques are discussed in detail.

SYNTHETIC DRESSINGS AND SKIN SUBSTITUTES

The skin has a vital role in the protection of underlying structures and functions as an evaporative and critical immunologic barrier. Disruption of skin continuity triggers a complex cascade of events, including hemostasis, inflammation, and wound healing via both re-epithelialization and contracture. Wounds occurring in several anatomic locations throughout the body are amenable to local wound care and healing via secondary intention; however, there are notable drawbacks to allowing a wound to heal in this manner. Healing via secondary intention is often slow. The duration of treatment carries both physiologic and economic disadvantages. A prolonged break in the continuity of the skin presents a potential portal for infection and may lead to desiccation of underlying structures. Wound care also carries a burden for both the patient and the health care system. Open wounds may lead to prolonged time away from work and other productive endeavors, and the cost of wound care, including home health provisions, is not trivial. Second, healing via secondary intention relies on wound contracture. Contracture may be tolerated in relatively immobile anatomic locations; however, even the slightest degree of contracture is often functionally limiting in regions of the body that require mobility. This principle is particularly pertinent when considering wound healing within the hand and upper extremity. Given the functional requirements of mobility within the hand, combined with the presence of superficially located critical structures, expeditious healing in the hand is paramount to the preservation of function.

Over the past 2 decades, tremendous research and bioengineering efforts have focused on developing ideal dressings and dermal substitutes that alter wound characteristics, expedite wound healing, minimize scarring, and seek to supplant or, at least enhance, autologous tissue reconstruction. Clinical research has suggested that maintaining moisture within a healing wound environment promotes both granulation and re-epithelialization.[1–3] A myriad of active wound coverings including both bioengineered skin and dermal substitutes have been developed and marketed. Hand surgeons have adapted these products for use in the hand in an attempt to provide potentially superior functional and aesthetic results and minimize donor morbidity. However, these products have only recently been formally evaluated in the context of soft tissue reconstruction of the hand. An understanding of the properties of these products as well as their relative attributes assists the reconstructive surgeon in making informed decisions regarding their use in hand reconstruction.

Synthetic Dressings

Synthetic dressings are designed to maintain a moist wound environment by minimizing evaporative loss, promoting autolytic wound debridement, minimizing the risk of infection, and promoting granulation and epithelialization. The simplest of these dressings consists of a polyurethane membrane, which functions as a simple evaporative barrier, whereas the most complex contain an array of biologically active materials that interact with and alter the wound environment (**Table 1**).

Biologically active dressings are specifically designed to alter the composition of matrix metalloproteinases (MMPs) within the healing wound. MMPs are critical enzymatic factors in wound remodeling; however, persistently high levels of MMPs are associated with prolonged healing.[3] In these circumstances, newly synthesized extracellular matrix components are degraded rather than allowed to contribute to wound healing. Collagen and oxidized regenerated cellulose or alginate fibers incorporated into these biologically active dressings chemically bind MMPs, inactivating them, thereby altering the physiologic balance of the healing wound. These dressings have shown efficacy in protecting local growth factors and extracellular matrix components from degradation by MMPs.[4,5]

In addition to inactivating MMPs through the incorporation of cellulose and alginate, collagen, and hyaluronic acids have been added in an effort to promote dermal regeneration and epithelialization. These components are hypothesized to act as chemotactic factors for macrophage and fibroblast migration and provide a temporary scaffold for tissue ingrowth.[5] Knowledge of these biologically active dressings primarily stems from their use in burn care and in the treatment of chronic venous ulcers.

Oasis Wound Matrix (Cook Biotech, West Lafayette, IN), composed of porcine intestinal submucosa, is a synthetic wound dressing that interacts with and is subsequently incorporated into a wound. The submucosal structure provides a scaffold for tissue ingrowth, and in vivo studies have shown enhanced angiogenesis and rapidity of wound healing in chronic leg ulcers.[6] Oasis, and wound matrices like it, has potential applicability in promoting granulation and healing, thereby bridging relatively avascular structures, including tendon and cortical bone. No studies exist showing the efficacy or applicability of any of these synthetic dressings in the hand and upper extremity, and their use remains primarily limited to the treatment of chronic, nonhealing leg wounds.

Skin Substitutes

The distinction between biologically active, synthetic wound dressings, and skin substitutes has become increasingly indistinct. Skin substitutes are defined by their bilaminar structure. Skin substitutes consist of a porous matrix layer containing a variable mixture of extracellular components (collagen, hyaluronic acid, fibronectin) and an overlying laminate (typically silicone) that serves as an evaporative barrier. This structure, in principle, recapitulates the structure of skin with its dermal and epidermal components (**Table 2**).

Biobrane

The first modern skin substitute, Biobrane (Smith & Nephew, Memphis, TN) was introduced in 1979 and has been widely used as a temporary wound cover. Biobrane can be used to promote re-epithelialization in superficial wounds with retained adnexal structures and granulation in deeper wounds, thereby providing a wound bed amenable for subsequent skin grafting. The structural component of Biobrane consists of porcine type I collagen covalently bound to a bilaminar membrane composed of nylon mesh and silicone. The collagen acts as a scaffold for angiogenesis and collagen deposition from fibroblasts. The nylon mesh acts as a semipermeable barrier, preventing wound desiccation and allowing limited fluid egress. This semipermeable barrier is removed before application of a split-thickness skin graft. The dressing acts as a biologically active dressing for superficial wounds, allowing for re-epithelialization and a skin substitute for deeper wounds, stimulating granulation via the collagen layer before split-thickness skin grafting.

Integra dermal regeneration template

Integra dermal regeneration template (Integra LifeSciences, Plainsboro, NJ) adheres to the bilayer model of skin substitutes, providing a scaffold for dermal regeneration and temporary wound coverage (**Fig. 1**). The structural matrix component

Table 1
Synthetic dressings

Type	Composition	Mechanism	Available Products
Film	Polyurethane membrane	Evaporative barrier	Opsite (Smith & Nephew, Memphis, TN), Tegaderm (3M, St Paul, MN)
Hydrocolloid	Carboxymethyl-cellulose	Moisture balance	Tegasorb (3M), Duoderm (ConvaTec, Skillman, NJ, Exuderm (Medline, Mundelein, IL)
Hydrogel	Polyethylene oxide/ acrylate/acrylamide, water	Moisture balance	IntraSite Gel (Smith & Nephew), Tegagel (3M), Restore Hydrogel (Hollister, Libertyville, IL)
Foams	Polyurethane foam	Moisture balance	Allevyn (Smith & Nephew), Mepilex (Molnlycke Health Care, Gothenberg, Sweden), Lyofoam (Molnlycke Health Care)
Alginates and hydrofibers	Calcium alginate fiber, carboxymethyl-cellulose fiber	Moisture balance, inactivation of MMPs	Aquacel Hydrofiber (ConvaTec), Medihoney (Derma Sciences, Toronto, Canada), Curasorb (Covidien, Mansfield, MA), Algisite (Smith & Nephew)
Extracellular matrix dermal scaffolds	Collagen, hyaluronic acids	Macrophage and fibroblast chemotaxis, biological scaffold	Terudermis (Terumo, Tokyo, Japan), Biostep (Smith & Nephew)

of Integra consists of cross-linked bovine collagen and shark chondroitin-6-sulfate characterized by a well-defined porosity and degradation rate. The dermal regeneration template is covered by a layer of polysiloxane (silicone) polymer, which serves as an evaporative barrier. The collagen-based scaffold acts as a template for the regeneration of a neodermis. This process generally takes 2 to 3 weeks. After this period of regeneration, the silicone layer is removed and the neodermis is grafted with a thin split-thickness skin graft, replicating the elasticity and durability of a thicker graft.

Histologic analysis of specimens obtained after reconstruction with Integra support its role as a true dermal regeneration template. In biopsies obtained 2 years after reconstruction, rete ridges were present at the junction between the epidermis and the dermis in 70%, collagen was routinely present in the dermal layer, and elastic fibers were present in all specimens.[7]

Integra is widely used in burn reconstruction and its use as a skin substitute has been expanded and used in hand surgery. Integra-based reconstruction offers the advantages of increasingly supple and durable wound healing compared with split-thickness skin grafting alone.[8] Reports of scar revision with Integra have shown increased functional range of motion and cosmetic improvement.[9] In addition to affording increased mobility by replicating native dermis, the neodermis allows for resurfacing with ultrathin skin grafts (0.076–0.203 mm [0.003–0.008 in]) containing little native dermal component. These thin grafts allow for more rapid healing of the donor site and provide for facile repeat harvesting from a donor site.[10]

Successful experiences with Integra use in burn reconstruction prompted several investigators to specifically examine its applicability for the reconstruction of complex wounds, including those with tendon and bone exposure. Weigert and

Table 2
Skin substitutes: synthetic bilayer dermal replacements and allogeneic acellular skin substitutes

	Composition	Properties
Synthetic Bilayer Acellular Dermal Replacements		
Biobrane (Smith & Nephew, Memphis, TN)	Silicone/nylon mesh, porcine collagen	Biosynthetic skin substitute Semipermeable Stimulation of granulation
Integra (Integra LifeSciences, Plainsboro, NJ)	Silicone, bovine collagen/chondroitin 6-sulfate	Biosynthetic skin substitute Scaffold for neodermis generation
Allogeneic Acellular Skin Substitutes		
Alloderm (Life Cell, Branchburg, NJ)	Decellularized, freeze-dried allogeneic dermis	Proprietary decellularization process Noncross-linked Stored at room temperature Requires rehydration (10–40 min) Aseptically processed (meets requirements for human tissue transplantation)
DermaMatrix (Synthes, Westchester, PA)	Decellularized, freeze-dried allogeneic dermis	Sodium chloride-based decellularization process Noncross-linked Stored at room temperature Requires rehydration Bacterially inactivated (meets US Pharmacopeia Standard 71 for sterility)
FlexHD (Mentor, Santa Barbara, CA)	Decellularized freeze-dried allogeneic dermis	Noncross-linked Stored at room temperature No rehydration required Bacterially inactivated (meets US Pharmacopeia Standard 71 for sterility)
Graftjacket (Wright Medical Technologies, Arlington, TX)	Decellularized freeze-dried allogeneic dermis	Noncross-linked Transported at ambient temperature, stored between 1 and 10°C Requires rehydration Aseptically processed (meets requirements for human tissue transplantation)

colleagues[11] reported the largest available series of complex hand wounds treated with an Integra-based reconstructive model. These investigators report successful engraftment in 13 of 15 patients. Thirteen patients had exposed tendons, devoid of paratenon. Three patients had exposed bone, devoid of periosteum, and 6 patients had exposed joint without intact capsule. The average time from injury to placement of Integra was 26 days. The average time from Integra placement to split-thickness skin grafting was 26 days as well. In Weigert and colleagues' experience, relatively large areas of exposed, nonvascularized tissue can be successfully bridged with Integra; however, they identify the importance of having a surrounding vascularized wound bed to serve as a foundation for integration and bridging of these nonvascularized structures. The investigators specifically identify some of the salient features of Integra-based reconstruction, including ease of use, immediate availability in large amounts, avoidance of donor site morbidity, restoration of a gliding plane for tendon excursion, and the generally acceptable functional and aesthetic results attained. Muangman and colleagues[12] reported a similar experience using Integra for the treatment of 10 patients with complex hand wounds. They reported engraftment rates of 98% ± 4%, along with the ability to provide

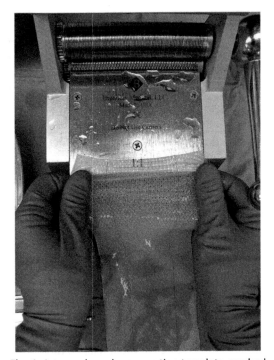

Fig. 1. Integra dermal regeneration template, meshed 1:1 to allow for fluid egress. Integra consists of cross-linked bovine collagen and shark chondroitin-6-sulfate covered by a layer of polysiloxane polymer.

successful wound healing over small areas of exposed bone and tendon. These investigators presented several salient techniques that improved engraftment rates, including the use of meshed (1:1) Integra, as well as the use of antibiotic-impregnated dressings in an effort to minimize bacterial colonization. When meshing Integra, it is important to use a noncrushing mesher (specifically one that does not use a carrier). Meshed Integra is now available from the manufacturer and allows for greater fluid egress. The use of antibiotic dressings (Acticoat [Smith & Nephew], V.A.C. Granu-Foam Silver sponge [Kinetic Concepts, San Antonio, TX]), and mafenide acetate soaks have helped minimize one of the major shortcomings of Integra, specifically its lack of intrinsic antimicrobial resistance during the period of neovascularization. In the burn population, rates of superficial infection are reported at 13%, with a 3% rate of invasive infection.[13] No specific reports addressing infection rates in extremity reconstruction exist. Rates of engraftment can be improved with the use of negative-pressure wound therapy as a bolster dressing.[14–16] This technique allows for reliable immobilization of the Integra and allows the product to conform to the contours of the wound bed. Specific reports using Integra for hand

reconstruction include the treatment of fingertip injuries and large dorsal hand wounds in patients with small areas of exposed tendons (**Fig. 2**).[17,18]

The advantages of supple restoration of skin cover, improved cosmetic appearance, the ability to bridge areas of exposed tendon or bone, and reduced split-thickness skin graft donor site morbidity must be weighed against the necessity for staged reconstruction, prolonged immobilization necessary to obtain engraftment, and an intrinsic lack of antimicrobial activity. Reconstruction requires 2 to 3 weeks of immobilization for engraftment, followed by 1 to 2 weeks of immobilization to allow for take of the split-thickness skin graft. This period of prolonged immobilization can result in considerable stiffness and functional loss in reconstruction of the hand. Given these considerations, use of Integra primarily limited to coverage of dorsal hand wound and scar revisions, particularly in patients who have no available local tissue options or are poor surgical candidates for more complex microvascular soft tissue reconstructions.

Allogeneic acellular substitutes

Allogenic acellular substitutes have become increasingly used throughout reconstructive surgery over the past 2 decades. These products are derived from cadaveric donors and differ in their method of processing, thickness, and sizes available. The precursor to these products is human cadaveric allograft. Allograft skin is harvested from highly screened tissue donors and is available in meshed and unmeshed forms. The skin may be stored in a refrigerated state for up to 1 week and frozen for more prolonged periods. The skin may be applied to a wound as a temporary, truly biologic dressing. The epidermis preserves hydration of the wound, and the dermal components stimulate neovascularization and granulation. The graft my even be used over exposed tendinous and bony structures as a temporary dressing before definitive reconstruction. The allograft skin is rejected by the host in 3 to 4 weeks, and definitive reconstruction with a skin graft or flap is typically performed before this time. Allograft skin is particularly useful in testing a marginally viable wound bed. If the allograft skin adheres, the bed is sufficient to support definitive skin grafting. Allograft skin is also useful as a temporary wound dressing while awaiting pathologic results after tumor resection and may be used to forestall reconstruction in patients who cannot tolerate immediate complex reconstruction such as unstable trauma patients. However, allograft skin does carry a risk, albeit low, of disease

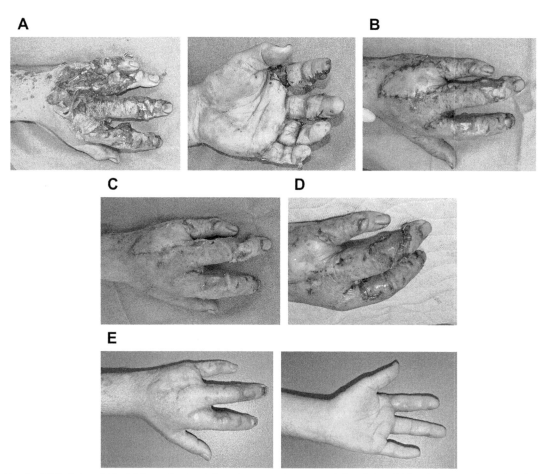

Fig. 2. (*A*) Left-hand blast injury obtained from homemade mortar. (*B*) Left-hand blast injury 14 days after filet flap of the ring finger and local wound care of the remaining index and long fingers. Note the small areas of exposed extensor tendon. (*C*) Left-hand blast injury immediately after application of Integra dermal regeneration template. (*D*) Left-hand blast injury 14 days after application of Integra dermal regeneration template, immediately before split-thickness skin grafting. Note the salmon color of the wound, indicating that the dermal template has incorporated into the underlying wound bed. (*E*) Left-hand blast injury 2 months after initial injury.

transmission, and these risks should be discussed with patients before application.[19,20]

Experience with allograft skin has provided the teleologic foundation for processed acellular dermal products. A host of these products are available, including Alloderm (Life Cell, Branchburg, NJ), DermaMatrix (Synthes, Westchester, PA), Neoform (Mentor, Santa Barbara, CA), and Graftjacket (Wright Medical Technologies, Arlington, TN). The products primarily differ in their method of processing, thickness, and US Food and Drug Administration-approved indications. All of these products are acellularized dermal scaffolds that may be placed in a wound to reconstitute the dermal structure. These scaffolds are neovascularized over time and, after revascularization, are amenable to skin grafting. These products remain expensive and carry the theoretic potential for disease transmission;

however, no cases of disease transmission have been reported in the medical literature.[21–25]

Acellular dermal products have been used in hand reconstruction in much the same manner as Integra. Reports of burn scar contracture release in the hand with application of dermal matrix and staged skin grafting have been reported. Askari and colleagues[26] reported on 9 patients undergoing hand burn scar contracture release with application of Alloderm and split-thickness skin grafts in 9 patients. Alloderm was applied to the hand and allowed to neovascularize for 10 to 14 days. The wound was then covered with a 0.305-mm (0.012-in) split-thickness skin graft and immobilized for an additional 2 weeks. Askari and colleagues reported an 83% gain in passive range of motion and an 89% gain in length of treated web spaces, and recommended the use of acellular dermal matrices in the treatment of difficult or recurrent scar contractures in the hand.

NEGATIVE-PRESSURE WOUND THERAPY

The use of negative-pressure wound therapy has dramatically altered the reconstructive landscape over the past 2 decades. This technology has been used throughout the body, and its relative applications and benefits have been refined. Despite its widespread applicability, the basic biological mechanisms underlying its usefulness remain poorly understood despite an increasing body of literature on the subject. Moues and colleagues[27] recently reviewed more than 400 articles addressing the use of negative-pressure wound therapy. The investigators distilled the mechanisms attributable to negative-pressure wound therapy to an increase in blood flow to the wound, stimulation of angiogenesis, a reduction in wound surface area, induction of cellular proliferation, and a reduction in inhibitory contents of the wound exudate. An increase in edema reduction and bacterial clearance, often ascribed to negative-pressure therapy, have not been convincingly established in the existing literature. Negative-pressure wound therapy, in its simplest form, provides for accelerated secondary wound healing via granulation and wound contracture. The technique has also been adapted and repurposed as an ideal bolster dressing over skin grafts, improving both skin graft take and enhancing re-epithelialization of graft interstices,[28–32] and has proved to increase incorporation of skin substitutes and acellularized dermal matrices.[33–35] Negative-pressure therapy has also been used as a temporary bridge to prevent desiccation and allow tissue demarcation before embarking on definitive soft tissue reconstruction.

Secondary healing within the hand and upper extremity of sufficiently large wounds to justify the use of negative-pressure wound therapy is rare; however, it is for these additional indications that the technique has found significant usefulness in the hand (**Fig. 3**). The hand is a difficult anatomic structure to bolster effectively given its irregularity and mobility. Negative-pressure dressings, applied over grafts and skin substitutes, facilitate fluid egress, minimize shear stress, and provide tight apposition to the underlying wound bed. Achieving a complete seal with these dressings is often challenging in the hand, but every effort should be made to incorporate only those structures immediately adjacent to the reconstructed area, and, when feasible, the fingers should be left free to allow for therapy and maintenance of mobility. When gliding structures such as extensor tendons must be immobilized temporarily to allow for incorporation of the reconstructed tissue, the hand should be splinted in a strict intrinsic plus posture to prevent collateral ligament shortening.

SUMMARY

The unique composition of the soft tissue envelope of the hand consisting of both glabrous palmar skin and thin pliable dorsal skin, combined with the large surface area, proximity of avascular structures to the skin surface, and the necessity for mobility of the hand create a reconstructive challenge for hand surgeons. Emphasis in reconstruction should be placed on providing stable, expeditious coverage of the vital structures of the hand and minimizing immobility. Under ideal circumstances, these objectives are most effectively met with autologous soft tissue reconstructions; however, in circumstances including polytrauma, and in patients with significant comorbid disease or vascular injuries that limit the surgeons' ability to perform more complex reconstruction, biologically active wound dressings, skin substitutes, and negative-pressure wound therapy provide essential adjuncts and alternative methods of reconstruction.

Skin substitutes have proved particularly useful in the reconstruction of scar contractures of the hand and in the coverage of dorsal hand wounds with small areas of exposed tendon. These products act to rebuild lost dermis and increase the pliability of soft tissue reconstruction, facilitating minimal donor site morbidity. Negative-pressure wound therapy has become widely used by hand surgeons as a temporary adjunct before definitive reconstruction and as an effective bolster dressing to facilitate the incorporation of skin substitutes and the overall take of skin grafts. These products and techniques continue to evolve. Additional skin substitutes, seeded with growth factors and antibiotic properties, are under development and likely will find additional usefulness in the soft tissue reconstructive algorithm of the hand. Innovative

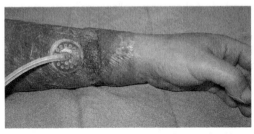

Fig. 3. Forearm wound V.A.C. used as a bridge to definitive reconstruction in a contaminated wound.

hand surgeons will continue to repurpose many of these tools, expanding their usefulness and indications.

REFERENCES

1. Winter GD. Formation of scab and the rate of epithelialization of superficial wounds in the skin of the young domestic pig. Nature 1962;193:293–4.
2. Hinman CD, Maibach HI. Effect of air exposure and occlusion on experimental human skin wounds. Nature 1963;200:377–8.
3. Ovington L. The art and science of wound dressings in the twenty-first century. In: Falabella A, Kirsner R, editors. Wound healing, 45. Boca Raton (FL): Taylor & Francis; 2005. p. P587–98.
4. Cullen B, Watt PW, Lundqvist C, et al. The role of oxidised regenerated cellulose/collagen in chronic wound repair and its potential mechanism of action. Int J Biochem Cell Biol 2002;34:1544–56.
5. Mian M, Beghe F, Mian E. Collagen as a pharmacological approach in wound healing. Int J Tissue React 1992;14:S1–9.
6. Mostow EN, Haraway GD, Dalsing M, et al. Effectiveness of an extracellular matrix graft (Oasis Wound Matrix) in the treatment of chronic leg ulcers: a randomized clinical trial. J Vasc Surg 2005;41: 837–43.
7. Moiemen N, Yarrow J, Hodgson E, et al. Long-term clinical and histological analysis of Integra dermal regeneration template. Plast Reconstr Surg 2011; 127:1149–54.
8. Fitton AR, Drew P, Dickson WA. The use of a bilaminate artificial skin substitute (Integra) in acute resurfacing of burns: an early experience. Br J Plast Surg 2001;54:208–12.
9. Stiefel D, Schiestl C, Mueli M. Integra burn scar revision in adolescents and children. Burns 2010;36: 114–20.
10. Klein MB, Engrav LH, Holmes JH, et al. Management of facial burns with a collagen/glycosaminoglycan skin substitute–prospective experience with 12 consecutive patients with large, deep facial burns. Burns 2005;31:257–61.
11. Weigert H, Choughri H, Casoli V. Management of severe hand wounds with Integra dermal regeneration template. J Hand Surg Eur Vol 2011;36:185–93.
12. Muangman P, Deubner H, Honari S, et al. Correlation of clinical outcome of Integra application with microbiologic and pathological biopsies. J Truama 2006; 61:1212–7.
13. Heimbach DM, Warden GD, Luterman A, et al. Multicenter postapproval clinical trial of Integra dermal regeneration template for burn treatment. J Burn Care Rehabil 2003;24:42–8.
14. Jescke MG, Rose C, Angele P, et al. Development of new reconstructive techniques: use of Integra in combination with fibrin glue and negative-pressure therapy for reconstruction of acute and chronic wounds. Plast Reconstr Surg 2004;113:525–30.
15. McEwan W, Brown TL, Mills SM, et al. Suction dressings to secure a dermal substitute. Burns 2004;30: 259–61.
16. Molnar JA, DeFranzo AJ, Hadaegh A, et al. Acceleration of Integra incorporation in complex tissue defects with subatmospheric pressure. Plast Reconstr Surg 2004;113:1339–446.
17. Taras JS, Sapienza A, Roach JB, et al. Acellular dermal regeneration template for soft tissue reconstruction of the digits. J Hand Surg (Am) 2010;35: 415–21.
18. Katrana F, Kostopoulos E, Delia G, et al. Reanimation of thumb extension after upper extremity degloving injury treated with Integra. J Hand Surg Eur Vol 2008;33:800–2.
19. Barnett JR, McCauley RL, Schutzler S, et al. Cadaveric donor discards secondary to serology. J Burn Care Rehabil 2001;22:124–7.
20. Mathur M, De A, Gore M. Microbiological assessment of cadaver skin grafts received in a skin bank. Burns 2008;35:104–6.
21. Wainwright DJ. Use of an acellular dermal matrix (Alloderm) in the management of full thickness burns. Burns 1995;21:243–8.
22. Munster AM, Smith-Meek M, Shalom A. Acellular allograft dermal matrix: immediate or delayed epidermal coverage? Burns 2001;27:150–3.
23. Brigido SA, Boc SF, Lopex RC. Effective management of major lower extremity wounds using an acellular regenerative tissue matrix: a pilot study. Orthopedics 2004;S27:145–9.
24. Rosales MA, Bruntz M, Armstrong DG. Gamma-irradiated human skin allograft: a potential treatment modality for lower extremity ulcers. Int Wound J 2004;1:201–6.
25. Onur R, Singla A. Solvent-dehydrated cadaveric dermis: a new allograft for pubovaginal sling surgery. Int J Urol 2005;12:801–5.
26. Askari M, Cohen MJ, Grossman PH, et al. The use of acellular dermal matrix in release of burn contracture scars in the hand. Plast Reconstr Surg 2011; 127:1593–9.
27. Moues CM, Heule F, Hovius SE. A review of topical negative pressure therapy in wound healing: sufficient evidence? Am J Surg 2011;201:544–56.
28. Blackburn JH II, Boemi L, Hall WW, et al. Negative pressure dressings as a bolster for skin grafts. Ann Plast Surg 1998;40:453–7.
29. Schneider AM, Morykwas MJ, Argenta LC. A new and reliable method of securing skin grafts to the difficult recipient bed. Plast Reconstr Surg 1998; 102:1195–8.
30. Scherer LA, Shiver S, Chang M, et al. The vacuum assisted closure device: a method of securing skin

grafts and improving graft survival. Arch Surg 2002; 137:930–3.

31. Moisidis E, Heath T, Boorer C, et al. A prospective, blinded, randomized, controlled clinical trial of topical negative pressure use in skin grafting. Plast Reconstr Surg 2004;114:917–22.

32. Llanos S, Danilla S, Barraza C, et al. Effectiveness of negative pressure closure in the integration of split thickness skin grafts: a randomized, double-masked, controlled trial. Ann Surg 2006;244:700–5.

33. Molnar JA. Applications of negative pressure wound therapy to thermal injury. Ostomy Wound Manage 2004;50:17–9.

34. Kim EK, Hong JP. Efficacy of negative pressure therapy to enhance take of 1-stage allodermis and a split thickness graft. Ann Plast Surg 2007;58:536–40.

35. Eo S, Kim Y, Cho S. Vacuum-assisted closure improves the incorporation of artificial dermis in soft tissue defects: Terudermis and Pelnac. Int Wound J 2011;8:261–7.

Nerve Glue for Upper Extremity Reconstruction

Raymond Tse, MD[a,b,]*, Jason H. Ko, MD[c]

KEYWORDS

• Peripheral nerve • Nerve glue • Nerve adhesive • Nerve reconstruction

KEY POINTS

- Nerve glue is an attractive alternative to sutures to improve the results of nerve repair.
- Improved axon alignment, reduced scar and inflammation, greater and faster reinnervation, and better functional results have been reported with the use of nerve glue.
- The current formulations of fibrin glue are routinely used for nerve grafts and transfers and may have a role in augmenting suture repairs. Polyethylene glycol sealants are currently being studied for their suitability as nerve glue.

INTRODUCTION

In the hand sensation is equal in value to motion.

— *Sterling Bunnell, 1946*[1]

Although great strides to produce consistently favorable outcomes in hand surgery have been made, peripheral nerve reconstruction remains a challenge. Patient and disease factors may account for much of the variability in functional results; however, the effectiveness of nerve repair for end target reinnervation underlies any functional result. Nerve glue for nerve repair is an attractive alternative to the current standard suture repair. Advantages of an adhesive for nerve repair include ease of use, less tissue trauma, maintenance of nerve architecture, and better fascicular alignment. Although the ideal nerve glue is not yet available, progress continues toward this end.

PROPERTIES OF THE IDEAL NERVE GLUE

"Glue" is a liquid or semiliquid substance that tightly adheres items together. In the setting of human peripheral nerve repair, the ideal glue should have specific biologic, mechanical, and technical properties as outlined in **Table 1**. Safety requires that the substance have minimal risk of disease transmission, antigenicity, or toxicity. The glue should not induce fibrosis that can lead to nerve compression and in the case of substance interposition between nerves, it should not act as a barrier to nerve regeneration. Application of the glue should preserve the normal nerve architecture and should facilitate ideal fascicular alignment. The glue should provide adequate mechanical strength to prevent gapping or rupture at the initial repair and during the postoperative period. It should be easy to use with minimal equipment and easy to apply thereby reducing operative time. Finally, the glue should be versatile

The authors have identified no professional or financial affiliations for themselves or their spouse/partner.
[a] Division of Plastic Surgery, Department of Surgery, University of Washington, WA 98105, USA; [b] Brachial Plexus Program, Pediatric Plastic Surgery, Seattle Children's Hospital, 4800 Sand Point Way Northeast, M/S W-7847, Seattle, WA 98105, USA; [c] Hand and Microvascular Surgery, Department of Orthopaedics and Sports Medicine, University of Washington, Seattle, WA 98105, USA
* Corresponding author. Pediatric Plastic Surgery, Seattle Children's Hospital, 4800 Sand Point Way Northeast, M/S W-7847, Seattle, WA 98105.
E-mail address: raymond.tse@seattlechildrens.org

Hand Clin 28 (2012) 529–540
http://dx.doi.org/10.1016/j.hcl.2012.08.006
0749-0712/12/$ – see front matter © 2012 Elsevier Inc. All rights reserved.

Table 1
Properties of the ideal nerve glue

	Biologic	Mechanical	Technical
Safety	No disease transmission No antigenic potential Nontoxic	Maintains tensile strength over time	No external energy sources for activation
Effectiveness and efficacy	Facilitates axon regeneration across coaptation Induces minimal or no inflammation or fibrosis	Facilitates fascicular alignment Maintains normal nerve architecture	Readily available Easy to use Reduces surgical time Versatile for different nerve repair scenarios

enough to be used in different clinical scenarios including primary nerve repair; nerve transfer (with single or multiple nerve elements); and nerve grafting (with single or multiple nerve elements).

DEVELOPMENT OF NERVE GLUE

Efforts to adhere nerves without suture date back to the 1940s when fibrin and clots were used for nerve coaptation.[2,3] Rapid absorption and low tensile strength produced disappointing results and efforts were not revived until the 1970s. Matras and coworkers[4,5] used a higher concentration of fibrinogen, factor XIII, calcium hydrochloride, and bovine thrombin to yield a longer lasting adhesive. Animal model studies demonstrated results similar to suture repair thereby prompting experimentation and development of nerve glues during the next several decades. Studies have examined various fibrin adhesives, platelet-rich plasma, cyanoacrylate, and laser solder welding. Because of ease of use, availability, and favorable results, fibrin sealants have been clinically used as nerve glue. The most recent candidate to be used as nerve glue is polyethylene glycol (PEG) hydrogel.

The different nerve glues are reviewed and evidence for or against their use is discussed with respect to the model used (animal, cadaver, or human) and the outcomes measured (biomechanics, histology, electrophysiology, and function). When interpreting results of animal and cadaver studies, it is important to recognize that clinical outcomes may not directly correlate. Currently, there are no commercially available products approved for use as nerve glue and any use is considered off-label.

FIBRIN GLUE

Fibrin is an end product of the coagulation cascade and building block of the hemostatic plug. The intrinsic and extrinsic coagulation pathways activate thrombin, which in turn cleaves fibrinogen to the fibrin monomers that polymerize to form a matrix. Factor XIII is also activated by thrombin and acts to covalently cross-link fibrin to form a stable clot.

The common components of fibrin sealants include fibrinogen, thrombin, and calcium chloride. Higher concentrations of fibrinogen increase strength, whereas higher concentrations of thrombin increase the rate of fibrinogen conversion. The addition of an antifibrinolytic can increase duration and addition of factor XIII may improve strength. Protein components can be human, bovine, or a combination and the antifibrinolytic agent is bovine or synthetic. When interpreting the results of studies using fibrin glue for nerve repair the formulation of the fibrin needs to be considered because the results may vary with different formulations.

Autologous fibrin glue has been produced by centrifuge and precipitation of fibrinogen from blood. When thrombin has been added to preparations, it is often from a bovine source because thrombin is not easily isolated. Production of truly autologous fibrin glue is limited by the need to add other components and the concentration of fibrinogen that can be made available is limited by the volume of plasma collected.

Generally, higher concentrations of fibrinogen are produced with commercially available fibrin sealants. **Table 2** summarizes the available products. Common to all of these products are concentrated fibrinogen and thrombin from a pooled human source that is treated with heat, detergent or solvent, and filtration to reduce the risks of disease transmission. The main distinguishing features are the antifibrinolytic agent or process. Tisseel (marketed as Tissucol in Europe) (Baxter, Westlake Village, CA) uses aprotinin that was previously of a bovine source but is now synthetic. Beriplast (CSL Behring, Kansas City, MO)

Table 2
Commercially available fibrin sealant preparations

	Human Fibrinogen (mg/mL)	Human Thrombin (U/mL)	Human Factor XIII (U/mL)	Antifibrinolytic Agent or Process	Shelf-Life After Thawing or Reconstitution
Tisseel Kit	15–115	500	N/A	Aprotinin (bovine) 3000 KU/mL	4 h
Tisseel Duo	70–110	500	None	Aprotinin (synthetic) 3000 KU/mL	36 h
Quixil	40–60	900–1100	N/A	Tranexamic acid (synthetic) 100 mg/mL	Immediate use but can be stored at 2°C–8°C for 30 d
Evicel	55–85	800–1200	9 U/mL	Plasminogen removed by chromatographic technique	24 h
Beriplast	90	500	60 U/mL	Aprotinin (bovine) 1000 KU/mL	8–24 h

Based on product guides and product reviews.

Data from Tredree R, Beierlein W, Debrix I, et al. Evaluating the differences between fibrin sealants: recommendations from an international advisory panel of hospital pharmacists. European Journal of Hospital Pharmacy Science 2006;12(1):3–9; and Dhillon S. Fibrin sealant (evicel [quixil/crosseal]): a review of its use as supportive treatment for haemostasis in surgery. Drugs 2011;71(14):1893–915.

continues to use bovine aprotinin. Quixil or Crosseal (Ethicon, Somerville, NJ) uses tranexamic acid, a synthetic competitive inhibitor of plasminogen, as a stabilizing agent. Tranexamic acid has potential central nervous system neurotoxicity when used in direct contact with cerebrospinal fluid or dura. The newer version of Quixil/Crosseal is called Evicel (Ethicon, Somerville, NJ). Rather than adding an antifibrinolytic, plasminogen is removed by a chromatographic technique thereby eliminating the tranexamic acid from their formulation. Most products are supplied as two frozen components that are thawed before application. Beriplast and Tisseel Kit are supplied in a powder form that is reconstituted with liquid solutions. Although the frozen (Tisseel Duo) and powder (Tisseel Kit) forms of Tisseel should be the same, differences in component concentrations[6] and strength have been noted. Povlsen[7] suggests that Tisseel Kit has a lower tensile strength as demonstrated by its 20% nerve repair dehiscence rate compared with 0% for Tisseel Duo.

Safety of Fibrin Glue for Nerve Repair

Autologous fibrin glue reduces the risk of disease transmission if bovine or pooled human thrombin is not used; however, tensile strength tends to be inadequate for consistent results. Commercially available fibrin glue from pooled human plasma undergoes multiple steps to eliminate potential pathogens. Although disease transmission is still possible the authors are not aware of any reported cases. Anaphylaxis to the bovine component of some fibrin glues has been reported; however, human thrombin has replaced bovine thrombin in most preparations and synthetic antifibrinolytics have replaced bovine aprotinin in other preparations.

Application of nerve glue inevitably places some of the glue between nerve ends. Nonetheless, fibrin glue is nontoxic and does not block axon regeneration.[8,9] In a rabbit sciatic nerve model, a 4-mm block of fibrin was interposed between nerve ends.[9] Eight weeks later normal axons were found distal to the interposed block with approximately 70% of the axon density. In a more recent study, a 10-mm segmental gap in a rat sciatic nerve model was bridged using either a nerve conduit or a nerve conduit filled with fibrin glue.[8] The nerve conduit filled with fibrin glue outperformed the nerve conduit alone on functional, electrophysiologic, and histologic outcomes. Not only does this study demonstrate that fibrin glue does not block reinnervation, it also suggests that the fibrin matrix may improve reinnervation.

Efficacy of Fibrin Glue Compared with Suture

Although the clinical use of fibrin glue for nerve repair has been well described,[10–19] there are few clinical studies that focus on the outcomes of using fibrin glue. A systematic review of fibrin glue for peripheral nerve repair revealed 14 animal studies, 1 cadaver study, and 1 human study that fit the study criteria.[20] Although some of the reported results were conflicting, most found fibrin glue repair to be equal or superior to suture repair. An appreciation of the different formulations, sources, and methods of applications may explain some of the conflicting results.

Fibrin Glue Versus Suture: Animal and Cadaver Studies

Variable results have been reported with autologous fibrin glue. Cruz and coworkers[21] reported dehiscence of 80% in addition to perineural fibrosis and inflammation when autologous fibrin glue was used without thrombin. In a study by Sames and coworkers,[22] bovine thrombin was used to ensure greater strength; however, dehiscence occurred in 20%. The fibrinogen concentration in these two studies is unclear and may have been inadequate. In a study by Feldman and coworkers,[23] the autologous fibrin glue was carefully prepared to mimic the fibrinogen concentration, adhesive strength, and degradation of commercially available fibrin glue. After the nerve repair, greater muscle bulk was found with glue repair compared with suture repair. Although there was axonal disorganization around each suture, there was maintenance of axon alignment and no evidence of inflammation with fibrin glue. Results with autologous fibrin glue rely on the specific preparation used.

Commercially available fibrin sealants are relatively consistent in terms of their concentration of fibrinogen and thrombin. Numerous studies have since reported equal[7,24–27] or better[28–34] results with fibrin glue versus suture repair. These results are based on histology,[7,29,32,33,35,36] electrophysiology,[26,28,31–33] and function.[26,28,32,34] Generally, less fibrosis and inflammation, better axonal alignment, and more axons across the repair site was seen with fibrin glue repairs. Suture granuloma, inflammation, fibrosis, and axonal disorganization were associated with suture repairs. Despite abundant reports of positive results with fibrin glue, several studies have reported suture repair to be superior.[37–41] Although none of these studies reported any difference in functional outcomes, the implications of each deserve careful consideration.

Boedts[41] used a model in which a segment of nerve was excised and the repair was performed under tension. In contrast, most models involve simply dividing and then repairing a nerve. Fibrin glue has limited strength and the inferior results suggest that fibrin sealants should not be used in the case of segmental nerve loss or significant tension. Farrag and coworkers[40] reported a model where fibrin glue was only applied between the cut ends of nerve. In contrast, most reports describe application of glue as a cuff along a length of the nerve repair. Inferior results with fibrin glue in this study may be related to the limited application of adhesive to the cut surfaces of nerve. Moy and coworkers[37] and Maragh and coworkers[39] reported inferior histology and electrophysiology but similar function in their models that compare fibrin glue to suture. Both studies were reported before 1990. All studies where fibrin was better were reported after 2000. It is possible that slight changes in fibrin sealant preparations during the three decades accounts for these differences. In addition, antigen response to bovine components may lead to inflammation and fibrosis. Most fibrin preparations have now reduced or eliminated bovine components. Junior and coworkers[38] found no difference in electrophysiology but slower and less axon regeneration with fibrin glue. No obvious reason for the negative result is apparent.

Although the balance of evidence suggests an advantage of fibrin glue over suture repair, concern about the lack of adequate tensile strength persists. A biomechanical study of rabbit sciatic nerve repair reported inferior load to failure and load to gapping with fibrin glue only relative to suture repair immediately after repair.[42] Similar inferior load to failure results have been found in a rat sciatic nerve model immediately and 7 days after repair. However, fibrin glue repair has been found to be equal in strength to suture repair after 14 and 28 days.[43] Maragh and coworkers[39] also found tensile strength at 2, 4, and 8 weeks after surgery to be the same for fibrin glue compared with suture repair. The results of these studies imply that if a nerve repair can be protected from tension for 2 weeks, the risk of disruption of the nerve repair is the same with fibrin glue and suture repair.

Suture Versus Suture Augmented with Fibrin Glue: Animal and Cadaver Studies

Given the low tensile strength during the first 2 weeks after nerve repair, a combined approach of suture repair with fibrin glue augmentation has gained popularity. One strategy is to add fibrin glue to a standard suture repair, whereas another strategy is to reduce the number of stitches used by augmenting the repair with fibrin glue. Farrag and coworkers[40] compared the same suture repair without and with fibrin glue in a rat facial nerve model. With the same number of stitches applied there was no advantage with fibrin glue (histology, electrophysiology, and function). Martins and coworkers[32] examined the other strategy and compared suture repair with four stitches against suture repair with one stitch plus fibrin glue. Although there were no differences in histology or function, nerve conduction velocities were better in the one stitch plus fibrin glue group. Menovsky and Beek[35] also reports advantages of fewer sutures and augmentation with fibrin glue. In a rat sciatic nerve model, suture repair with four to six stitches was compared with repair with two stitches plus fibrin glue. Although no difference was demonstrated in function there was less scarring and better axonal alignment in the group with fewer stitches. Taken together, augmenting suture repair with fibrin glue seems to offer no advantage but using fibrin glue to reduce the number of stitches may ultimately lead to better outcomes.

Isaacs and coworkers[44] recently reported a biomechanical study that compared suture repair with suture repair augmented with fibrin glue in a fresh-frozen cadaver model. All groups underwent repair with two stitches. The addition of fibrin glue improved resistance to gapping but did not change load to failure.

Fibrin Glue Versus Sutures: Human Studies

There are few clinical studies that directly compare fibrin glue with sutures for nerve repair. Egloff and Narakas[19] reported a large series of peripheral nerve reconstructions that used fibrin glue. Fifty-six cases were reported spanning free functional muscle transfer, brachial plexus reconstruction, major peripheral nerve reconstruction, and digital nerve reconstruction. The nerve glue was formed as a cylinder around the repair site rather than being applied between opposed nerve surfaces. Multiple cable graft reconstruction of the brachial plexus involved proximal stump coaptation with fibrin glue only and distal target coaptation with a combination of fibrin glue and suture. The multiple cable grafts were bundled together with fibrin glue and then sutured to the distal targets. For primary repair of major peripheral nerves, fibrin glue was used to augment suture repair and for secondary repair with nerve grafts, fibrin glue was used alone. No primary digital nerve repairs were reported but secondary digital repair with nerve graft used fibrin glue alone. The heterogeneity of clinical scenarios makes comparison with reported results of suture repair difficult; however, the results seem to compare favorably.

Narakas[45] followed his initial report with a comparison of suture repair and fibrin glue repair in major peripheral nerves. Most cases involved nerve grafts but some direct repairs were also performed. Heterogeneity of clinical scenarios precluded rigorous statistical analysis, but results of fibrin glue repair compared favorably.

CYANOACRYLATES

Cyanoacrylates (esters of cyanoacrylic acid) are synthetic, resorbable adhesives that harden by polymerization on contact with weak basic substances. Cyanoacrylates have sparked much interest as tissue adhesives because of their mechanical strength and fast cure rates.[46] However, cyanoacrylate polymers yield formaldehyde and cyanoacetate as by-products of hydrolysis, which are toxic to surrounding tissues. Significant inflammation and fibrosis have led to poor results when short-chain acrylates have been used for vessel anastomoses or nerve coaptations.[47–49] Although formaldehyde production can be reduced with longer-chain derivatives,[50–52] the tensile strength is generally weaker.[53] Thus far, the use of cyanoacrylates as nerve glue has been limited to animal experimentation.

Early animal studies with octyl-2-cyanoacrylate (Dermabond; Ethicon, Inc, Somerville, NJ) demonstrated adverse tissue reactions[54,55] in addition to obliteration of electrical activity when butyl cyanoacrylate (Histoacryl; B. Braun, Melsungen, Germany) is injected directly into a nerve gap.[56] If cyanoacrylate seeps into the nerve coaptation site, the adhesive can incite a significant tissue reaction, and the foreign body response tends to push the glue fragments inward rather than outward, preventing axonal regeneration.[49] Although butyl cyanoacrylate (Glubran; GEM, S.r.l. Viareggio, Italy) has been shown to decrease nerve diameter significantly,[47] a study by Choi[57] demonstrated that butyl cyanoacrylate provided minimal tissue reactivity without inhibiting axonal regeneration compared with sutures. Piñeros-Fernandez[46] reported improvements in motor recovery and axonal regeneration with octyl-2-cyanoacrylate (Dermabond) versus sutures. Landegren and coworkers[58] also found that ethyl-cyanoacrylate (Evobond; Tong Shen Enterprise Co., Ltd., Lin-Yuan, Taiwan) provided comparable results to sutures in terms of tensile strength, nerve histology, and functional recovery. However, the authors also note that application of ethylcyanoacrylate was time-consuming and induced an increased inflammatory response.[59]

Cyanoacrylates vary considerably in tissue toxicity and mechanical properties. For example, the breaking strength of octyl-2-cyanoacrylate is reported to be three times that of butyl cyanoacrylate and comparable with the breaking strength of

5–0 nylon sutures for skin closure.[60] Balanced against the great tensile strength are robust inflammation and fibrosis and the fact that cyanoacrylates can be a barrier to axonal regeneration if interposed between nerve ends. Future formulations of cyanoacrylates may strike a better balance between toxicity, biocompatibility, and mechanical strength but at this time cyanoacrylates are not good candidates for clinical use as nerve glue.

LASER WELDING

Fischer and coworkers[61] reported successful nerve coaptation by laser welding in 1985; however, this was followed by reports of frequent dehiscence of 12% to 41%.[62–64] To prevent dehiscence, one or two stay sutures can be placed before laser welding[61,65,66]; however, nylon stay sutures lose their tensile strength when irradiated with a CO_2 laser.[67] More recently, protein solders have been melted onto the outer surface of the nerve coaptation site to create stronger constructs.[68,69] The protein solder hardens immediately when it absorbs the energy of the laser, creating a sleeve over the nerve that is mechanically stronger than a simple edge-to-edge coaptation. The solder may also bridge small gaps in the coaptation, thereby reducing the need for stay sutures. In addition, the solder may protect the underlying nerve tissue from any potential damaging thermal effects of the laser-welding process.[35]

Numerous animal studies have evaluated the efficacy of laser-welded nerve coaptations. Studies by Hwang and coworkers[70,71] and Menovsky and Beek[35] demonstrated similar results for histologic and functional[35] outcomes when comparing laser-welding with suture repair. Studies by Happak and coworkers[72] demonstrated superior results for histologic and functional outcomes when comparing laser-welding with suture repair. Laser-welded nerves seemed to heal with less cellular response and less scar tissue than sutured nerves.[69] In addition, axon alignment, intraneural scarring, and distal nerve segment regeneration were more favorable in soldered nerves. The use of solder with CO_2 laser produces better histologic results than CO_2 laser alone.

Although CO_2 laser-welded nerve adhesion has demonstrated favorable results in animal models, its clinical use can be cumbersome and its versatility is limited. The safety of laser-welded nerve adhesion requires further study and no benefit over other methods of nerve coaptation has been proved. It is difficult to justify the use of laser coaptation when other simpler and more versatile nerve glue is available.

POLYETHYLENE GLYCOL

PEG has great potential for use as nerve glue. It has previously been used in attempts at axon fusion and has more recently been studied for its application as a nerve adhesive. Early experimentation with PEG aimed to fuse severed axons to maintain their electrophysiologic function immediately after repair.[73] This strategy differs from more common strategies aimed at optimizing nerve regeneration. Preliminary studies have been promising[74] and a recent study reported that compound action potentials could be recorded distal to a 10-mm nerve graft repair up to 7 days after surgery.[75] The mechanism of this phenomenon and its implications require further investigation.

Application of PEG as nerve glue has primarily involved DuraSeal (Confluent Surgical, Inc, Waltham, MA), a commercially available product that was developed to help seal dura in neurosurgical procedures. DuraSeal consists of a PEG ester solution and a trilysine amine solution. When mixed together these solutions form a strongly adherent hydrogel sealant that naturally absorbs within 4 to 8 weeks and is cleared by the kidneys.[76] The two precursors are applied using a double syringe holder that mixes them within the applicator to form a firm, rubbery, gellike substance.

PEG hydrogel demonstrates adhesive power without being neurotoxic.[77,78] In a rat sciatic nerve model, Lin and coworkers[79] created a 5-mm nerve defect as a model of nerve coaptation under tension and repaired the nerve with 10–0 nylon epineural sutures, fibrin glue, or PEG hydrogel. Nerve continuity and myelination achieved by PEG hydrogel approached that of suture repair at 1 and 8 weeks. Similarly, motor function and electrophysiologic parameters were comparable between PEG hydrogel and sutures. The placement of PEG hydrogel over the coaptation site did not induce an appreciable elevation in inflammation or escalation of Schwann cell apoptosis over the injured area. Interestingly, nerve gapping occurred in the nerves repaired with fibrin glue but not in the suture or PEG hydrogel groups, making PEG hydrogel potentially superior to fibrin glue in areas of increased tension, such as the hand and upper extremity. To directly compare the biomechanical performance of several available nerve glues, Isaacs and colleagues[44] transected and repaired 57 fresh-frozen cadaveric nerve specimens with two 8–0 nylon epineural sutures. The nerve repairs were subsequently augmented with autologous fibrin glue, Tisseel fibrin glue, Evicel fibrin glue, DuraSeal, or no glue. Resistance to gapping was greater for the Tisseel, Evicel, and DuraSeal groups compared with the group with no glue; however, there were no significant differences in stiffness among any of the nerve glues. Further study by Isaacs and coworkers[80] compared suture repair of sciatic nerves augmented with either fibrin or PEG hydrogel. Although there was no difference in force of muscular contraction and nerve diameter, the PEG hydrogel was associated with reduced scar thickness.

PEG may be superior to fibrin glue because of its greater tensile strength and long duration before breakdown (4 weeks). Mixture of DuraSeal does not generate any appreciable heat and the hydrogel sets up in approximately 2 seconds. PEG is nontoxic and biocompatible and does not induce a significant inflammatory response. What may be an additional advantage is that it may have adhesion-inhibiting properties that prevent perineural scarring.[81,82] PEG hydrogel is a promising candidate as nerve glue; however, further study is necessary. Specifically, the effect of PEG interposition between nerve ends on axon regeneration needs to be examined. Just as with fibrin glue,[8,9] PEG needs to be shown to not act as a barrier to axon regeneration.

DISCUSSION

Nerve repair by suture requires manipulation and placement of stitches that persist as foreign bodies and can potentially distort axonal alignment. Different patterns of scarring and inflammation have been observed with absorbable and nonabsorbable sutures[83–85] and increased scarring has been shown to impede regeneration at peripheral nerve repair sites.[86] Although a dose-response to sutures has not been demonstrated, Martins and coworkers[87] found that a six-stitch repair results in more scarring and unfavorable electrophysiologic outcomes compared with a three-stitch repair. In addition, traumatic nerve manipulation for suture repair and differences in surgical skill can result in nerve trauma, scarring, and fascicular malalignment.[88] Any alternative to the current standard of suture repair of nerves must be shown to be equal or better in use and outcome.

Nerve glue is an attractive alternative to suture repair because it allows better maintenance of nerve architecture, better fascicular alignment, and reduced tissue trauma. Nerve glue is easy and rapid to use, requires less tissue handling than suture repair, and eliminates the foreign body reaction associated with sutures. The ability to manipulate and align nerve elements makes it versatile for various clinical situations and ideal for targeted reinnervation. Nerve glue is indispensible in the setting of brachial plexus reconstruction where grafts are insert into from nerve roots at or within the bony vertebral foramen.

Whitlock and coworkers[88] nicely demonstrated the advantages of glue in a mouse sciatic nerve graft repair model. Fibrin glue was compared with suture repair by both naive and experienced surgeons. Overall, fibrin glue was associated with shorter surgical time and more myelinated fibers across the repair. In the hands of the naive surgeons, the results of suture repair were inferior to those of experienced surgeons, whereas the results of fibrin glue repair were similar to those of experienced surgeons. They conclude that glue mitigates the learning curve of microsurgical repair.

Despite the advantages of fibrin glue, surgeons must be cautious with the use of fibrin glue in the clinical setting. Given the low tensile strength, its use alone should be limited to nerve graft or nerve transfer reconstruction when there is no tension on the nerve ends. Fibrin glue may be used to augment suture repair in a variety of situations; however, the surgeon must be aware that fibrin glue only reduces load to gap and not load to failure. Adequate size and number of sutures must be used if there is any tension on the nerve repair.

The longest and greatest experience with nerve glue is in brachial plexus reconstruction. In this setting, fibrin glue has been indispensible. Narakas reported significantly reduced operative times[19,45] and the ability to perform nerve repairs in areas where it was previously not possible. Nerve glue allows repairs to be performed at or immediately within the bony foramen of a proximal nerve root where quality suture repair is not possible (**Fig. 1**A, B). The ability to trim nerves to healthier proximal stumps improves the quality of axons for reinnervation. Other advantages relate to the ability to tailor multiple cable graft reconstruction. Cables can be placed on the face of a proximal nerve root according to known topography and trajectory (see **Fig. 1**C–E). The cable graft reconstruction can also be adjusted according to the findings of the explorations (ie, multiple root avulsions or varying quality of the proximal nerve root stumps). Fine adjustments of the epineurium can also be made to accommodate for slight mismatches of nerve diameter or for mismatches in the nerve stumps and available nerve graft (see **Fig. 1**F, G).

Technical details using fibrin glue for brachial plexus application can be applied to other situations

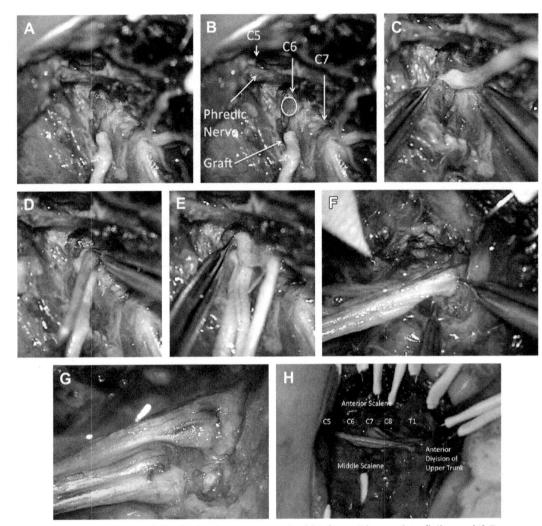

Fig. 1. Nerve grafting for birth brachial palsy in a 4-month-old infant with complete flail arm. (*A*) Exposure of cervical roots after excision of upper trunk neuroma, middle trunk rupture, C8 rupture, and T1 avulsion. (*B*) Grafts have been secured to the deeper proximal C7 stump while the C6 stump is exposed to receive cable grafts. The phrenic nerve obscures exposure of the C5 root. (*C–E*) The epineurium is manipulated to facilitate the best match and the cables are glued along the normal trajectory of the brachial plexus. Each cable is accurately secured from deep to superficial. (*F, G*) Cable grafts are secured to their distal targets while manipulating the epineurium to accommodate for size mismatch. (*H*) The final reconstruction illustrating the importance of sequencing from deep to superficial and the benefits of nerve glue.

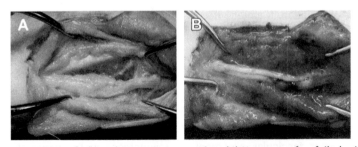

Fig. 2. Secondary reconstruction of a low ulnar nerve transection. (*A*) Neuroma after failed primary repair. (*B*) The neuroma has been excised and multiple sural nerve cable grafts have been interposed. The wrist was positioned in full extension and the grafts were trimmed to include some redundancy. Repair was performed with fibrin glue. There was no tension on any repair site with wrist and elbow range of motion.

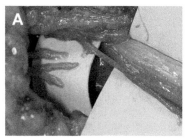
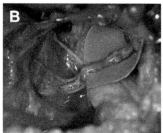

Fig. 3. Nerve transfers for isolated deficits of elbow extension and elbow flexion. (*A*) Isolated lack of elbow extension in a 9-year-old boy caused by traumatic brachial plexus palsy with C7 avulsion. The third, fourth, and fifth intercostals were harvested and tunneled across the axilla for coaptation to the radial nerve branch to the long head of the triceps. Neurolysis of the radial nerve branch proximally allows tension-free end-to-end nerve repair. (*B*) Reconstruction of elbow flexion in an infant with total brachial plexus palsy and previous nerve graft reconstruction of the brachial plexus. The third, fourth, and fifth intercostals have been glued in an end-to-end fashion to the musculocutaneous nerve.

and are worthy of mention. Before reconstruction the patient should be positioned so that nerves are on maximal stretch. The length of each cable graft should incorporate some redundancy to ensure there is no tension on the repair (**Fig. 2**). Likewise, in the case of a nerve transfer, donor and recipient nerves should be adequately mobilized so that there is no tension and, ideally, some redundancy (**Fig. 3**). Progress is greatly facilitated by working from deep to superficial and from proximal to distal. Meticulous hemostasis with cautery or topical vasoconstrictors makes application of the fibrin glue much easier. Nerve surfaces need to be wiped dry of excess fluids to ensure optimal adherence. After nerve repair, the fibrin should be left to polymerize and cross-link for several minutes before irrigation. Finally, the upper extremity should be brought through a range of motion to verify that there is no tension on any of the repairs. After reconstruction, patients are immobilized for 3 to 4 weeks to ensure an ideal environment for axon regeneration.

Fibrin sealants have a proven track record as safe and effective nerve glue. Cyanoacrylates may be toxic and laser coaptation is cumbersome. PEG demonstrates the greatest promise as a future alternative. It is synthetic, strong, and durable and it may outperform fibrin glue.

SUMMARY

The outcome of upper extremity reconstruction depends on functional nerve recovery. Nerve glue is an attractive alternative to suture repair of nerves for upper extremity reconstruction. Fibrin sealants have made an impact on the quality of nerve reconstruction with nerve grafts and nerve transfers. However, the currently available nerve glues are inadequate in strength for primary nerve repair and only play a role in augmenting suture repair. With ongoing development

and testing of biomaterials the need for better nerve glue may one day be fulfilled.

REFERENCES

1. Bunnell S. Plastic problems in the hand. Plast Reconstr Surg 1946;1(3):265–70.
2. Young J, Homes W, Sanders F. Fibrin suture of peripheral nerves: measurement of the rate of regeneration. Lancet 1940;236(6101):128–30.
3. Seddon HJ, Medawar PB. Fibrin suture of human nerves. Lancet 1942;240(6204):87–90.
4. Matras H, Dinges HP, Mamoli B, et al. Non-sutured nerve transplantation (a report on animal experiments). J Maxillofac Surg 1973;1(1):37–40.
5. Matras H, Braun F, Lassmann H, et al. Plasma clot welding of nerves (experimental report). J Maxillofac Surg 1973;1(4):236–47.
6. Tredree R, Beierlein W, Debrix I, et al. Evaluating the differences between fibrin sealants: recommendations from an international advisory panel of hospital pharmacists. Eur J Hosp Pharm 2006;12(1):3–9.
7. Povlsen B. A new fibrin seal in primary repair of peripheral nerves. J Hand Surg Br 1994;19(1): 43–7.
8. Rafijah G, Dolores C, Bowen, A. Fibrin glue augmentation of nerve repair does not impede neurological recovery in an animal model. [abstract MHS Outstanding Paper]. In: Program Book for American Association for Hand Surgery Annual meeting Las Vegas: 2012. p. 153. 2012
9. Palazzi S, Vila-Torres J, Lorenzo JC. Fibrin glue is a sealant and not a nerve barrier. J Reconstr Microsurg 1995;11(2):135–9.
10. Kozin SH. Nerve transfers in brachial plexus birth palsies: indications, techniques, and outcomes. Hand Clin 2008;24(4):363–76, v.
11. Borrero JL. Surgical technique. In: Gilbert A, editor. Brachial plexus injuries. London: Martin Dunitz Ltd. 2001. p. 189–204.

12. Hentz VR. Adult and obstetrical brachial plexus injuries. In: Slutsky DJ, Hentz VR, editors. Peripheral nerve surgery. 1st edition. Philadelphia: Churchill Livingstone Elsevier; 2006. p. 299–317.

13. Stevanonvic M, Sharpe FE. Nerve transfer for restoration of elbow flexion: the modified Oberlin procedure. In: Slutsky DJ, editor. Upper extremity nerve repair - tips and techniques: a master skills publication. Rosemont (IL): American Society for Surgery of the Hand; 2008. p. 193–204.

14. Borschel GH, Clarke HM. Obstetrical brachial plexus palsy. Plast Reconstr Surg 2009;124(Suppl): 144e–55e.

15. Malessy MJ, van Duinen SG, Feirabend HK, et al. Correlation between histopathological findings in C-5 and C-6 nerve stumps and motor recovery following nerve grafting for repair of brachial plexus injury. J Neurosurg 1999;91(4):636–44.

16. Bahm J, Ocampo-Pavez C, Noaman H. Microsurgical technique in obstetric brachial plexus repair: a personal experience in 200 cases over 10 years. J Brachial Plex Peripher Nerve Inj 2007;2:1.

17. Liverneaux PA, Diaz LC, Beaulieu JY, et al. Preliminary results of double nerve transfer to restore elbow flexion in upper type brachial plexus palsies. Plast Reconstr Surg 2006;117(3):915–9.

18. Gilbert A, Pivato G, Kheiralla T. Long-term results of primary repair of brachial plexus lesions in children. Microsurgery 2006;26(4):334–42.

19. Egloff DV, Narakas A. Nerve anastomoses with human fibrin. Preliminary clinical report (56 cases). Ann Chir Main 1983;2(2):101–15.

20. Sameem M, Wood TJ, Bain JR. A systematic review on the use of fibrin glue for peripheral nerve repair. Plast Reconstr Surg 2011;127(6):2381–90.

21. Cruz NI, Debs N, Fiol RE. Evaluation of fibrin glue in rat sciatic nerve repairs. Plast Reconstr Surg 1986; 78(3):369–73.

22. Sames M, Blahos J, Rokyta R, et al. Comparison of microsurgical suture with fibrin glue connection of the sciatic nerve in rabbits. Physiol Res 1997; 46(4):303–6.

23. Feldman MD, Sataloff RT, Epstein G, et al. Autologous fibrin tissue adhesive for peripheral nerve anastomosis. Arch Otolaryngol Head Neck Surg 1987;113(9):963–7.

24. Smahel J, Meyer VE, Bachem U. Glueing of peripheral nerves with fibrin: experimental studies. J Reconstr Microsurg 1987;3(3):211–20.

25. Becker CM, Gueuning CO, Graff GL. Sutures or fibrin glue for divided rat nerves: Schwann cell and muscle metabolism. Microsurgery 1985;6(1):1–10.

26. Povlsen B. A new fibrin seal: functional evaluation of sensory regeneration following primary repair of peripheral nerves. J Hand Surg Br 1994;19(2):250–4.

27. Hadlock T. Research in facial paralysis. [Invited lecture]. In: Program book for American Society for Peripheral Nerve Annual meeting Las Vegas: 2012. p. 68

28. Ornelas L, Padilla L, Di Silvio M, et al. Fibrin glue: an alternative technique for nerve coaptation. Part I. Wave amplitude, conduction velocity, and plantar-length factors. J Reconstr Microsurg 2006;22(2): 119–22.

29. Ornelas L, Padilla L, Di Silvio M, et al. Fibrin glue: an alternative technique for nerve coaptation. Part II. Nerve regeneration and histomorphometric assessment. J Reconstr Microsurg 2006;22(2):123–8.

30. Suri S. Design features and simple methods of incorporating nasal stents in presurgical nasoalveolar molding appliances. J Craniofac Surg 2009; 20(Suppl 2):1889–94.

31. Martins RS, Siqueira MG, Silva CF, et al. Electrophysiologic assessment of regeneration in rat sciatic nerve repair using suture, fibrin glue or a combination of both techniques. Arq Neuropsiquiatr 2005; 63(3A):601–4.

32. Martins R, Siqueira M, Dasilva C, et al. Overall assessment of regeneration in peripheral nerve lesion repair using fibrin glue, suture, or a combination of the 2 techniques in a rat model. Which is the ideal choice? Surg Neurol 2005;64:S10–6.

33. Inalöz SS, Ak HE, Vayla V, et al. Comparison of microsuturing to the use of tissue adhesives in anastomosing sciatic nerve cuts in rats. Neurosurg Rev 1997;20(4):250–8.

34. Faldini A, Puntoni P, Magherini PC, et al. Comparative neurophysiological assessments of nerve sutures performed by microsurgical methods and with fibrin glue: experimental study. Ital J Orthop Traumatol 1984;10(4):527–32.

35. Menovsky T, Beek JF. Laser, fibrin glue, or suture repair of peripheral nerves: a comparative functional, histological, and morphometric study in the rat sciatic nerve. J Neurosurg 2001;95(4):694–9.

36. Suri A, Mehta VS, Sarkar C. Microneural anastomosis with fibrin glue: an experimental study. Neurol India 2002;50(1):23–6.

37. Moy OJ, Peimer CA, Koniuch MP, et al. Fibrin seal adhesive versus nonabsorbable microsuture in peripheral nerve repair. J Hand Surg 1988;13(2):273–8.

38. Junior E, Valmasedacastellon E, Gayescoda C. Facial nerve repair with epineural suture and anastomosis using fibrin adhesive: an experimental study in the rabbit. J Oral Maxillofac Surg 2004;62(12):1524–9.

39. Maragh H, Meyer BS, Davenport D, et al. Morphofunctional evaluation of fibrin glue versus microsuture nerve repairs. J Reconstr Microsurg 1990;6(4):331–7.

40. Farrag TY, Lehar M, Verhaegen P, et al. Effect of platelet rich plasma and fibrin sealant on facial nerve regeneration in a rat model. Laryngoscope 2007; 117(1):157–65.

41. Boedts D. A comparative experimental study on nerve repair. Arch Otorhinolaryngol 1987;244(1):1–6.

42. Temple CL, Ross DC, Dunning CE, et al. Resistance to disruption and gapping of peripheral nerve repairs: an in vitro biomechanical assessment of techniques. J Reconstr Microsurg 2004;20(8):645–50.

43. Nishimura M, Mazzer N, Barbieri C, et al. Mechanical resistance of peripheral nerve repair with biological glue and with conventional suture at different postoperative times. J Reconstr Microsurg 2008; 24(05):327–32.

44. Isaacs JE, McDaniel CO, Owen JR, et al. Comparative analysis of biomechanical performance of available "nerve glues." J Hand Surg 2008;33(6):893–9.

45. Narakas A. The use of fibrin glue in repair of peripheral nerves. Orthop Clin North Am 1988;19(1):187–99.

46. Piñeros-Fernández A, Rodeheaver PF, Rodeheaver GT. Octyl 2-cyanoacrylate for repair of peripheral nerve. Ann Plast Surg 2005;55(2):188–95.

47. Wieken K, Angioi-Duprez K, Lim A, et al. Nerve anastomosis with glue: comparative histologic study of fibrin and cyanoacrylate glue. J Reconstr Microsurg 2003;19(1):17–20.

48. Lerner R, Binur NS. Current status of surgical adhesives. J Surg Res 1990;48(2):165–81.

49. Hurwitz PJ, Magora A, Gonen B, et al. Microsurgical techniques and the use of tissue adhesive in the repair of peripheral nerves. J Surg Res 1974;17(4): 245–52.

50. Toriumi DM, Raslan WF, Friedman M, et al. Histotoxicity of cyanoacrylate tissue adhesives. A comparative study. Arch Otolaryngol Head Neck Surg 1990; 116(5):546–50.

51. Toriumi DM, Raslan WF, Friedman M, et al. Variable histotoxicity of histoacryl when used in a subcutaneous site: an experimental study. Laryngoscope 1991;101(4 Pt 1):339–43.

52. Ang ES, Tan KC, Tan LH, et al. 2-octylcyanoacrylate-assisted microvascular anastomosis: comparison with a conventional suture technique in rat femoral arteries. J Reconstr Microsurg 2001;17(3):193–201.

53. Vote BJ, Elder MJ. Cyanoacrylate glue for corneal perforations: a description of a surgical technique and a review of the literature. Clin Experiment Ophthalmol 2000;28(6):437–42.

54. Braun RM. Comparative studies of neurorrhaphy and sutureless peripheral nerve repair. Surg Gynecol Obstet 1966;122(1):15–8.

55. Ferlic D, Goldner J. Evaluation of the effect of methyl-2-cyanoacrylate on peripheral nerves. Southern Medical Journal 1965;58:679–85.

56. Włodarczyk J. Effects of tissue glues on electrical activity in isolated nerve. Polim Med 1991;21(3–4): 37–41.

57. Choi B. Microneural anastomosis using cyanoacrylate adhesives. Int J Oral Maxillofac Surg 2004; 33(8):777–80.

58. Landegren T, Risling M, Brage A, et al. Long-term results of peripheral nerve repair: a comparison of nerve anastomosis with ethyl-cyanoacrylate and epineural sutures. Scand J Plast Reconstr Surg Hand Surg 2006;40(2):65–72.

59. Landegren T, Risling M, Persson JKE. Local tissue reactions after nerve repair with ethyl-cyanoacrylate compared with epineural sutures. Scand J Plast Reconstr Surg Hand Surg 2007;41(5):217–27.

60. Penoff J. Skin closures using cyanoacrylate tissue adhesives. Plastic Surgery Educational Foundation DATA Committee. Device and Technique Assessment. Plast Reconstr Surg 1999;103(2):730–1.

61. Fischer DW, Beggs JL, Kenshalo DL, et al. Comparative study of microepineurial anastomoses with the use of CO_2 laser and suture techniques in rat sciatic nerves: part 1. Surgical technique, nerve action potentials, and morphological studies. Neurosurgery 1985;17(2):300–8.

62. Maragh H, Hawn RS, Gould JD, et al. Is laser nerve repair comparable to microsuture coaptation? J Reconstr Microsurg 1988;4(3):189–95.

63. Huang TC, Blanks RH, Berns MW, et al. Laser vs. suture nerve anastomosis. Otolaryngol Head Neck Surg 1992;107(1):14–20.

64. Ochi M, Osedo M, Ikuta Y. Superior nerve anastomosis using a low-output CO_2 laser on fibrin membrane. Lasers Surg Med 1995;17(1):64–73.

65. Bailes JE, Cozzens JW, Hudson AR, et al. Laser-assisted nerve repair in primates. J Neurosurg 1989; 71(2):266–72.

66. Beggs JL, Fischer DW, Shetter AG. Comparative study of rat sciatic nerve microepineurial anastomoses made with carbon dioxide laser and suture techniques. Part 2. A morphometric analysis of myelinated nerve fibers. Neurosurgery 1986;18(3):266–9.

67. Menovsky T, Beek JF, van Gemert MJ. Effect of the CO_2 milliwatt laser on tensile strength of microsutures. Lasers Surg Med 1997;20(1):64–8.

68. Menovsky T, Beek JF, van Gemert MJ. CO_2 laser nerve welding: optimal laser parameters and the use of solders in vitro. Microsurgery 1994;15(1):44–51.

69. Menovsky T, Beek JF. Carbon dioxide laser-assisted nerve repair: effect of solder and suture material on nerve regeneration in rat sciatic nerve. Microsurgery 2003;23(2):109–16.

70. Hwang K, Kim SG, Kim DJ. Facial-hypoglossal nerve anastomosis using laser nerve welding. J Craniofac Surg 2006;17(4):687–91.

71. Hwang K, Kim SG, Kim DJ. Hypoglossal-facial nerve anastomosis in the rabbits using laser welding. Ann Plast Surg 2008;61(4):452–6.

72. Happak W, Neumayer C, Holak G, et al. Morphometric and functional results after CO(2) laser welding of nerve coaptations. Lasers Surg Med 2000; 27(1):66–72.

73. Krause TL, Bittner GD. Rapid morphological fusion of severed myelinated axons by polyethylene glycol. Proc Natl Acad Sci U S A 1990;87(4):1471–5.

74. Donaldson J, Shi R, Borgens R. Polyethylene glycol rapidly restores physiological functions in damaged sciatic nerves of guinea pigs. Neurosurgery 2002; 50(1):147–56 [discussion: 156–7].

75. Sexton KW, Del Corral GA, Britt JM, et al. Hydrophillic polymers allow immediate physiologic function of severed nerves after interposition grafting. [Scientific Paper Session 5]. In: Program book for American Society for Peripheral Nerve Annual meeting. Las Vegas: 2012. p. 177.

76. Boogaarts JD, Grotenhuis JA, Bartels RH, et al. Use of a novel absorbable hydrogel for augmentation of dural repair: results of a preliminary clinical study. Neurosurgery 2005;57(Suppl 1):146–51 [discussion: 146–51].

77. Glickman M, Gheissari A, Money S, et al. A polymeric sealant inhibits anastomotic suture hole bleeding more rapidly than gelfoam/thrombin: results of a randomized controlled trial. Arch Surg 2002;137(3):326–31 [discussion: 332].

78. Leng LZ, Brown S, Anand VK, et al. "Gasket-seal" watertight closure in minimal-access endoscopic cranial base surgery. Neurosurgery 2008;62(5 Suppl 2):ONSE342–3 [discussion: ONSE343].

79. Lin KL, Yang DY, Chu IM, et al. DuraSeal as a ligature in the anastomosis of rat sciatic nerve gap injury. J Surg Res 2010;161(1):101–10.

80. Isaacs J, Klumb I, McDaniel C. Preliminary investigation of a polyethylene glycol hydrogel "nerve glue." J Brachial Plex Peripher Nerve Inj 2009;4(1):16.

81. Ferland R, Mulani D, Campbell PK. Evaluation of a sprayable polyethylene glycol adhesion barrier in a porcine efficacy model. Hum Reprod 2001; 16(12):2718–23.

82. Preul MC, Bichard WD, Spetzler RF. Toward optimal tissue sealants for neurosurgery: use of a novel hydrogel sealant in a canine durotomy repair model. Neurosurgery 2003;53(5):1189–98 [discussion: 1198–9].

83. Cham RB, Peimer CA, Howard CS, et al. Absorbable versus nonabsorbable suture for microneurorrhaphy. J Hand Surg 1984;9(3):434–40.

84. Lee S, de Macedo AR, Hweidi SA, et al. Efficacy of polyglycolic acid (Dexon) microsutures in peripheral nerve anastomoses in the rat: 2. Perineural suture. Microsurgery 1984;5(3):123–6.

85. Lee S, deMacedo AR, Chan E, et al. Efficacy of polyglycolic acid (Dexon) microsutures in peripheral nerve anastomoses in the rat: 1. Epineural suture. Microsurgery 1983;4(2):120–3.

86. Atkins S, Smith KG, Loescher AR, et al. Scarring impedes regeneration at sites of peripheral nerve repair. Neuroreport 2006;17(12):1245–9.

87. Martins RS, Teodoro WR, Simplício H, et al. Influence of suture on peripheral nerve regeneration and collagen production at the site of neurorrhaphy: an experimental study. Neurosurgery 2011;68(3):765–72.

88. Whitlock EL, Kasukurthi R, Yan Y, et al. Fibrin glue mitigates the learning curve of microneurosurgical repair. Microsurgery 2010;30(3):218–22.

Advanced Imaging and Arthroscopic Management of Shoulder Contracture After Birth Palsy

Scott H. Kozin, MD[a,b,*], Dan A. Zlotolow, MD[a,c]

KEYWORDS

- Imaging • Arthroscopic management • Shoulder contracture • Birth palsy

KEY POINTS

- Persistent nerve injury frequently results in muscle imbalance about the shoulder.
- Shoulder internal rotations contracture leads to glenohumeral joint dysplasia.
- Arthroscopic capsular release rebalances the joint and promotes glenohumeral joint remodeling.

INTRODUCTION

The incidence of brachial plexus birth palsy has changed little over the past few decades. Shoulder dystocia caused by fetal-pelvic disproportion remains the primary cause of birth injury to the brachial plexus. Due to inherent errors in prenatal ultrasonography, fetal size is difficult to predict near term. Gauging the changes in pelvic anatomy during pregnancy also has considerable error given the current inability to accurately predict hormonal relaxation of the maternal pelvis.[1] This combination makes the prediction of shoulder dystocia problematic. Babies may be becoming bigger as the prevalence of maternal obesity and diabetes mellitus rises.[2] Uncontrolled diabetes leads to changes in a baby's size and proportion, resulting in heavier birth weights and wider shoulder diameters. This combination is a recipe for shoulder dystocia, which leads to subsequent brachial plexus birth palsy in 25% of cases.

The most common pattern of brachial plexus birth palsy is an isolated injury to C5 and C6 (upper trunk). With shoulder dystocia during the birthing process, the upper trunk is stretched beyond its physiologic limits. This strain directly correlates with reduction of intraneural blood flow; for example, a 15% elongation of the nerve reduces blood flow by 80% to 100%[3–5] The extrinsic neural vascular system (longitudinal vessels in the epineurium) seems more susceptible to stretch compared with the intrinsic neural circulation (endoneurial vascular network).[4] Continued elongation leads to overt ischemia and interruption of nerve metabolism. Persistent traction eventually disrupts nerve continuity. Therefore, nerve traction can cause a spectrum of nerve injury beginning with a temporary disruption in nerve fiber conduction (neuropraxia) to more severe injury, resulting in discontinuity of the nerve sheath and axons (axonotmesis and neurotmesis).

Neuropraxic injuries demonstrate considerable recovery within the first 2 months as the segmental demyelination reverses. Because there is maintenance of nerve fiber and axonal sheath continuity, these injuries favor full recovery.[6] Axonotmesis

[a] Department of Orthopaedic Surgery, Temple University, Philadelphia, PA, USA; [b] Shriners Hospitals for Children, 3401 North Broad Street, Philadelphia, PA 19140, USA; [c] Upper Extremity Center of Excellence, Shriners Hospitals for Children, Philadelphia, PA, USA
* Corresponding author.
E-mail address: skozin@shrinenet.org

Hand Clin 28 (2012) 541–550
http://dx.doi.org/10.1016/j.hcl.2012.08.004
0749-0712/12/$ – see front matter © 2012 Published by Elsevier Inc.

injuries begin to show recovery between 3 and 6 months. Axonotmesis consists of disruption of nerve fiber integrity with preservation of the epineurial sheath and structure. Distal to the site of injury, wallerian degeneration occurs and extends to the motor endplate. The cell bodies (motor and sensory) switch from a mainly signaling role to one that promotes nerve cell growth.[7–9] Axonal sprouts emerge from the first node of Ranvier proximal to the injury with many axon collaterals (5–20) entering the distal nerve stump.[7] Incorrect collaterals are pruned and the majority of motor neurons project their axons to muscle.[8] Axonal regeneration from the proximal stump into inappropriate distal pathways is a contributing factor to poor functional recovery. Axonal regeneration occurs slowly at a rate of 1 mm to 3 mm per day. Neurotmesis injuries fail to show signs of recovery, which implies complete disruption of the nerve fiber and axonal sheath. The prognosis is bleak without microsurgical reconstruction. The standard procedure consists of resection of the intervening neuroma and nerve reconstruction using interposition grafts.

THE SHOULDER

The shoulder is prone to posterior subluxation after brachial plexus birth palsy, especially after an axonotmesis to the upper trunk. The human shoulder has an innate propensity for internal rotation, which is exacerbated by upper trunk injury and subsequent axonal regeneration. The shoulder's predilection for internal rotation remains a perplexing question with uncertain evolutionary importance. The quantity and strength of the muscles that internally rotate the shoulder (subscapularis, pectoralis major, lattisimus dorsi, and teres major muscles) far outweigh the number and power of the muscles that externally rotate the shoulder (infraspinatus and teres minor muscles).

After an axonotmetric injury to C5·C6 (upper trunk), the shoulder is disposed to further imbalance. Immediately after the injury, the muscles that internally rotate the shoulder maintain part of their innervation, including the sternocostal portion of the pectoralis major (C7, C8, and T1), lower portion of the subscapularis (C7), latissimus dorsi (C7), and teres major (C7). In contrast, the muscles that externally rotate the shoulder are completely denervated, including the infraspinatus (C5 and C6) and the teres minor (C5 and C6). As nerve regeneration progresses from proximal to distal, the more proximal internal rotators are reinnervated before the more distal external rotators. Axonal dropout becomes more pronounced as

nerve regeneration travels the additional distance necessary for reinnervation of the infraspinatus and teres minor, which can lead to incomplete recovery or even a complete lack of reinnervation.[8] If the regenerating nerve does not reach its target muscle within 18 to 24 months, motor endplate degradation and muscle fibrosis occur.

After birth, the normal glenoid is in approximately 10° of retroversion. Over the first decade of life, the glenoid remodels toward neutral version (simply stated as −10 to 0 by 10 years of age).[10] In the normal shoulder, the transverse axis of the scapular body bisects the humeral head. In neonates with brachial plexus injuries, constant internal rotation of the shoulder applies a disproportionate load to the cartilaginous posterior glenoid and anterior humeral head. The cartilage responds according to the Heuter-Volkmann law with decreased growth of the posterior glenoid and deformation of the humeral head.[11] The glenoid becomes retroverted, the head becomes ovoid, and the humeral head subluxates posteriorly.

In a screening study of infants with brachial plexus birth palsy, the mean age at which posterior humeral head subluxation was first detected was 6 months, with a range from 3 to 10 months.[12] In a separate prospective study, most children younger than 5 months of age had a normal-appearing glenoid (5 of 7 shoulders), whereas in children between 5 and 12 months of age, a significant minority had normal-appearing shoulders (only 2 of 10 shoulders were normal).[13] Both studies support the idea that the deformity occurs early and often, highlighting the need for early screening to diagnose and prevent glenohumeral dysplasia.

The proximal humeral epiphysis begins to ossify between birth and 4 months of age but can be delayed in children with brachial plexus birth palsy.[14] Glenohumeral dysplasia can occur as early as 3 months; because the proximal humerus remains largely cartilage, plain radiographs are ineffective as a screening tool. Earlier studies using traditional radiographs, therefore, likely underestimated the prevalence of glenohumeral joint dysplasia.[15]

ULTRASOUND

Ultrasound can be performed via a variety of views and angles.[16] The posterior portal is the most useful in infants with brachial plexus birth palsy (**Fig. 1**). A high-frequency linear transducer with the ability to capture images is placed behind the glenohumeral joint just inferior to the scapular spine. If the humeral head is subluxated posteriorly, it is prominent and easy to visualize (**Fig. 2**). The head is primarily hypoechoic cartilage with

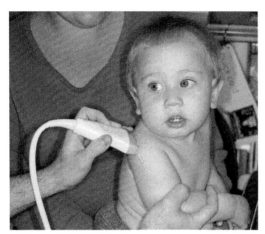

Fig. 1. The posterior portal is the most useful in infants with brachial plexus birth palsy. (*Courtesy of* Shriners Hospital for Children, Philadelphia.)

specular echoes (ossification centers) within the cartilage. The glenoid can be seen at the junction between the posterior aspect of the bony scapular body and the humeral head, and is itself cartilage. The glenoid version can be estimated by the angle of the subchondral bone medial to the glenoid physis against the scapular body. Humeral head subluxation can be estimated using 2 ultrasound measurements.[17] The SGH or α-angle is the angle formed by the intersection of a line along the posterior scapular margin and a line tangent to the humeral head passing through the posterior osseous lip of the glenoid (**Fig. 3**). The percentage of the humeral head posterior to the axis of the posterior scapular margin dictates the amount of

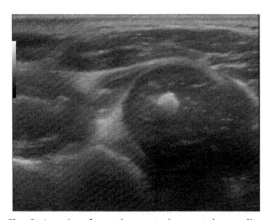

Fig. 2. Imaging from the posterior portal revealing a normal shoulder with the hypoechoic cartilage surrounding the ossification centers that is located within anterior to the axis of the posterior scapular margin within the glenoid. (*Courtesy of* Shriners Hospital for Children, Philadelphia.)

posterior displacement of the humeral head. This is calculated by measuring the distance from the posterior scapular line to the posterior margin (numerator) divided by the greatest diameter of the humeral head (denominator), expressed as a percentage (**Fig. 4**). The ultrasound measurement of humeral head position has been found reliable with reference to intraobserver and interobserver variability but has not been evaluated for validity.[17]

The benefits of ultrasound include the absence of ionizing radiation, lack of need for sedation, decreased cost compared with MRI, and ability to perform a dynamic examination. Because ultrasound is a real-time examination, it provides some assessment of whether the posteriorly subluxated humeral head is reducible (**Fig. 5**). The disadvantage of ultrasound is the decreased ability to visualize glenoid version and deformity.[17,18]

MRI

MRI is performed with a child sedated and monitored by electrocardiography, oxygen-saturation measurements, and observation by several medical staff. MRI of the affected shoulder is obtained using cartilage-sensitive axial images with a minimal interslice gap.[11] The authors prefer 3-D axial gradient-echo and axial T2 images (2.5-mm section thickness with 0 spacing) along with fast spin-echo T1-weighted and T2-weighted images with fat saturation (3-mm section thickness with 0 spacing) in the axial plane. The exact sequence, however, may vary according to the institution.

MRI allows complete evaluation of the pediatric cartilaginous glenohumeral joint.[19] Any deformities of the humeral head and glenoid are clearly visualized and can be graded. The disadvantages of MRI compared with ultrasound include the cost, the need for sedation, and the inability to obtain dynamic images.

CLASSIFICATION

Glenohumeral joint deformity has been classified from grades 1 through 5 and likely represents a continuum of deformation over time from mild to severe (**Table 1**).[19] A simpler method is to describe the glenoid (concave, flat with retroversion, biconcave, and a false glenoid) and to quantify the amount of posterior humeral head subluxation.[20]

The current standard for evaluation of the glenohumeral joint is based on an axial cross-sectional image on a cartilage sensitive MRI sequence. To improve the reproducibility and decrease the variability in glenoid deformity classification, the axial image chosen should be inferior to the coracoid

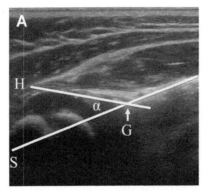
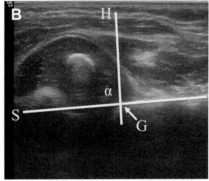

Fig. 3. The SGH or α-angle from the posterior portal. (*A*) The SGH or α-angle of normal shoulder with humeral head within glenoid. (*B*) The SGH or α-angle of dysplastic shoulder with humeral head far posterior to the scapular margin. (*Courtesy of* Shriners Hospital for Children, Philadelphia.)

apophysis and spinoglenoid notch, preferably visualizing the subscapularis tendon and the tip of the coracoid.[11] Using this image, the glenoscapular angle (the degrees of version) and the percentage of humeral head anterior to the middle of the glenoid fossa (PHHA) can be measured (**Fig. 6**).[19,21,22]

The glenohumeral joint parameters are determined as follows. A line is drawn along the labral surfaces of the glenoid between the anterior and posterior lips. A bisecting line is drawn from the medial margin of the scapula to the middle of the glenoid fossa. The posterior medial quadrant angle is calculated by subtracting 90° from the angle measured to determine the glenoid version (see **Fig. 6**). A negative value means that the glenoid is retroverted, whereas a positive value indicates anteversion.[19,21] When the humeral head no longer articulates with the true glenoid due to posterior dislocation, it comes to rest on a concavity formed on the posterior scapular body, termed a *pseudoglenoid* (see **Fig. 6**B).[19,20] The angle of retroversion

is determined by measuring the slope of the posterior concavity. The PHHA is calculated by measuring the amount of humeral head anterior to the axis of the scapula (numerator) divided by the anteroposterior diameter of the humeral head (denominator) expressed as a percentage (see **Fig. 6**A). A lower value for PHHA indicates that less of the humeral head is anterior to the axis of the scapula and therefore implies greater posterior humeral head subluxation.

Another measure of internal rotation is the biceps angle, which is the angle between the biceps tendon and a line perpendicular to the axis of the scapula. Progressive shoulder internal rotation is associated with a more acute biceps angle.[23]

ADDITIONAL IMAGING TECHNIQUES

Arthrography allows visualization and categorization of the glenohumeral joint.[20] Arthrography is an invasive study that can be performed at the time of

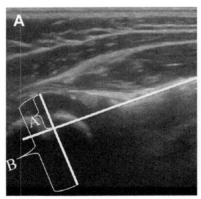
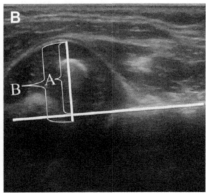

Fig. 4. Humeral head subluxation measured as the percentage of the humeral head posterior to the axis of the posterior scapular margin (A/B × 100). (*A*) Normal shoulder with the percentage of the humeral head posterior to the axis of the posterior scapular margin. (*B*) Dysplastic shoulder with substantial humeral head subluxation. (*Courtesy of* Shriners Hospital for Children, Philadelphia.)

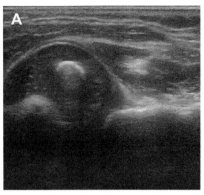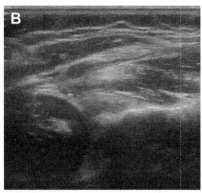

Fig. 5. Real-time assessment using ultrasound to assess reducibility of humeral head subluxation. (*A*) Internal rotation with profound humeral head subluxation. (*B*) External rotation with marked improvement in humeral head position relative to the axis of the posterior scapular margin. (*Courtesy of* Shriners Hospital for Children, Philadelphia.)

surgery but has largely been supplanted by MRI. CT provides the best assessment of the bony deformity but fails to visualize the cartilaginous structures of the infant. In addition, sedation is required and a high dose of radiation is administered.[18]

DIAGNOSIS

The diagnosis of glenoid dysplasia and posterior shoulder subluxation is primarily a clinical one. The sine qua non is loss of passive external rotation of the glenohumeral joint.[11] External rotation must be assessed with the arm placed in adduction and the scapula stabilized. The elbow is flexed to

Table 1 Classification of glenohumeral joint deformity	
Type or Grade	**Glenohumeral Joint**
I	Normal glenoid (<5° retroversion compared with contralateral normal)
II	Minimal deformity (<5° retroversion compared with contralateral normal)
III	Moderate deformity (posterior humeral head subluxation)
IV	Severe deformity (posterior humeral head subluxation with false glenoid)
V	Severe flattening of humeral head ± complete dislocation
VI	Infantile glenohumeral dislocation
VII	Proximal humeral growth arrest

Adapted from Waters PM, Smith GR, Jaramillo D. Glenohumeral deformity secondary to brachial plexus birth palsy. J Bone Joint Surg Am 1998;80:668–77.

90° to tighten the medial collateral ligament. The forearm is rotated to endpoint with firm stabilization of the scapula to prevent scapulothoracic motion. External rotation less then neutral is practically pathognomonic of glenohumeral joint dysplasia (**Fig. 7**).[11,24] Additional clinical findings include asymmetry of skin folds about the axilla or within the proximal arm, apparent shortening of the arm (humeral segment), a palpable humeral head in the posterior shoulder, and a palpable and/or audible click during shoulder manipulation.[12] In the authors' practice, ultrasound serves as an excellent tool for confirming and quantifying clinical findings. MRI remains the authors' modality of choice for visualizing glenohumeral morphology, in particular glenoid version and shape.

EARLY MANAGEMENT OF SHOULDER CONTRACTURE
Prevention

Botulinum toxin type A (Botox) blocks the release of acetylcholine at the presynaptic neuromuscular junction, which temporarily weakens the injected muscle.[24] When used in the appropriate dosage and carefully injected, Botox has a high safety profile. A maximum total dose of 10 U/kg is given. Although use in brachial plexus birth palsy is off-label and should be discussed with parents beforehand, the efficacy of Botox in the treatment of posterior shoulder subluxation in neonatal brachial plexus palsy has been well established.[24]

Botox injection is indicated in patients who present with an internal rotation contracture of the shoulder with a posteriorly subluxated but reducible humeral head. Ultrasound examination is essential to confirm that the joint is reducible. If the joint cannot be reduced, even under general anesthesia, an open or arthroscopic reduction

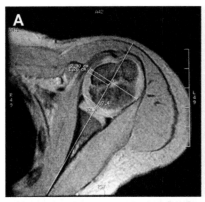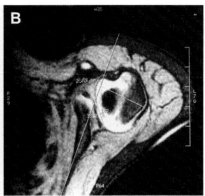

Fig. 6. Cartilage-sensitive MRI sequence of pediatric shoulders. (*A*) MRI of normal shoulder. The glenoscapular angle (version) is −7.5° and PHHA is 43%. (*B*) MRI of dyplastic shoulder. The humeral head articulates with a posterior articular concavity that is markedly retroverted (51°) and the humeral head scarcely crosses the midportion of the glenoid (PHHAS = .21 cm/2.7 cm or 7.7%). (*Courtesy of* Shriners Hospital for Children, Philadelphia.)

should be performed, and concomitant tendon transfers may be necessary.

Technique for Botox Injection

Botox injection is performed under general anesthesia in the operating room. Typically a child is

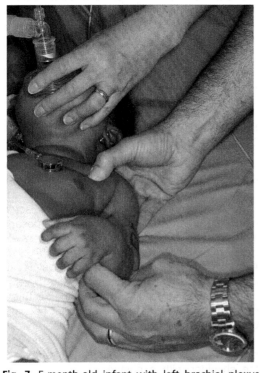

Fig. 7. 5-month-old infant with left brachial plexus palsy and tightening of her shoulder external rotation assessed with the arm placed in adduction and the scapula stabilized. (*Courtesy of* Shriners Hospital for Children, Philadelphia.)

mask ventilated by the anesthesia team with adjunctive intravenous medication, and a definitive airway is not required. The patient is then placed in a lateral decibitus position with the affected side up. The ultrasound is then performed with one examiner and one assistant. The examiner stabilizes the scapula with one hand while the other hand holds the ultrasound transducer against the posterior shoulder; the posterior approach visualizes the humeral head and its relationship to the posterior surface of the scapula. The degree of posterior humeral head subluxation is assessed before shoulder manipulation. Retroversion or pseudoglenoid formation can be inferred from a flat and posterior sloping glenoid.

After obtaining the static images, the authors proceed to the dynamic portion of the examination. Again, the examiner stabilizes the scapula with one hand while the other hand holds the ultrasound transducer against the posterior shoulder; the assistant then externally rotates the arm while the shoulder is held in adduction and the elbow is flexed to 90°. A slow steady force may be necessary to accomplish the closed reduction. On successful reduction, the head of the humerus typically disappears from view. If the shoulder is reducible, the child is placed supine for the Botox injections (**Fig. 8**). The Botox is prepared by diluting it with preservative-free saline. An insulated needle connected to an electrical stimulation unit is inserted into the target muscle. Placement within the correct muscle is verified by stimulation before injection. The pectoralis major, subscapularis, and teres major/latissiumus dorsi complex are injected with 3 equal aliquots of the diluted toxin. After injection, the child is placed into a shoulder spica cast with the shoulder positioned in adduction and

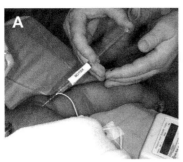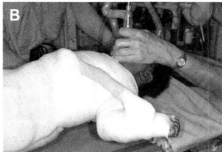

Fig. 8. 5-month-old infant with left brachial plexus palsy depicted in **Fig. 7** treated with closed reduction and Botox injections. (*A*) Botox injection into pectoralis major. (*B*) Shoulder spica casting. (*Courtesy of* Shriners Hospital for Children, Philadelphia.)

external rotation. The cast is removed at three weeks and therapy is re-instituted.

DELAYED MANAGEMENT OF SHOULDER CONTRACTURE

A fixed deformity requires surgical joint reduction to realign the humeral head onto the glenoid. Extra-articular tendon transfers improve range of motion and helps stabilize the joint after reduction but fails to realign the joint.[25,26]

Technique of Arthroscopic Glenohumeral Reduction

Arthroscopic reduction is performed in the operating room under general anesthesia. The child is placed in a lateral decubitus position with the affected side up, and the body is stabilized with a beanbag and all pressure points are padded. Dynamic ultrasound imaging is used to confirm that the shoulder is not reducible. Under sterile conditions, a spinal needle is inserted into the posterior soft spot and the joint is filled with saline. The posterior portal is established after making a small stab incision. A 2.7-mm arthroscope is inserted and the anterior capsule is visualized. The anterior portal is made under direct visualization using an 18-gauge spinal needle just inferior to the biceps tendon. An electrocautery wand is introduced through the anterior portal. The cautery is used to release the thickened superior glenohumeral ligament, the middle glenohumeral ligament, and the tendinous upper one-half to two-thirds (rolled border) of the subscapularis. The tendinous portion of the subscapularis transitions into a more muscular portion as the release continues in an inferior direction. The muscle of the subscapularis is left intact while the capsule is divided past the axillary pouch. The inferior capsule is released with an arthroscopic punch to avoid thermal damage to the axillary nerve. After

release, the arthroscopic equipment is removed from the joint and the glenohumeral joint is manipulated into external rotation, with the shoulder in adduction and the elbow in 90° of flexion. Marked improvement in external rotation is usually noted with accompanying joint reduction. Inability to reduce the joint or passive external rotation less than 45° requires additional arthroscopic release of the capsule and/or subscapularis.

In children undergoing concomitant tendon transfers, the posterior portal is extended into a posterior axillary incision. The latissimus dorsi and teres major tendons are released from the humerus with a periosteal sleeve. The tendons are then transferred superficial to the long head of the triceps to the superior-posterior rotator cuff and secured via transosseous sutures placed through the humeral head. The authors recommend against the use of newer braided nonabsorbable sutures, such as FiberWire (Arthrex, Inc.), because these have a tendency to saw through the cartilage of the humeral head.

After wound closure and application of a sterile dressing, a shoulder spica cast with the glenohumeral joint positioned in 45° to 60° of external rotation is applied. The amount of abduction varies according to whether or not concomitant tendon transfers were performed. The arm is positioned in 30° to 40° of abduction after isolated release and 100° to 120° of abduction after release combined with tendon transfer. Spica casting is maintained for 3 weeks after isolated release and then the child is free to move without restrictions. After tendon transfer, the child is maintained in the shoulder spica cast for 4 to 5 weeks and then is transitioned to a brace for an additional 4 weeks except during therapy.

OUTCOMES
Botulinum Toxin

There are few reports of using Botox in the treatment of posterior shoulder subluxation in neonatal brachial plexus palsy. Ezaki and colleagues[24] reported the efficacy of this technique in 35 infants. The average age at time of injection was approximately 6 months. Six patients required a second injection. At an average follow-up of slightly greater than 3 years, shoulder reduction was maintained in 24, or 69%, of the infants. There were no complications related to the injection of botulinum toxin.

Price and colleagues[27] use Botox as an adjunct to the surgical treatment of the internal rotation deformity of the shoulder in birth injuries of the brachial plexus. In a retrospective review, they found better results in the cohort of children (n = 13) who underwent surgery and Botox injection compared with surgery alone (n = 13). The investigators suggest the benefits of Botox may be both at the surgical site and at the sensorimotor cortex related to cortical plasticity.

Arthroscopic Joint Reduction

Pearl and colleagues[28,29] initially described an arthroscopic technique for contracture release in children with brachial plexus birth palsy. Forty-one children underwent arthroscopic release of the anterior capsule and subscapularis tendon. The mean age of the children at the time of surgery was 3.5 years. Eighteen children were treated with arthroscopic release only and 23 children underwent concomitant latissimus dorsi transfer. Restoration of passive external rotation was achieved in 40 of the 41 children. The only patient who did not attain external rotation was 12 years of age and had advanced glenoid deformity. The status of the glenohumeral joint was not evaluated after surgery.

Pearl[28] subsequently reported on the first 33 children followed for a minimum of 2 years. Nineteen children (mean age of 1.5 years) underwent arthroscopic contracture release only and 14 children (mean age of 6.7 years) also underwent simultaneous latissimus dorsi transfer. Prior to surgery, passive external rotation averaged −2° for the children who underwent isolated arthroscopic contracture release and −24° for those children treated with release and transfer. The internal rotation contracture recurred in 4 children who had undergone an isolated release. Repeat arthroscopic release and concomitant latissimus dorsi transfer were performed on these patients. No child who underwent combined release and transfer required additional shoulder surgery. At follow-up, the mean passive external rotation was increased by 67° in the 15 children with a successful arthroscopic release only and 81° in those treated with release and transfer. Internal

rotation was noted to have decreased substantially after surgery. MRI performed before surgery displayed a pseudoglenoid deformity in 18 of the children. At 2 years, MRI in 12 of 15 of those children showed marked remodeling.

The authors' initial arthroscopic series consisted of 20 children (average age 46 months) who underwent preoperative MRI, arthroscopic surgery, and postoperative imaging in their spica cast.[6] Preoperative mean PHHA was 16.9% and the mean glenoid version was −39°. After surgery, the postoperative mean PHHA corrected to 41.4% and the mean glenoid version improved to −12°. Based on these results, the authors determined that arthroscopic capsular release and subscapularis tenotomy successfully reduced the glenohumeral joint subluxation in all patients.

The authors then followed 44 patients who underwent arthroscopic release only or arthroscopic release combined with tendon transfer.[30,31] Twenty-eight children underwent isolated release and 16 children underwent release and transfer of the latissimus dorsi and teres major tendons. MRI and clinical measurements were obtained at 1 year and 3 years postoperatively.[31] Data analysis showed that retroversion improved from −34° before surgery to −19° at 1 year and −14° at 3 years (P<.001). Similarly, PHHA improved from 19% before surgery to 33% at 1 year and was maintained at 36% at 3 years. Passive external rotation improved from −26° before surgery to 48° at 1 year and was sustained at 49° at 3 years. Likewise active abduction improved from 112° preoperatively to 130° at 1 year and 132° at 3 years (P<.01). Individual Mallet score components were significantly improved (P<.001) for external rotation, hand to neck, and hand to mouth when comparing preoperative scores to those at 1 and 3 years. No change was noted in Mallet abduction or hand to spine. All improvements were maintained between 1 and 3 years but no significant improvement was noted over this time. Most importantly, superior outcomes were associated with younger age and less severe deformity, consistent with the principle that prompt recognition and timely intervention result in improved joint alignment and ultimately better shoulder motion.

SUMMARY

Modern imaging techniques applied to the pediatric glenohumeral joint have advanced understanding of the anatomic changes that occur secondary to muscular imbalance after brachial plexus birth palsy. A better understanding of the progression and timing of glenohumeral dysplasia has also increased awareness and vigilance of this problem. Early detection of glenohumeral joint subluxation is now possible, allowing for prompt treatment with closed, arthroscopic, or open joint reduction with and without tendon transfers. Dynamic ultrasound imaging, Botox, and arthroscopic techniques have expanded treatment options, providing minimally invasive methods to successfully manage glenohumeral joint dysplasia.

REFERENCES

1. Nahum GG, Stanislaw H. Ultrasonographic prediction of term birth weight: how accurate is it? Am J Obstet Gynecol 2003;188:566–74.
2. Ludwig DS, Janet Currie J. The association between pregnancy weight gain and birthweight: a within-family comparison. Lancet 2010;376:984–90.
3. Clark WL, Trumble TE, Swiontkowski MF, et al. Nerve tension and blood flow in a rat model of immediate and delayed repairs. J Hand Surg Am 1992;17:677–87.
4. Kitamura T, Takagi K, Yamaga M, et al. Brachial plexus stretching injuries: microcirculation of the brachial plexus. J Shoulder Elbow Surg 1995;4:118–23.
5. Lundborg G, Rydevik B. Effects of stretching the tibial nerve of the rabbit. A preliminary study of the intraneural circulation and the barrier function of the perineurium. J Bone Joint Surg Br 1973;55:390–401.
6. Pedowitz DI, Gibson B, Williams GR, et al. Arthroscopic treatment of posterior glenohumeral joint subluxation. J Shoulder Elbow Surg 2007;16:6–13.
7. Brushart TM, Gerber J, Kessens P, et al. Contributions of pathway and neuron to preferential motor reinnervation. J Neurosci 1998;18:8674–81.
8. Fu SY, Gordon T. Contributing factors to poor functional recovery after delayed nerve repair: prolonged denervation. J Neurosci 1995;15:3886–95.
9. Fu SY, Gordon T. The cellular and molecular basis of peripheral nerve regeneration. Mol Neurobiol 1997;14:67–116.
10. Mintzer GM, Waters PM, Brown DJ. Glenoid version in children. J Pediatr Orthop 1996;6:563–6.
11. Kozin SH. Correlation between external rotation of the glenohumeral joint and deformity after brachial plexus birth palsy. J Pediatr Orthop 2004;24:189–93.
12. Moukoko D, Ezaki M, Wilkes D, et al. Posterior shoulder dislocation in infants with neonatal brachial plexus palsy. J Bone Joint Surg Am 2004;86:787–93.
13. van der Sluijs JA, van Ouwerkerk WJ, de Gast A, et al. Deformities of the shoulder in infants younger than 12 months with an obstetric lesion of the brachial plexus. J Bone Joint Surg Br 2001;83:551–5.
14. Clarke S, Chafetz RS, Kozin SH. Ossification of the proximal humerus in children with residual brachial

plexus birth palsy: a magnetic resonance imaging study. J Pediatr Orthop 2010;30:60–6.
15. Torode I, Donnan L. Posterior dislocation of the humeral head in association with obstetric paralysis. J Pediatr Orthop 1998;18:611–5.
16. Grissom LE, Harcke HT. Infant shoulder sonography: technique, anatomy, and pathology. Pediatr Radiol 2001;31:863–8.
17. Vathana T, Rust S, Mills J, et al. Intraobserver and interobserver reliability of two ultrasound measures of humeral head position in infants with neonatal brachial plexus palsy. J Bone Joint Surg Am 2007;89:1710–5.
18. Zhang S, Ezaki M. Sonography as a preferred diagnostic tool to asses shoulder displacement in brachial plexus palsy. J Diagnostic Medical Sonography 2008;24:339–43.
19. Waters PM, Smith GR, Jaramillo D. Glenohumeral deformity secondary to brachial plexus birth palsy. J Bone Joint Surg Am 1998;80:668–77.
20. Pearl ML, Edgerton BW. Glenoid deformity secondary to brachial plexus birth palsy. J Bone Joint Surg Am 1998;80:659–67.
21. Friedman RJ, Hawthorne KB, Genez BM. The use of computerized tomography in the measurement of glenoid version. J Bone Joint Surg Am 1992;74:1032–7.
22. Randelli M, Gambrioli PL. Glenohumeral osteometry by computed tomography in normal and unstable shoulders. Clin Orthop 1986;208:151–6.
23. Clarke SE, Kozin SH, Chafetz RS. The biceps tendon as a measure of rotational deformity in residual brachial plexus birth palsy. J Pediatr Orthop 2009;29:490–5.
24. Ezaki M, Malungpaishrope K, Harrison RJ, et al. Onabotulinum toxinA injection as an adjunct in the treatment of posterior shoulder subluxation in neonatal brachial plexus palsy. J Bone Joint Surg Am 2010;15(92):2171–7.
25. Kozin SH, Chafetz RS, Shaffer A, et al. Magnetic resonance imaging and clinical findings before and after tendon transfers about the shoulder in children with residual brachial plexus birth palsy: a 3-year follow-up study. J Pediatr Orthop 2010;30:154–60.
26. Waters PM, Bae DS. Effect of tendon transfers and extra-articular soft-tissue balancing on glenohumeral development in brachial plexus birth palsy. J Bone Joint Surg Am 2005;87:320–5.
27. Price AE, Ditaranto P, Yaylali I, et al. Botulinum toxin type A as an adjunct to the surgical treatment of the medial rotation deformity of the shoulder in birth injuries of the brachial plexus. J Bone Joint Surg Br 2007;89:327–9.
28. Pearl ML. Arthroscopic release of shoulder contracture secondary to birth palsy: an early report on findings and surgical technique. Arthroscopy 2003;19:577–82.
29. Pearl ML, Edgerton BW, Kazimiroff PA, et al. Arthroscopic release and latissimus dorsi transfer for shoulder internal rotation contractures and

glenohumeral deformity secondary to brachial plexus birth palsy. J Bone Joint Surg Am 2006;88:564–74.

30. Kozin SH, Boardman MJ, Chafetz RS, et al. Arthroscopic treatment of internal rotation contracture and glenohumeral dysplasia in children with brachial plexus birth palsy. J Shoulder Elbow Surg 2010;19:102–10.

31. Kozin SH, Abzug J, Zlotolow DA, et al. Arthroscopic treatment of internal rotation contracture and glenohumeral dysplasia in children with brachial plexus birth palsy—3 year follow-up. Presented at the Annual American Academy of Orthopaedic Surgeons. San Francisco, February 7-11, 2012.

Advances in the Management of Dupuytren Disease
Collagenase

Vincent R. Hentz, MD[a],*, Andrew J. Watt, MD[b],
Shaunak S. Desai, MD[a], Catherine Curtin, MD[c]

KEYWORDS

- Dupuytren disease • Collagenase • Myofibroblasts • Connective tissue disorder

KEY POINTS

- Dupuytren disease is a benign, generally painless connective tissue disorder affecting the palmar fascia that leads to progressive hand contractures.
- Mediated by myofibroblasts, the disease most commonly begins as a nodule in the palm or finger.
- If the disease progresses, pathologic cords form leading to progressive flexion deformity of the involved fingers, commonly of the metacarpal-phalangeal and proximal interphalangeal joints, but also of the distal interphalangeal joint, and the first web space.

INTRODUCTION

Dupuytren disease (DD) is a benign, generally painless connective tissue disorder affecting the palmar fascia that leads to progressive hand contractures. Mediated by myofibroblasts, the disease most commonly begins as a nodule in the palm or finger. If the disease progresses, pathologic cords form leading to progressive flexion deformity of the involved fingers, commonly of the metacarpophalangeal (MCP) and proximal interphalangeal (PIP) joints, but also of the distal interphalangeal joint, and the first web space. The palmar skin overlying the cords may become excessively calloused and contracted and involved joints may develop periarticular fibrosis. This is particularly true of the PIP joints. Although there is as yet no cure, the sequellae of this affliction can be corrected.

TREATMENT OF DD AND THE OUTCOMES OF TREATMENT

Treatment for DD was first described by Henry Cline[1] in the late seventeenth century and involved sectioning the pathologic cords, later known as fasciotomy or aponeurotomy. Since then surgical intervention traditionally has been the most effective and widely accepted treatment for progressive contracture. Today's surgical options include limited percutaneous needle aponeurectomy, open versus percutaneous fasciotomy, and the more commonly performed open fasciectomy. Until recently, nonsurgical interventions, such as injectable corticosteroids or verapamil, have proved to be largely ineffective for the treatment of contractures and rejected clinically. Collagenase *Clostridium histolyticum* (CCH) was introduced to the literature slightly more than

Drs Hentz and Curtin are Co-Principal Investigator for a postinjection study sponsored by Auxilium Pharmaceuticals.

[a] Robert A. Chase Center for Hand and Upper Limb Surgery, Stanford University, Stanford, CA 94304, USA;
[b] Division of Plastic Surgery, Stanford University, Stanford, CA 94304, USA; [c] Division of Plastic Surgery, Robert A. Chase Center for Hand and Upper Limb Surgery, Stanford University, Stanford, CA 94304, USA
* Corresponding author. 770 Welch Road, Suite 400, Palo Alto, CA 94304.
E-mail address: vrhentz@stanford.edu

Hand Clin 28 (2012) 551–563
http://dx.doi.org/10.1016/j.hcl.2012.08.003
0749-0712/12/$ – see front matter Published by Elsevier Inc.

15 years ago[2] as a potential minimally invasive, nonsurgical option to treat Dupuytren contractures. This has ultimately led to completion of phase 3 clinical trials and its recent US Food and Drug Administration (FDA) approval for clinical use under the marketed name Xiaflex. In Europe, the drug is marketed as Xiapex. The remainder of this article focuses on the role of collagen in DD and the development of a collagen-specific enzymatic treatment for DD contractures and early post-FDA product release results.

THE ROLE OF COLLAGEN IN DD

Luck[3] described the pathogenesis of Dupuytren contracture in pathologic terms consisting of proliferative, involutional, and residual phases. The proliferative phase is characterized by nodule formation within the palmar fascia. Fibroblasts differentiate into myofibroblasts and comprise most of the nodular architecture. Myofibroblasts are fibroblastic in origin; however, they contain actin microfilaments that communicate with the extracellular matrix fibronectin, thereby allowing transmission of intracellular contractile forces to the extracellular tissues.

Marked nodular thickening and early joint contracture characterize the involutional phase. A preponderance of type III collagen is synthesized and the myofibroblasts reorient along the lines of tension within the palm. Type III collagen is a hallmark of the disease because it is not typically observed within the mature palmar fascia of patients unaffected by DD.[4,5]

Myofibroblasts have largely disappeared by the residual phase, resulting in a relatively hypocellular amalgam of type I and type III collagen.[3,6,7] This process results in the conversion of normal palmar and digital fascial structures into fibrotic Dupuytren cords, which are clinically manifested as contractures of the joints of the hand. This evolution in the understanding of the molecular pathogenesis of DD has provided a host of potential nonsurgical therapeutic clinical targets for treatment.

ENZYMATIC FASCIOTOMY

The concept of targeting abnormal collagen was first reported by Bassot[8] in 1965, with his technique of "exerese pharmodynamique," which used a mixture of trypsine, alphachymotrypsin, hyaluronidase, thiomucase, and lignocaine and degraded the proteinaceous component of the pathologic cords, allowing for rupture. Bassot's[9] results in 1969 showed an impressive correction of severe contractures in 34 patients. In 1971, Heuston[10] reported his experience with trypsin,

hyaluronidase, and marcaine, achieving favorable initial results. McCarthy[11] reported his experience with enzymatic fasciotomy in 14 patients, noting recurrence of initial contracture in 75% of patients at an average of 2- to 3-year follow-up. He expressed concern regarding the possibility of tendon rupture and neurovascular injury as a consequence of nonspecific enzymatic degradation of the palmar tissues, although no frank ruptures or neurologic sequelae were reported.

COLLAGENASE *CLOSTRIDIUM HISTOLYTICUM*

CCH, long available and frequently used in laboratory research, emerged as a potential therapeutic option for the treatment of DD in 1996, offering the potential advantage of target specificity. CCH, first discovered in the culture media of *C histolyticum* and reported by Maclennon and coworkers in 1953,[12] is one of several matrix metalloproteinase enzymes responsible for the degradation of extracellular matrix components. CCH, structurally and functionally related to endogenous human collagenase enzymes, is encoded in two distinct genes: *ColG* and *ColH*. Seven distinct enzyme isoforms have been recognized belonging to two separate classes, designated class I (*ColG*) and class II (*ColH*).

Pharmacokinetics

Commercially available CCH consists of a defined mixture of a class I collagenase (termed Aux I by the manufacturer) and class II collagenase (termed Aux II) isoforms that work synergistically on all types of collagen, with the exception of type IV collagen (**Fig. 1**). Type IV collagen is the primary collagen component of basement membranes of neurovascular structures and ex vivo studies have demonstrated preservation of arterioles, nerves, and epithelia after local injection of collagenase.[2,13,14]

There is limited systemic absorption after local injection suggesting the ability of the renal system to concentrate and excrete collagenase. The remainder of the injected collagenase is thought to bind to endogenous serum proteins that are subsequently eliminated by the liver. In vitro studies and in vivo clinical experience suggests that most CCH activity is confined to the region of local tissue infiltration and that its catalytic activity against collagen persists for less than 24 hours.[2]

CLINICAL STUDIES IN DD

Topical application of collagenase has been performed for more than four decades and its use in

A

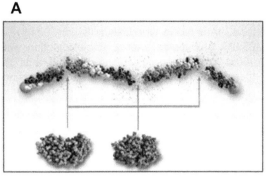

B

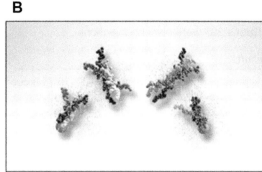

Fig. 1. (*A, B*) Cartoon illustrating the complimentary effects of the two enzyme subtypes that cleave the collagen molecule at different sites thus hastening molecule lysis.

the treatment of chronic ulcers and burns is well tolerated and widely accepted.[15] Since 1982, 13 clinical studies have been conducted on injectable CCH to treat Peyronie disease or DD. Currently, a large body of literature exists regarding the safety, efficacy, and initial long-term outcomes for the treatment of DD with injectable CCH.

The initial phase 1 and 2 studies focused on establishing a safety profile, appropriate dosing, and refining injection techniques. The initial study[16] was conducted as an open-label trial in 35 subjects with DD. Six were ineffectively treated with various lower levels of drug. The remaining subjects received an injection dose of 10,000 units of CCH. A total of 28 (82%) out of 34 MCP joints corrected to normal extension within 2 weeks of injection, whereas 4 (44%) out of 9 PIP joints corrected to normal extension within 2 weeks of injection. Within this patient population there were two treatment failures.

This was followed by a multicenter, double-blind, placebo-controlled phase IIb trial[17] designed to examine dose response, pharmacokinetics, and clinical outcomes. A total of 80 subjects were enrolled and randomized to receive either a placebo or a 2500-, 5000-, or 10,000-unit dose of CCH. A total of 18 out of 23 subjects who received

10,000 units of collagenase achieved normal extension at 1 month compared with 10 of 22 who received 5000 units and 9 out of 18 who received 2500 units. No response to placebo injection was seen in any subject. Hazard function analysis demonstrated a 90% success rate in patients with MCP contractures and 70% in patients with PIP contractures (**Table 1**).

The initial double-blind, placebo-controlled phase III clinical trial involved 33 subjects.[18] A total of 21 out of 23 subjects achieved correction of contracture to within 0 to 5 degrees of full extension with a mean of 1.4 injections. Correction was achieved in 12 (86%) out of 14 primary MCP joints and in 9 (100%) out of 9 PIP joints. No major adverse events were reported. Five subjects were noted to have recurrence after 24-month follow-up.

This initial phase III clinical trial was followed by the largest randomized, double-blind, placebo-controlled study phase III trial, whose results were reported in the *New England Journal of Medicine* in 2009.[19] Sixteen centers enrolled 308 subjects with MCP or PIP contracture of 20 degrees. Success was defined as a reduction of joint contracture to 0 to 5 degrees of full extension within 30 days of the last injection. Up to three injections spaced 1 month apart could be given

Table 1
Summary of phase II clinical trials

Clinical Study Y	Study Design	Patients Enrolled (n)	MCP Contracture (n)	PIP Contracture (n)
Hurst et al,[19] 2000	Open label	35	28/34 (82%)[a]	4/9 (44%)[a]
Hurst et al,[19] 2007	Double-blind, placebo-controlled	80	12/14 (86%)[b]	9/9 (100%)[b]

[a] Clinical success defined as correction to normal extension within 2 weeks of injection, single injection.
[b] Clinical success defined as correction to normal extension within 1 month of final injection, patient received up to three injections.

to treat the target joint. A total of 741 injections were performed, 444 of which were with CCH, whereas 297 were placebo injections.

Results

The primary end point was met in 102 (76.7%) out of 133 patients with MCP joint contractures and in 28 (40%) out of 70 with PIP joint contractures (**Fig. 2**). The percent change in contracture from baseline was 87.1%. Subjects presenting with more severe contractures were significantly less likely to attain the primary end point. Specifically, 88.9% of collagenase-injected MCP joints with a baseline contracture of 50 degrees or less met the primary end point, compared with 57.7% of such joints with a baseline contracture of more than 50 degrees. In total, 80.9% of the collagenase-injected PIP joints with a baseline contracture of 40 degrees or less met the primary end point, compared with 22.4% of such joints with a baseline contracture of less than 40 degrees (**Table 2**).

ADVERSE EVENTS AND IMMUNOLOGIC CONSEQUENCES

Adverse events were documented in 97% of subjects receiving collagenase injection, mostly local reaction to injection including peripheral edema (72.5%); contusion (51%); injection site hemorrhage (37.3%); injection site pain (32.4%); and skin laceration with manipulation (10.8%). Three experienced major adverse events including one subject with complex regional pain syndrome after injection and two subjects who experienced flexor tendon ruptures after collagenase injection. Serum assay for antibodies to type I (Aux I) and type II (Aux II) were positive in 85.8% of patients after a single injection, with 100% of patients exhibiting positive antibody titers after three injections. Despite this immune recognition, no hypersensitivity reactions were reported (**Table 3**).

SUMMARY OF CLINICAL TRIALS TO DATE

All results from published and unpublished phase I, II, and III trials were combined in Auxillium's FDA report.[20] In total, 2630 collagenase injections were performed on 1780 cords in 1082 patients. In all studies, MP joints responded significantly better than PIP joints.

No clinically significant difference in the incidence of adverse outcomes was noted among subgroups (age, weight, gender, diabetes mellitus, location of injection) or in patients receiving multiple sequential objections. Although adverse events were noted in nearly all subjects receiving collagenase injection, the incidence of major adverse outcomes was low. Most of these complications may be categorized as self-limited, periprocedural complications including peripheral edema, ecchymosis, injection site pain, skin tears with manipulation, and adenopathy.

Major treatment-related events included three subjects with flexor tendon ruptures (0.27%) and a single subject who developed complex regional pain syndrome after injection (0.09%). The three flexor tendon ruptures were attributed to CCH injection into the flexor tendon sheath. These

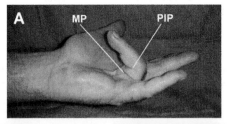

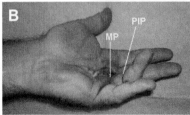
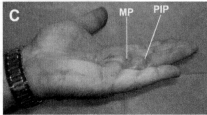

Fig. 2. (*A–C*) Phase III subject who presented with MCP and PP joint contractures. (*A*) Postmanipulation appearance of the digit after the initial injection into the pretendinous cord. (*B*) The MCP joint is now fully extended, whereas the PIP joint remains contracted. (*C*) The finger after the second injection (third total) given to correct the PIP joint contracture. (*Courtesy of* Dr Larry Hurst, Stony Brook, NY.)

Table 2
Summary of phase III clinical trials

Clinical Study Y	Study Design	Patients Enrolled (n)	MCP Contracture	Mean Change in MCP Range of Motion	PIP Contracture (n)	Mean Change in PIP Range of Motion
Hurst et al,[19] 2009; CORD I	Multicenter, double-blind, placebo-controlled	308	102/133 (76.7%)[a]	40.6 degrees	28/70 (40%)[a]	29 degrees
Gilpin et al,[26] 2010; CORD II	Multicenter, double-blind, placebo-controlled	66	13/20 (65%)[a]	42 degrees	7/25 (28%)[a]	32.2 degrees

Abbreviation: CORD, Collagenase Option for Reduction of Dupuytren's.
[a] Clinical success defined as correction of contracture to within 0–5 degrees of full extension within 30 days of last injection, patient received up to three injections.

subjects ultimately required staged flexor tendon reconstruction.

RECURRENCE

DD is characterized by recurrence and disease progression irrespective of the treatment method. Acknowledging that recurrence is inconsistently defined across nearly all published reports, recurrence after palmar fasciectomy ranges from 41% to 54% at 5 years,[21–24] and 15% of these patients require reoperation to address disease recurrence.[22] Disease recurrence rates after percutaneous aponeurotomy have not been definitively established; however, recurrence rates seem to be in the range of 50% to 60%.[25]

Table 3
Incidence of adverse reactions experienced in the phase III trial

Adverse Reaction	All Patients Collagenase (n = 272)
Edema peripheral	75.7%
Contusion	50%
Injection site pain	39%
Injection site hemorrhage	34.9%
Pain in extremity	31.3%
Ecchymosis	23.2%
Tenderness	22.8%
Injection site swelling	21.7%
Lymphadenopathy	15.1%
Pruritus	12.1%

Data regarding the long-term efficacy and durability of CCH injection are scarce. A total of 645 of 950 joints treated in multiple phase III trials[19,26] were currently enrolled in a 5-year study to assess recurrence after successful release of contracture by CCH injection. For this study, recurrence is defined as the presence of a palpable cord associated with an increase of at least 20 degrees of joint contracture compared with baseline. **Table 4** features data from the initial 3 years of the study. The overall recurrence rate at years 1, 2, and 3 was 3%, 20%, and 35%, respectively. **Table 4** also includes a compilation of two studies. The first study by Rijssen are data from a prospective randomized study comparing the incidence of recurrence after needle aponeurotomy or limited fasciectomy, and the Year 3 data regarding collagenase. In Rijssen's groups, recurrence has been defined as an increase of at least 30 degrees of total passive extension deficit, whereas recurrence for collagenase is defined as an increase of at least 30 degrees over the immediate post-treatment joint angle. Although the criteria for the groups is different, these data suggest that the incidence of recurrence for CCH falls closer to that seen after limited fasciectomy and is dissimilar to the rapid recurrence rates published for needle aponeurotomy.

Currently, only a single published study has ventured to quantify the long-term efficacy of collagenase injection.[27] This study followed a subset of the patients enrolled in the phase II dose-response clinical trial at 8 years after initial treatment. Recurrence was stringently defined as any increase in the degree of contracture compared with maximal extension achieved after injection. Recurrence was noted in four (66%) out of six patients treated for MCP contracture

Table 4
Upper data: Incidence of recurrence in successfully treated contractures from phase III trial, at 2 and 3 years posttrial completion. Lower data: Unpublished results from a randomized study comparing incidence of recurrence after either needle aponeurotomy or limited fasiectomy and using the Year 3 postcollagenase data with recurrence defined as increase in joint angle ≥30 degrees

	All Joints	MCP	PIP
All phase III (950)	1568	820	648
Enrolled (364)	1065	641	424
Successfully Rx	623	451	172
Recurrence[a] Year 2	119/623 (19.3%)	61/446 (13.6%)	58/172 (34%)
Recurrence[a] Year 3	217/623 (35%)	86/446 (27%)	96/172 (56%)
Recurrence[a] by severity	Low	High	
MCP	28%	18%	
PIP	50%	71%	
43 of 623 successfully treated joints have had further intervention			

Rx	No.	Recurrence[b]	Interval (y)
Needle aponeurotomy	60	85%	2.3
Limited fasciectomy	52	24%	3.7
Collagenase	623	19%	3

[a] Recurrence defined as change from baseline of 20 degrees associated with a palpable cord.
[b] Recurrence defined as increase in treated finger ≥30 degrees.

with an average contracture of 22 degrees. Two patients with an average preinjection contracture of 45 degrees had recurrence with an average contracture of 60 degrees. No patients had chosen further intervention on the treated finger. Patient satisfaction with injection was high, with seven out of eight patients stating that they would pursue collagenase injection for the treatment of recurrent or progressive disease.

CURRENT STATUS OF CCH

CCH has been approved by the FDA and European Medical Agency for the treatment of Dupuytren contracture and is marketed in the United States under the trade name Xiaflex and in Europe under the trade name Xiapex. In the United States, CCH is currently under postmarket surveillance and is only available to physicians who have completed focused training in drug dosing and injection technique. In Europe, regulatory issues for Xiapex are occurring on a country-by-country basis.

GENERAL CLINICAL INDICATIONS

FDA and manufacturer treatment guidelines include the presence of a palpable cord causing at least a 20-degree contracture of an MCP or PIP joint, and no evidence of sensitivity to the drug. Only a single dose can be administered at any one time and the dose must be injected

directly into the specific (targeted) cord. The patient returns the following day or days to allow time for the collagenase to digest and lyse the collagen within the cord. An extension force is then applied to the involved finger to rupture the already weakened cord. FDA and manufacturer guidelines state that no more than three injections given at no less than monthly intervals may be used to affect improvement for the targeted joint.

Dosage and Injection Guidelines

CCH is supplied as a lyophilized powder with each vial containing 0.9 mg of CCH. Just before injection the drug is reconstituted with sterile diluent consisting of 0.3 mg/mL of calcium cloride dihydrate and 0.9% sodium chloride. For MCP joint contractures, a volume of 0.39 mL of sterile diluent is used for reconstitution and 0.58 mg of CCH in a total volume of 0.25 mL is injected into the targeted cord. For PIP joint contractures, 0.31 mL of sterile diluent is used for reconstitution and 0.58 mg of CCH in a total volume of 0.20 mL is injected into the targeted cord. Once reconstituted, CCH may be stored at room temperature for 1 hour or refrigerated for up to 4 hours.

Injection is performed with a 1-mL syringe and a 0.5-in, 27-gauge needle. Local anesthesia is not recommended at the time of injection because of distortion of the soft tissue anatomy and to obviate the risk of intraneural injection. The practitioner's nondominant hand is used to apply gentle extension to the finger undergoing injection, displacing the cord superficially away from the underlying flexor tendon mechanism. The needle is inserted perpendicularly through the skin into the underlying cord. The tissue should be firm and resist easy passage of the needle. Passive manipulation of the PIP or distal interphalangeal joint ensures that the needle has not been improperly positioned within the underlying flexor tendon. Inject one-third of the volume. The needle is withdrawn slightly and inclined distally and reinserted into the cord, approximately 3 mm from the site of the first aliquot. Proper positioning is confirmed and one-third of the dose is administered. The needle is then repositioned 2 to 3 mm proximal to the initial injection and the final one-third of the dose is administered (**Fig. 3**). The pretendinous cord causing an MCP contracture should be injected where the cord is displaced the farthest from the MP joint and underlying flexor sheath (**Fig. 4**). This is typically midway between the distal palmar and palmodigital creases. Avoid injecting at the site of callosities because the skin is likely to tear on manipulation. Cords causing PIP contractures should be injected just distal to the palmodigital crease. Care should be taken to avoid injection more than 4 mm distal to the palmodigital crease because injection in this region maintains a higher risk of intratendinous injection.

Manipulation

The manufacturer advises performing manipulation 24 hours after injection. The authors have varied the interval between injection and manipulation from 1 day to 1 week without seemingly altering the rate of success (**Table 5**). Digital or wrist blocks may be used at the time of manipulation to facilitate patient comfort. Manipulation of MCP joint contractures is performed by applying gentle passive extension, holding the finger in maximal extension for 10 to 20 seconds. Up to three attempts may be performed. For PIP contractures, the MCP joint is flexed before application of gentle, passive extension across the PIP joint. Patients are then placed in nighttime extension splinting for 4 weeks and instructed in passive extension exercises. No splint is worn during the day and patients often return to active use of the hand within 3 to 5 days depending on comfort.

AUTHORS' EXPERIENCE AND TECHNICAL TIPS

The authors were fortunate to be involved in the 1999 to 2000 phase II (34 subjects) and the 2007 to 2008 phase III trials (39 subjects, >100 injections) and have performed 140 injections in 84 patients since the FDA released the drug for general use. **Box 1** summarizes this clinical experience. Their clinical results mirror almost perfectly the results of the phase III trial, except for several notable differences, especially concerning PIP contractures. Recall that the phase III study called for up to three injections into the target cord to achieve a nearly straight joint. Many study patients with PIP contractures had multiple injections. Most of the authors' post-FDA release patients with PIP joint contractures do not want a second injection if they had a notable response to the first injection.

As they gained experience, the authors learned that most patients with either MCP or PIP joint contractures are very satisfied with almost any

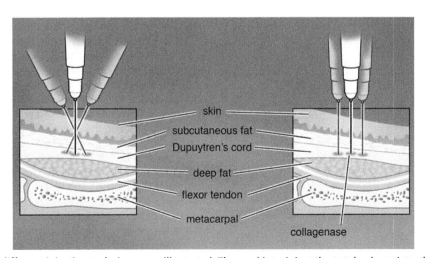

Fig. 3. Two different injection techniques are illustrated. The goal is to inject the total volume into the cord over a distance of 5 to 6 mm.

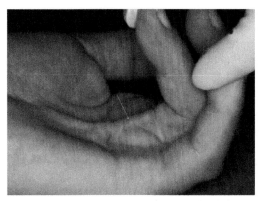

Fig. 4. A good candidate has an easily palpable pretendinous cord. The optimum site for injection is indicated by the *arrow*.

notable improvement and rarely ask to have a second injection. Their indications have broadened and narrowed, as discussed later. The following discussion is based on this still growing experience.

General Rules

1. You must have one clearly palpable cord as the target for injection and some degree of fixed joint contracture, meaning that you cannot fully passively extend the joint. Even if the patient cannot fully actively extend, if you can passively fully extend the joint, the cord may not respond to injection because at the time of manipulation you may not be able to exert sufficient force to rupture the now-weakened cord.

Table 5 Comparision of 25 joints manipulated at 24 hours postinjection with 25 joints manipulated at 7 days postinjection time		
	1 Day	**7 Days**
No. of MCP joints	14	13
Pre-Rx angle	47 degrees	46 degrees
Post-Rx angle	11 degrees	9 degrees
No. of PIP joint	11	12
Pre-Rx angle	56 degrees	53 degrees
Post-Rx angle	25 degrees	16 degrees
Spontaneous ruptures (no manipulation)		
7-day group: 7/12 MCP joints	1-day group: 1/14 MCP joints	
4/12 PIP joints	0/11 PIP joints	
Skin tears = 0	Skin tears = 3	

Box 1
Post-FDA release clinical experience

84 patients received 140 injections (average, 1.7 injections per patient)

130 different affected joints injected (average, 1.5 joints per patient)

Number of affected joints injected per patient (1–5)

Number of injections per patient (1–6)

    One injection = 50 patients

    Two injections = 23 patients

    Three injections = 8 patients (6 patients with thumb, natatory cord)

Second injection to same joint: 8

(average injections per joint = 1.1)

    Seven patients had second injection to same joint

    One patient had third injection to same joint

2. Although the needle is small and sharp, you should be able to distinguish the resistance caused by the cord.
3. Most cords are no more than 3 to 4 mm deep to the skin. Develop a sense of topographic anticipation regarding cord location and needle depth.
4. A surprising amount of force may be needed to inject the fluid into the dense collagen of the mature cord. It is safer to use both hands during the actual injection (**Fig. 5**). The authors prefer to passively extend the finger with the ulnar side of one hand. They control the syringe with the thumb and index finger of this hand to help maintain the exact depth of the needle while the second hand pushes the plunger of the syringe. This reduces the risk of the needle advancing deeper into the tissues as the plunger is depressed and resistance to the flow of fluid is encountered. This also reduces the risk of suddenly encountering no resistance to fluid flow and inadvertently injecting the entire volume in one place.
5. Often it is easier and safer to make three separate skin punctures, 2 to 3 mm apart, rather than inclining the needle as the manufacturer's guidelines suggest.
6. Give the patient some take-home information regarding the very common side effects, such as pain, swelling, bruising, and also the less common side effects, such axillary lymphangitis. Reproduce some photographs of postinjection hands so that the patient is fully

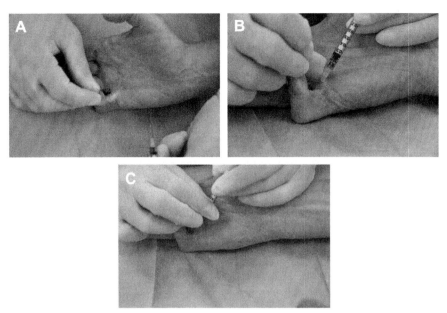

Fig. 5. (*A–C*) The preferred two-handed injection technique is illustrated. See text for description. The cord is delineated by palpation (*A*), the needle is inserted into the cord while tension is applied to the cord (*B*), and both hands support the syringe while the plunger is pressed (*C*).

informed. Prescribe analgesics. This avoids midnight telephone calls from the patient (**Fig. 6**).

7. The period between injection and manipulation can be varied considerably without negatively influencing the outcome (see **Table 5**). The cord remains weak for a still yet to be defined period of time postinjection.

8. When the patient comes for manipulation, examine the hand before injecting local anesthesia. The cord may have spontaneously ruptured.

9. The authors have operated on four former study patients who either had an inadequate response to injection or a recurrence. At surgery performed at least 1 year after

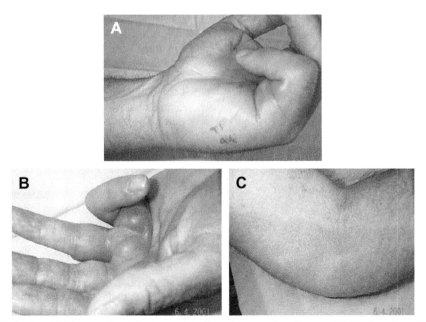

Fig. 6. (*A, B*) The hand 24 hours after injection. Note the edema and erythema. (*C*) The lymphangitis that some patients may experience.

injection, normal tissue planes were observed. It did not appear as if the injection had caused any residual scarring or alteration in the expected anatomy.

10. Review the billing and coding recommendations from the manufacturer, or those suggested by the American Society for Surgery of the Hand. There are now two specific CPT-4 codes created for this treatment. Obtain insurance preauthorization for patients who have private insurance. Be prepared for patient sticker-shock because the US manufacturer's current charge for one vial (ie, one injection) is $3200.

MCP Joint Contractures

1. MCP joint contractures almost always respond adequately to one injection. Rarely is a second injection needed, unless the first injection misses the cord. If the cord ruptures (or stretched notably) and the contracture corrects to a level of 60% to 75%, (usually <15 degrees of residual contracture) no patient has asked for a second injection to correct the remaining few degrees of residual contraction. Patients are very happy with this outcome. It is unwise to talk them into a second injection. Typically, not much more extension is gained unless they have a joint contracted by its pretendinous cord and also by a natatory cord arising from an adjacent digit's contracted pretendinous cord. In this case, the Y-shaped cord first should have been injected as described next.

2. If a Y-shaped cord is present and second adjacent digits are involved, inject at the confluence of the Y. You may achieve two corrected digits for the price and effort of a single injection (**Fig. 7**).

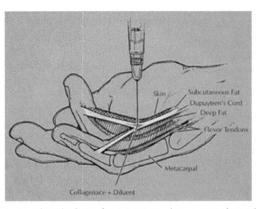

Fig. 7. The ideal site for injection when a "Y"-shaped cord is causing contracture of two adjacent digits is at the confluence of the "Y."

3. A tight natatory cord can be successfully treated. These can be more bothersome to piano players than pretendinous cords. Although technically off-label, natatory cords do not require 0.58 mg of drug. Look for another, possibly narrow cord causing a contracture and consider splitting the dose.

4. The skin often tears with MCP joint contractures greater than 50 degrees, particularly if the skin overlying the cord is calloused. Prepare the patient (and yourself) for this eventuality. All such tears have healed with simple wound care within 7 to 10 days. The authors have experienced far fewer skin tears when the interval between injection and manipulation is extended to 7 days.

PIP Contractures

1. All tendon ruptures experienced in the clinical trials occurred after injections for fifth finger PIP contractures, usually for central cords. For a central cord, do not inject more than 4 mm distal to the palmodigital crease and consider inserting the needle more horizontally (from the side of the finger) rather than vertically or perpendicular to the palmar plane. Patients must understand this risk and practitioners must appreciate the implications of tendon rupture and reconstruction before incorporating collagenase injection into their practice.

2. The abductor digiti minimi cord is the most frequent cause of fifth finger PIP contractures. It is easily palpable and a good target for injection. It is always wide in the palmar to dorsal direction and you need to vary the depth of the three aliquots in this plane. The cord is well away from the flexor sheath and can be safely injected.

3. Lateral digital cords present good targets. Occasionally, radial and ulnar lateral digital cords coexist and cause PIP joint contracture. Weaken one and the other remains to maintain the joint contracted and resistant to manipulation. Consider splitting the dose and injecting both cords. This is also technically off-label.

4. Periarticular fibrosis is unaffected by CCH. However, if the offending cord ruptures or softens and is no longer palpable, try dynamic splinting postinjection.

5. The PIP joint contracture associated with a huge nodule that practically fills the proximal phalanx does not respond to collagenase. The authors explain to the patient that injecting a tiny volume of drug is akin to pouring a teacup of boiling water on the top of a glacier; a little ice melts but the glacier remains.

6. The recurrent PIP contracture associated with shrunken, scarred skin over the proximal phalanx is a poor candidate for CCH (**Fig. 8**).
7. The extensor mechanism over the PIP joint becomes elongated in contractures that achieve 60 degrees. The contracted PIP joint may, after injection and manipulation, be nearly fully passively correctable but the patient is unable to actively fully extend the joint and the contracture recurs to some degree rather quickly.

DISCUSSION

CCH represents the first commercially available, clinically efficacious option for the nonoperative treatment of DD. In the authors' experience, CCH has proved to be a safe and effective, office-based treatment for contractures caused by DD occurring at any level in the hand and digit. Definitive indications for CCH injection have not been clearly established and it is reasonable to extrapolate well-established operative indications as a basis for this nonoperative treatment. MCP joint contractures respond dramatically, whereas PIP contractures respond to a lesser but still satisfactory (to the patient) level. There is a role for CCH in patients who are not generally considered good operative candidates because of inability to tolerate a general anesthetic, sedation, or regional anesthesia required to perform an open operation.

It is clear that neither collagenase injection nor percutaneous fasciotomy or open fasciectomy, provide a cure for DD. Recurrence and progression are to be expected irrespective of the treatment path chosen; however, these interventions differ with respect to ease of treatment, periprocedural course, inherent risk of intervention, complications, and durability of the correction (see

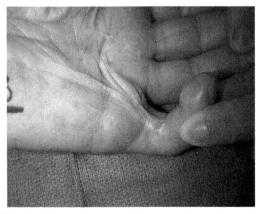

Fig. 8. A severe recurrent PIP contracture with badly scarred and contracted skin is a poor candidate for collagenase treatment.

Table 4). These are the factors that must be considered by the treating physician and the patient.

Phase II and III clinical trials of CCH have demonstrated relative safety in the hands of well-trained physicians with a clear understanding of the anatomy and pathoanatomy of DD. Although minor complications associated with injection are common, major complications including complex regional pain syndrome and flexor tendon rupture are rare and occur at rates comparable with those observed in open fasciectomy.

Currently, patients with multiple or severe contractures and those with recurrent disease are ideal candidates for open fasciectomy, whereas those with isolated contractures of moderate severity are candidates for either percutaneous fascioctomy or collagenase injection. The relative advantages and disadvantages of needle aponeurotomy or CCH over fasciotomy remain speculative and there exists a role for all of these treatments. For example, the authors have had the experience in two patients of injecting CCH and achieving a notable although not total correction after the administration of local anesthesia and manipulating a contracted MCP joint. However, there remained a tight, narrow, unruptured cord paralleling the target cord that was not palpable before rupturing the target cord. Because the palm had been anesthetized as part of the manipulation procedure, the authors chose to perform a simple percutaneous needle aponeurotomy of this remaining cord and achieved full extension of the joint.

Further delineating the role of CCH and defining the safety and efficacy profile in general clinical practice provides avenues for further research. To date, injection protocols in all studies have been performed by fellowship-trained hand surgeons, instructed in proper injection technique. Familiarity with the surgical anatomy of DD and formal training has likely mitigated many of the potential complications of CCH injections. There is the risk that use of CCH in the hands of less skilled practitioners may lead to a greater incidence of serious complications. Postmarketing surveillance will provide an accurate assessment of the efficacy and safety profiles as the drug is administered by a broader group of practitioners.

PERSONAL PERSPECTIVES

As practitioners become more familiar with CCH injection, the indications for injection will most likely expand. Current indications are reflective of surgical practices. Over time, the indications for collagenase injection will evolve to reflect the balance between the relative risk of injection in relation to the functional limitations imparted by the degree of contracture. CCH injection of contractures may potentially forestall the need for operative intervention. Application to multiple, simultaneous contractures will likely occur and clinical trials exploring the risks of simultaneously injecting more than one cord are underway.

Palmodigital fasciectomy remains the gold standard. The initial outcome is, in the authors' experience, far more predictable than either percutaneous needle aponeurotomy or CCH. It is also a more durable treatment. It is also what hand surgeons have been trained to do in the operative playing field. They did not spend years learning how to plunge a needle up and down like a sewing machine or inject a few tenths of a milliliter of liquid just under the skin. Percutaneous needle aponeurotomy and CCH can be conceptualized as similar procedures; one uses a needle and the other an enzyme to weaken a cord sufficient to be able to rupture it and thus straighten a contracted joint. Both are less invasive and the hand is quick to recover. Both procedures are equally initially effective. CCH seems to offer greater durability. However, few hand surgeons experience the same degree of satisfaction after performing either of these procedures as he or she experiences at the end of a successful fasciectomy. Keep in mind that although surgeons enjoy performing surgery, for the patient surgery is misery to one degree or another. Today's patients often come better educated and seeking a particular type of treatment, particularly effective nonoperative treatment. Pharmaceutical companies now market directly and effectively to the patient and this strategy and Internet use is likely to result in an increase in the number of patients searching for practitioners willing and capable of administering collagenase treatment.

REFERENCES

1. Elliot D. The early history of contracture of the palmar fascia. J Hand Surg 1988;13B:246–53.
2. Starkweather K, Lattuga S, Hurst L, et al. Collagenase in the treatment of Dupuytren's disease: an in vitro study. J Hand Surg Am 1996;21(3):490–5.
3. Luck JV. Dupuytren's contracture. A new concept of the pathogenesis correlated with the surgical management. J Bone Joint Surg Am 1959;40(4):635–64.
4. Kloen P, Jennings CL, Gebhardt MC, et al. Transforming growth factor-b: possible roles in Dupuytren's contracture. J Hand Surg Am 1995;20(1):101–8.
5. Kloen P. New insights in the development of Dupuytren's contracture: a review. Br J Plast Surg 1999; 52(8):629–35.
6. Brickley-Parsons D, Glimcher MJ, Smith RJ, et al. Biochemical changes in the collagen of the palmar fascia in patients with Dupuytren's disease. J Bone Joint Surg Am 1981;63:787–97.
7. Tomasek JJ, Schultz RJ, Episalla CW, et al. The cytoskeleton and extracellular matrix of the Dupuytren's disease myofibroblast: an immunofluorescence study of a non-muscle cell type. J Hand Surg Am 1986;11:365–71.
8. Bassott J. Treatment of Dupuytren's disease by isolated pharmacodynamic "exeresis" or "exeresis" completed by a solely cutaneous plastic step. Lille Chir 1965;20:38–44.
9. Bassot J. Traitment de la maladie de Dupuytren par exerese pharmaco-dynamique: bases physiobiologiques; technique. Gaz Hop 1969;20:557.
10. Hueston JT. Enzymic fasciotomy. Hand 1971;3: 38–40.
11. McCarthy DM. The long term results of enzymatic fasciotomy. J Hand Surg Br 1992;17:356.
12. Maclennon J, Mandl I, Howes E. Bacterial digestion of collagen. J Clin Invest 1953;32(12):1317–22.
13. Toyoshima T, Matsushita O, Minami J, et al. Collagen-binding domain of a Clostridium histolyticum collagenase exhibits a broad substrate spectrum both in vitro and in vivo. Connect Tissue Res 2001;42(4):281–90.
14. Gelbard MK, Walsh R, Kaufman JJ. Collagenase for Peyronie's disease experimental studies. Urol Res 1982;10(3):135–40.
15. Mandl I. Collagenase comes of age. In: Mandel I, editor. Collagenase. New York: Gordon & Breach Science Publishers; 1972. p. 1–16.
16. Badalamente MA, Hurst LC. Enzyme injection as nonsurgical treatment of Dupuytren's disease. J Hand Surg Am 2000;25(4):629–36.
17. Badalamente MA, Hurst LC, Hentz VR, et al. Collagen as a clinical target: nonoperative treatment of Dupuytren's disease. J Hand Surg Am 2002;27(5): 788–98.
18. Badalamente MA, Hurst LC. Efficacy and safety of injectable mixed collagenase subtypes in the treatment of Dupuytren's contracture. J Hand Surg Am 2007;32(6):767–74.
19. Hurst LC, Badalamente MA, Hentz VR, et al. Injectable collagenase Clostridium histolyticum for Dupuytren's contracture. N Engl J Med 2009;361(10):968–79.
20. United States FDA Report. Briefing document for collagenase Clostridium histolyticum (AA4500) in the treatment of advanced Dupuytren's disease. Arthritis Advisory Committee Meeting. September 16, 2009 Available at: www.fda.gov/downloads/advisorycommittees/committeesmeetingmaterials/drugs/arthritisdrugsadvisorycommittee/ucm182015.pdf.
21. Tonkin MA, Burke FD, Varian JP. Dupuytren's contracture: a comparative study of fasciectomy

and dermofasciectomy in one hundred patients. J Hand Surg Br 1984;9(2):156–62.

22. Foucher G, Medina J, Malizos K. Percutaneous needle fasciotomy in Dupuytren's disease. Tech Hand Up Extrem Surg 2001;5(3):161–4.

23. Bryan AS, Ghorbal MS. The long-term results of closed palmar fasciotomy in the management of Dupuytren's contracture. J Hand Surg Br 1988; 13(3):254–6.

24. Rodrigo JJ, Niebauer JJ, Brown RL, et al. Treatment of Dupuytren's contracture: long-term results after fasciotomy and fascial excision. J Bone Joint Surg Am 1976;58:380–7.

25. LeBourg M, Raimbeau G, Fouque P, et al. Devenir a 5 ans de la maladie de Dupuytren traitee par aponevrotomie precutanee. Etude prospective de 106 cas consecutifs. Presented at 37th Meeting of the French Society for Surgery of the Hand (GEM). Paris, May 18, 19, 2001.

26. Gilpin D, Coleman S, Hall S, et al. Injectable collagenase clostridium histolyticum: a new nonsurgical treatment for Dupuytren's disease. J Hand Surg Am 2010;35(12):2027–38.

27. Watt AJ, Curtin CM, Hentz VR. Collagenase injection as nonsurgical treatment of Dupuytren's disease: 8-year follow-up. J Hand Surg Am 2010;35(4):534–9.

Modern Tendon Repair Techniques

Steve K. Lee, MD

KEYWORDS

- Tendon repair • Hand • Upper extremity • Flexor • extensor

KEY POINTS

- Digital tendon repair is one of the most common issues in hand surgery and also one of the most vexing.
- A repair must withstand the forces imparted on it during early motion.
- A specific goal of zone II repairs is one where there is minimal increase in work of flexion.
- Repair of tendons that have flat morphology present a particular challenge to achieving a strong repair while maintaining the native tendon shape.

Digital tendon repair is one of the most common issues in hand surgery and also one of the most vexing. The surgeon and patient are in a literal race for tendon healing while retaining motion: a healed tendon with no motion may render the entire hand dysfunctional because there are interconnections between multiple tendons in the hand and wrist. Essentially each institution and surgeon has their own particular preferences for repair; indeed, which techniques are best is a quintessentially controversial topic in hand surgery. A recent PubMed search for "tendon" and "hand" returned more than 2500 scientific articles. Despite the controversy, some common themes do exist.

Early motion after repair is paramount. Classic articles that support this include a clinical article by Strickland and Glogovac[1] and a basic science study by Gelberman and colleagues.[2] Strickland and Glogovac[1] compared two patient cohorts after flexor tendon repair; one cohort was immobilized postoperatively and the other underwent an early motion protocol. There were better ultimate results with early motion.[1] In a canine study, Gelberman and colleagues[2] studied 3 groups: one group was immobilized following tendon repair, a second group underwent delayed mobilization, and the third group underwent early mobilization. The groups performed progressively better with regard to angular motion and ultimate strength when motion was started earlier postoperatively.

A repair must withstand the forces imparted on it during early motion, to avoid not only the catastrophic rupture that unfortunately still occurs in 4% to 10% of cases,[3] but also to avoid excessive gapping, which has deleterious effects on outcome such as increased adhesions and increased gliding resistance, leading to poor motion.[4] While the amount of allowable gapping ranges from 2 to 3 mm,[4,5] the goal is to have as little gapping as possible. Gelberman and colleagues,[5] in a canine study, repaired the tendons and demonstrated that if the gap exceeded 3 mm, biological healing over time was compromised.

How much force the flexor tendon must withstand is not completely known because studies that have been previously performed were either in normal hands or in cadaveric specimens. The effects of bulkiness of repairs, postoperative edema, adhesions, and joint stiffness have not been measured and evaluated. Powell and Trail[6] performed studies on patients with force transducers while they were undergoing elective carpal

Hospital for Special Surgery, Weill Cornell Medical College, 535 East 70th Street, New York, NY 10021, USA
E-mail address: leest@hss.edu

Hand Clin 28 (2012) 565–570
http://dx.doi.org/10.1016/j.hcl.2012.08.012
0749-0712/12/$ – see front matter © 2012 Elsevier Inc. All rights reserved.

tunnel releases. The results suggest that during passive motion, flexor tendons are subjected to forces of less than 20 N. For active motion against 300 g, this increased to up to 50 N.[6] Strickland[7] produced a table that attempted to take into account postoperative edema and other factors, and summarized that for active motion the tendon must withstand 30 to 50 N of force. For strong grasp, this increases to 70 N.

Common clinical scenarios that challenge the hand surgeon are flexor tendon injuries in zone II, zone I, and extensor tendons. Repair of tendons that have flat morphology present a particular challenge to achieving a strong repair while maintaining the native tendon shape. When faced with these problems, there are several very specific issues for repair methods that affect the quality of repair and therefore the eventual outcome. Questions include: What type of suture method is best? Locking or grasping method? How many core sutures in a zone II repair? What kind of circumferential repair? What type of suture material? How far from the lacerated end of the tendon to place the sutures?

The following is a description of the author's approach to these problems with a rationale for the specifics.

ZONE II

Zone II flexor tendon repairs are particularly difficult secondary to the anatomic constraints of the region. The flexor digitorum profundus (FDP) and flexor digitorum superficialis (FDS) tendons run in a common flexor sheath, rendering very little room for added bulk of repair. The area is fraught with possible complications of tendon adhesions, resulting in poor motion. Zone II was named "no man's land" by Bunnell, referring to an area within which no man should operate. The name was derived from the land between two opposing forces in war: land that no man controlled. Repairs in this area should be strong enough to allow early motion without gapping or rupturing, yet not be bulky. Increased bulk is biomechanically seen as an increase in work of flexion.

An optimal repair would therefore be one that is strong enough to allow for early motion and smooth enough to allow for easy gliding. The ultimate repair would be one whereby a patient would be allowed to move the finger and hand postoperatively with minimal therapy requirements. Sandford and colleagues[8] showed that two-thirds of patients were noncompliant with splint use after flexor tendon repairs. Elliot stated "in approximately half of these patients (where the repair fails), tendon rupture followed acts of stupidity."[9] Even in the most compliant patient, all normal humans move during sleep.

The questions therefore to be answered are: what kind of core suture method should be used, with how many strands, using which suture method, with what distance of suture span (distance of the suture purchase from the ends of the injured tendons). For the circumferential suture, similar questions are: what suture method, which suture, and what suture span?

There are many methods from which to choose. The author presents a method that combines several these parameters that have been shown to optimize the strength and minimize the bulk. This method is known as the cross-locked cruciate–interlocking horizontal mattress (CLC-IHM) repair, which combines the cross-locked cruciate core suture method using 3-0 Fiberwire (Arthrex, Naples, FL) at a suture span of 10 mm and an interlocking horizontal mattress suture method with 6-0 Prolene (Ethicon, Somerset, NJ) with a suture span of 2 mm (**Fig. 1**).[10] These specifics originate from a history of work dating back to the 1990s.[11–15] The cross-locked cruciate suture method has been shown to be an excellent 4-strand biomechanical repair.[16] Fiberwire has been shown to be an optimal material when compared with other common suture materials.[17] Suture span of 10 mm has been shown to be the optimal distance with regard to strength and work of flexion.[10,18] The interlocking horizontal mattress repair has been shown to be the best circumferential repair when compared with other common methods,[19] and a 2-mm suture span for the circumferential portion has been shown to be the optimal distance.[20] This combination repair has ultimate strength of 111 N, 2-mm gap force of 90 N, and only a 5% increase in work of flexion, the lowest increase in work of flexion reported to date.[10] Concerns have arisen regarding 10 mm being too great a distance requiring large exposure. The 7-mm suture span was very close to 10 mm in the tested parameters, and therefore in practice the author uses 7 mm as the minimum suture span.

Some specifics of the CLC-IHM are as follows. The repair may be technically demanding at first, but the benefits of a strong repair with minimal bulk are undoubtedly worth the effort. The author recommends preoperative practice in the laboratory, with human cadaveric hands, but another option is porcine feet, which have tendons similar in size to human hands.[16] The author sketches out the repair on the operating-room drapes before each repair. The core suture should start in the center and dorsally; this assures that the suture knot will not protrude out of the repair site and

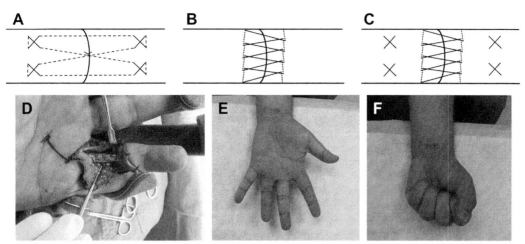

Fig. 1. (*A*) Cross-locked cruciate repair. (*B*) Interlocking horizontal mattress repair. (*C*) Cross-locked cruciate–interlocking horizontal mattress combination repair. (*D*) Clinical intraoperative photograph of the cross-locked cruciate–interlocking horizontal mattress combination repair. Note that there is no bunching (trumpeting) of the repair. (*E*) Three months postoperatively demonstrating motion, open hand. (*F*) Three months postoperatively demonstrating motion, fist. (*From* Lee SK, Goldstein RY, Zingman A, et al. The effects of core suture purchase on the biomechanical characteristics of a multistrand locking flexor tendon repair: a cadaveric study. J Hand Surg Am 2010;35(7):1165–71.)

catch on pulleys. The tendon ends must be perfectly opposed before starting the suturing; this is accomplished with 25-gauge needles placed in both tendon ends approximately 15 to 20 mm from the cut ends of the tendon. Once the second cross lock is placed and tightened, the tendon ends will hold their position, and the ends cannot be "overopposed," which bulges the tendon ends. This bulging effect was termed trumpeting by Joseph Boyes. On the other hand, the tendons cannot be opposed if they are gapped at the beginning of the suture process. Each cross lock should be cinched tightly like shoestrings as the surgeon proceeds; the author cinches and re-cinches each cross lock during the procedure. The knots are tied as tightly as the surgeon desires, tying perpendicular to the tendon. Because the suture is cross locked, there will be no bunching of the tendon ends when tying strong knots, as opposed to other techniques that do not lock. Six knots should be placed (initial surgeon's knot plus 4 half hitches); this has been shown to be the number of knots required for knot stability (Lee and colleagues, American Academy of Orthopedic Surgeons [AAOS] 2007).

At the end of the repair, it may be disconcerting to the surgeon that the inside of the repair may be seen. Suture material is exposed within the tendon ends, and because the suture purchase is 7 to 10 mm, there is 14 to 20 mm of suture material that may be seen if the tendon ends are everted. Use of a circumferential suture is therefore imperative. It also adds up to 50 N of strength. After the

core suture is placed, but before the circumferential suture is placed, any loose ends are debrided from the tendon ends to debulk the repair site. This technique is especially necessary if the repair is performed after a few days from the injury, when the tendon ends have become "mop-ended." The interlocking horizontal mattress suture is placed with 6-0 Prolene with a suture purchase of 2 mm. A technical tip is for the suture bites to be taken in a direction slightly away from the lacerated tendon end so that the suture does not eventually converge. Another technical tip is that the first suture pass is tied to itself in case the circumferential suture cannot be placed all of the way around the tendon for technical reasons. This situation usually arises in cases where there is difficulty with exposure because of the pulleys. In this case, the suture may then be tied at the furthest place around the tendon as possible. One further technical tip is that the pulley system should only be opened at the site that is necessary to gain exposure. This opening is not necessarily between the A2 and A4 pulleys; this window may be moved more proximally or more distally depending on where the injury is. To gain better exposure, pulleys may be partially vented. A2 or A4 may be vented by 50% safely. Tang and colleagues[21,22] showed in a chicken model that pulley venting may decrease tendon rupture rates and resistance to gliding.

With this repair method, patients may begin rehabilitation early. A 90-N 2-mm gap force far exceeds the strength of 70 N needed for strong grasp.[10] The strength of the repair in an early motion protocol increases from time zero; only when tendons are immobilized postoperatively do they get weaker temporarily before getting stronger (the "softening" effect). Cao and Tang[23] have shown in a chicken model that edema and resistance is high immediately after repair and that the optimal time to start postoperative motion is at 4 to 7 days. The author strives to have patients start motion at 4 to 5 days after surgery. Wrist tenodesis place-and-hold position and hook fist position are key exercises with regard to tendon motion and intertendinous (between FDP and FDS) motion. (Yoon and colleagues, AAOS 2012). The author has patients perform wrist tenodesis active digital extension, wrist tenodesis active fist followed by tip to palm place and hold, hook fist, and intrinsic plus exercises at 4 to 5 days. Blocking exercises start at 4 weeks, strengthening at 8 weeks, unrestricted regular activity at 6 months, and contact sports at 9 months.

ZONE I

Zone I injuries occur as an avulsion (Jersey finger) or laceration distal to the FDS insertion. Despite the original recommendations by Leddy and Packer,[24] all of these injuries should be treated as soon as possible because there is the possibility that there is a fracture plus a tendon avulsion from the bone fragment,[25,26] rendering the tendon in the palm. Delay in treatment would allow the pulleys to collapse and would not allow the passage of the tendon back through the pulley system.

For repairs of the FDP back to the distal phalanx and tendon transfers or tendon grafts to the distal phalanx, secure fixation of the tendon to bone is imperative. Among common methods described are the classic button technique first described by Bunnell,[27] and the anchor technique, which has had several proponents. The advantages of the button technique are that it can be very strong because the fixation is across a bony tunnel. The disadvantages of the button technique are that the fixation point (button) is a great distance from

the tendon to bone contact, which may allow for a "bungee effect" and gapping of the tendon off the bone.[28] Others have advocated anchors, with an advantage of less gapping because the fixation point is close to the tendon-to-bone interface.[29,30] A disadvantage of the anchor technique is that it fails through anchor to bone pullout, especially in weaker bone.[31] The author has combined these 2 common methods to create the anchor button (AB) technique, which combines the strength of the button method and the stiffness (resistance to gapping) of the anchor technique (**Fig. 2**).[32] The details of this technique are as follows. Once the FDP tendon, transferred tendon, or tendon graft is in placed near the distal phalanx, the distal phalanx is prepared by removing the tendon remnant and other soft tissue off of the palmar aspect of the distal phalanx distal to the volar plate. The radial and ulnar aspects of the distal phalanx should be visualized as well as the distal extent of the volar plate and two-thirds of the distal phalanx. Sutures are then placed into the tendon end. A Krakow suture is placed (running lock) on the dorsal half of the tendon with 3 locks on each side (radial and ulnar) of the tendon with 3-0 Fiberwire. A Bunnell suture is placed on the palmar side of the tendon end with 3 passes on each side using 2-0 Prolene. The Fiberwire sutures are then threaded through 2 different MicroMitek bone suture anchors (Depuy Mitek, Somerset, NJ) and these anchors are placed in the proximal portion of the distal phalanx just distal to the volar plate, aiming slightly toward the midline of the phalanx and slightly retrograde. This retrograde trajectory has been shown to be biomechanically superior.[30] A Keith needle is then drilled distal to these anchors in the midline, exiting the dorsal nail bed and nail plate through the sterile matrix, avoiding the germinal matrix. The 2-0 Prolene suture ends are then placed in the Keith needle eyelet and the needle is advanced dorsally. The anchor sutures are then tied over a bone bridge brought on the same side under the Keith needle sutures. The 2-0 Prolene suture is then tied over a button.

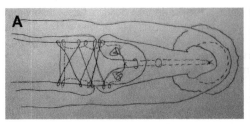
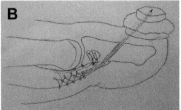

Fig. 2. (*A*) Anchor button (AB) repair of the tendon to the distal phalanx (anteroposterior view). (*B*) AB repair of the tendon to the distal phalanx (lateral view). (*From* Lee SK, Fajardo M, Kardashian G, et al. Repair of flexor digitorum profundus to distal phalanx: a biomechanical evaluation of four techniques. J Hand Surg Am 2011;36(10):1604–9.)

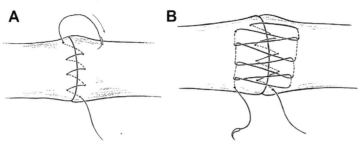

Fig. 3. (*A*) Running-interlocking horizontal mattress repair method. The first half of the repair is a running suture. (*B*) Running-interlocking horizontal mattress repair method. The second half of the repair adds the interlocking horizontal mattress suture in the opposite direction to the running suture. (*From* Lee SK, Dubey A, Kim BH, et al. A biomechanical study of extensor tendon repair methods: introduction to the running-interlocking horizontal mattress extensor tendon repair technique. J Hand Surg Am 2010;35(1):19–23.)

Secure button fixation is achieved by the following technique. Two-ply cotton is placed underneath the button. The convex side of the button is placed on the nail plate, making sure that no portion of the button is pressing on the eponychium. After the suture is tied, a piece of Xeroform dressing (Kendall Covidien, Mansfield, MA) folded lengthwise in thirds is wrapped 2 to 3 times between the button and the nail plate. A 2-0 silk tie is wrapped around the Xeroform 2 to 3 times to snug the Xeroform and keep it in place. This action increases the stability of the button-suture-nail complex. The postoperative rehabilitation is similar to that of a zone II repair because the AB technique is extremely strong, with a failure at 115 N.[32]

EXTENSOR TENDON REPAIR

Relative to flexor tendon research, there is a relative paucity of extensor tendon research. Several studies have compared repair techniques.[33–36] The author has devised a strong, stiff construct with minimal shortening of the tendon that is quick to perform, called the running-interlocking horizontal mattress (R-IHM) method, which is particularly designed for extensor tendons where there is a flat morphology (**Fig. 3**).[37] It is performed with a 3-0 or 4-0 Fiberwire suture, and starts with a running suture in one direction and ends with an interlocking horizontal mattress suture on the way back. Tested against other previously touted repairs, it is biomechanically superior.[37] It is particularly useful in combination injuries of flexor and extensor tendons whereby early motion must be started. It is strong enough for immediate gentle, active assisted range of motion.

SUMMARY

Modern digital tendon repair techniques have several common themes: multistrand locking repairs and early active motion. The author recommends the CLC-IHM technique for zone II flexor

tendon injuries. For zone I flexor tendon injuries and also for fixation of tendon grafts and transfers to the distal phalanx, the AB technique is recommended. For extensor tendon injuries, the R-IHM technique is the preferred technique. These techniques are biomechanically tested repair methods with superior characteristics that allow for early motion with low chance of rupture. The author's early clinical experience with all of these repair methods has shown clinical success of improved motion and no known ruptures.

REFERENCES

1. Strickland JW, Glogovac SV. Digital function following flexor tendon repair in Zone II: a comparison of immobilization and controlled passive motion techniques. J Hand Surg Am 1980;5(6):537–43.
2. Gelberman RH, Woo SL, Lothringer K, et al. Effects of early intermittent passive mobilization on healing canine flexor tendons. J Hand Surg Am 1982;7(2):170–5.
3. Tang JB. Clinical outcomes associated with flexor tendon repair. Hand Clin 2005;21(2):199–210.
4. Zhao C, Amadio PC, Tanaka T, et al. Effect of gap size on gliding resistance after flexor tendon repair. J Bone Joint Surg Am 2004;86-A(11):2482–8.
5. Gelberman RH, Boyer MI, Brodt MD, et al. The effect of gap formation at the repair site on the strength and excursion of intrasynovial flexor tendons. An experimental study on the early stages of tendon-healing in dogs. J Bone Joint Surg Am 1999;81(7):975–82.
6. Powell ES, Trail IA. Forces transmitted along human flexor tendons during passive and active movements of the fingers. J Hand Surg Br 2004;29(4):386–9.
7. Strickland JW. Development of flexor tendon surgery: twenty-five years of progress. J Hand Surg Am 2000;25(2):214–35.
8. Sandford F, Barlow N, Lewis J. A study to examine patient adherence to wearing 24-hour forearm

thermoplastic splints after tendon repairs. J Hand Ther 2008;21(1):44–52 [quiz: 53].

9. Harris SB, Harris D, Foster AJ, et al. The aetiology of acute rupture of flexor tendon repairs in zones 1 and 2 of the fingers during early mobilization. J Hand Surg Br 1999;24(3):275–80.

10. Lee SK, Goldstein RY, Zingman A, et al. The effects of core suture purchase on the biomechanical characteristics of a multistrand locking flexor tendon repair: a cadaveric study. J Hand Surg Am 2010; 35(7):1165–71.

11. McLarney E, Hoffman H, Wolfe SW. Biomechanical analysis of the cruciate four-strand flexor tendon repair. J Hand Surg Am 1999;24(2):295–301.

12. Barrie KA, Tomak SL, Cholewicki J, et al. Effect of suture locking and suture caliber on fatigue strength of flexor tendon repairs. J Hand Surg Am 2001; 26(2):340–6.

13. Barrie KA, Tomak SL, Cholewicki J, et al. The role of multiple strands and locking sutures on gap formation of flexor tendon repairs during cyclical loading. J Hand Surg Am 2000;25(4):714–20.

14. Barrie KA, Wolfe SW. The relationship of suture design to biomechanical strength of flexor tendon repairs. Hand Surg 2001;6(1):89–97.

15. Barrie KA, Wolfe SW, Shean C, et al. A biomechanical comparison of multistrand flexor tendon repairs using an in situ testing model. J Hand Surg Am 2000;25(3): 499–506.

16. Croog A, Goldstein R, Nasser P, et al. Comparative biomechanic performances of locked cruciate four-strand flexor tendon repairs in an ex vivo porcine model. J Hand Surg Am 2007;32(2):225–32.

17. Lawrence TM, Davis TR. A biomechanical analysis of suture materials and their influence on a four-strand flexor tendon repair. J Hand Surg Am 2005; 30(4):836–41.

18. Tang JB, Zhang Y, Cao Y, et al. Core suture purchase affects strength of tendon repairs. J Hand Surg Am 2005;30(6):1262–6.

19. Dona E, Turner AW, Gianoutsos MP, et al. Biomechanical properties of four circumferential flexor tendon suture techniques. J Hand Surg Am 2003; 28(5):824–31.

20. Merrell GA, Wolfe SW, Kacena WJ, et al. The effect of increased peripheral suture purchase on the strength of flexor tendon repairs. J Hand Surg Am 2003;28(3):464–8.

21. Tang JB, Cao Y, Wu YF, et al. Effect of A2 pulley release on repaired tendon gliding resistance and rupture in a chicken model. J Hand Surg Am 2009; 34(6):1080–7.

22. Cao Y, Tang JB. Strength of tendon repair decreases in the presence of an intact A2 pulley: biomechanical study in a chicken model. J Hand Surg Am 2009; 34(10):1763–70.

23. Cao Y, Tang JB. Resistance to motion of flexor tendons and digital edema: an in vivo study in a chicken model. J Hand Surg Am 2006;31(10): 1645–51.

24. Leddy JP, Packer JW. Avulsion of the profundus tendon insertion in athletes. J Hand Surg Am 1977; 2(1):66–9.

25. Langa V, Posner MA. Unusual rupture of a flexor profundus tendon. J Hand Surg Am 1986;11(2): 227–9.

26. Trumble TE, Vedder NB, Benirschke SK. Misleading fractures after profundus tendon avulsions: a report of six cases. J Hand Surg Am 1992;17(5):902–6.

27. Bunnell S. Surgery of the hand. J.B. Lippincott Company; 1944.

28. Schreuder FB, Scougall PJ, Puchert E, et al. Effect of suture material on gap formation and failure in type 1 FDP avulsion repairs in a cadaver model. Clin Biomech (Bristol, Avon) 2006;21(5):481–4.

29. Brustein M, Pellegrini J, Choueka J, et al. Bone suture anchors versus the pullout button for repair of distal profundus tendon injuries: a comparison of strength in human cadaveric hands. J Hand Surg Am 2001;26(3):489–96.

30. Schreuder FB, Scougall PJ, Puchert E, et al. The effect of Mitek anchor insertion angle to attachment of FDP avulsion injuries. J Hand Surg Br 2006;31(3): 292–5.

31. Matsuzaki H, Zaegel MA, Gelberman RH, et al. Effect of suture material and bone quality on the mechanical properties of zone I flexor tendon-bone reattachment with bone anchors. J Hand Surg Am 2008;33(5):709–17.

32. Lee SK, Fajardo M, Kardashian G, et al. Repair of flexor digitorum profundus to distal phalanx: a biomechanical evaluation of four techniques. J Hand Surg Am 2011;36(10):1604–9.

33. Newport ML, Blair WF, Steyers CM Jr. Long-term results of extensor tendon repair. J Hand Surg Am 1990;15(6):961–6.

34. Newport ML, Pollack GR, Williams CD. Biomechanical characteristics of suture techniques in extensor zone IV. J Hand Surg Am 1995;20(4):650–6.

35. Howard RF, Ondrovic L, Greenwald DP. Biomechanical analysis of four-strand extensor tendon repair techniques. J Hand Surg Am 1997;22(5): 838–42.

36. Woo SH, Tsai TM, Kleinert HE, et al. A biomechanical comparison of four extensor tendon repair techniques in zone IV. Plast Reconstr Surg 2005; 115(6):1674–81 [discussion: 1682–3].

37. Lee SK, Dubey A, Kim BH, et al. A biomechanical study of extensor tendon repair methods: introduction to the running-interlocking horizontal mattress extensor tendon repair technique. J Hand Surg Am 2010;35(1):19–23.

Nerve Transfers

A.H. Wong, MD[a,b],*, T.J. Pianta, MD[a], D.J. Mastella, MD[a]

KEYWORDS

- Nerve transfers • Peripheral nerve • Reconstruction • Sensory • Motor

KEY POINTS

- There is a time and place for each option on the reconstructive ladder, and, when appropriately selected, nerve transfers have been shown to restore function in cases previously deemed difficult or impossible.
- If the goal is to achieve motor function, the donor nerve should be as purely motor as possible. The same is true for sensory function.
- The functional loss from transferring the donor nerve should be less than the expected functional gain of the recipient nerve.

INTRODUCTION

Several options currently exist for the treatment of peripheral nerve injuries. Similar to planning a strategy for soft tissue coverage, repair of nerve injuries may be thought of as a reconstructive ladder. At the bottom of the ladder, nonoperative treatment is selected for self-resolving nerve insults such as neurapraxia. If the nerve is transected and a tension-free anastomosis is possible, primary repair is chosen. If the repair cannot be performed without tension, then the treatment options diverge depending on the patient and the type of injury.

The concept of nerve transfers is not new, but the technique is evolving and has gained acceptance over the years. There is a time and place for each option on the reconstructive ladder and, when appropriately selected, nerve transfers have been reliably shown to restore function in cases previously deemed difficult or impossible. This article discusses a brief history of nerve transfers, general principles, and some specific transfers, and provides an overview of postoperative rehabilitation following motor and sensory transfers.

HISTORY

Nerve transfers have been performed since the 1900s to treat root avulsion and other difficult nerve injuries. As early as 1921, Harris[1] described a radial to median nerve transfer to treat a low median nerve injury suffered during World War I; the patient's sensation gradually improved over the next 3 months. Pollock and Davis[2] were skeptical of the procedure, stating that "a complete return of physiologic function does not occur" after transfer. Despite this dismissal of the technique, Turnbull[3] reported on 4 radial to median nerve transfers in 1948. In his initial report, Turnbull[3] described return of sensation "of a 'crude' quality" in each of his 4 patients. He then examined these patients 16 years later and confirmed appropriate localization in 3 of the original 4 patients, although he again described their sensory results as "crude."[4] He concluded that these were better results than were previously thought possible, especially in otherwise irreparable nerve injuries.[3,4]

Despite these relative successes, nerve transfers still did not gain wide acceptance until the introduction of the microscope for nerve repairs in the 1960s.[5] In 1974, Sunderland[6] cited unpredictable and largely unsuccessful results with the radial to median nerve transfer, stating that using the superficial radial nerve for the procedure would remove too much sensation from the thumb, index, and middle fingers; he therefore proposed transfer of dorsal rami of the ulnar nerve to the median nerve instead. To further investigate

a University of Connecticut Combined Hand Surgery Fellowship Program, Farmington; Hartford Hospital, Hartford, CT, USA; b University of Miami Plastic Surgery Residency Program, Miami, FL, USA
* Corresponding author.
E-mail address: anselm.wong@gmail.com

Hand Clin 28 (2012) 571–577
http://dx.doi.org/10.1016/j.hcl.2012.08.007
0749-0712/12/$ – see front matter © 2012 Elsevier Inc. All rights reserved.

these criticisms, Chacha and colleagues[7–9] performed both Turnbull's[3] and Sunderland's[6] nerve transfers in monkeys. Certain enzymes, such as cholinesterase, are absent in cases of neuropathy and increase with intact nerve function. Chacha and colleagues[7] used these principles to show increased enzymatic activity and therefore nerve regeneration in the thumb, index, and middle fingers after both procedures.

In 1983, Bedeschi and colleagues[10] duplicated Turnbull's[3] and Sunderland's[6] transfers in human patients. Out of their 5 patients, 3 had excellent recovery at their 5-year follow-up. This result led them to confirm that nerve transfers were a reasonable surgical solution for long-standing median nerve injuries. Matloubi[11] built on these results by performing the transfers in 37 patients, and showed satisfactory to excellent results in all but 3 of his patients.

Around the same time as Turnbull's[3] work in the late 1940s, Alexander Lurje[12] treated a patient with Erb palsy by combining several transfers, including transferring the long thoracic nerve to the suprascapular nerve, the anterior thoracic to the musculocutaneous nerve, and the radial to the axillary nerve. In 1948, he showed good follow-up results in his patient; pectoralis and triceps function had improved, and the patient's atrophy of her deltoid, biceps, and scapular muscles disappeared.[12] However, for several decades afterward, further experimentation with transfers was delayed because of the great successes of Millesi and colleagues[13,14] with nerve grafts.[15] It was not until the 1970s and 1980s that interest in nerve transfers was revived. Even with Millesi and colleagues[13,14] advancement of nerve grafting techniques, loss of biceps function caused by brachial plexus injuries was too difficult to treat with nerve grafts alone.

One of the early revivals of transfers for biceps restoration was performed in the 1980s by Brandt and Mackinnon,[16] in which the medial pectoral nerve was transferred to the musculocutaneous nerve, and the lateral antebrachial cutaneous directly to the biceps muscle. Another transfer from the early 1990s for biceps flexion was the eponymous Oberlin transfer, in which a portion of the ulnar nerve was sutured to the motor nerve of the biceps.[17] Although modifications to this transfer have been described since, the procedure is still successful and has reproducible results.

Because of the increasingly reliable success with various nerve transfers, the concept and procedures have gained greater acceptance as a viable treatment strategy. Standard nerve transfers have been used more frequently, and innovative nerve transfers have been developed to treat a variety of deficits. The development and refinement of these procedures continues.

INDICATIONS

The benefits of nerve transfers are well described.[18] In most cases, as in the Oberlin transfer, there is only 1 neurorrhaphy site; with nerve grafts, there are 2. In addition, nerve transfers minimize the distance over which a nerve has to regenerate. Given that nerves regenerate approximately 1 mm/d, the distance involved in proximal nerve injuries is too great to expect significant recovery. A nerve transfer converts a high proximal nerve injury to a more distal nerve injury, which may accelerate muscle reinnervation.[19] For an elderly patient or patient with significant scarring, a nerve transfer is a good choice compared with a nerve graft requiring more extensive dissection.[20–22] In addition, with modern nerve stimulator technology, it is easier to ensure that a motor nerve is anastomosed to a motor nerve, and a sensory nerve to a sensory nerve. As Brenner and colleagues[23] have shown, this yields better results than if a mixed motor-sensory nerve is anastomosed to a pure motor nerve.

Although tendon transfers are common procedures in the setting of prolonged nerve deficits, nerve transfers require less dissection and postoperative immobilization.[24] Guelinckx and colleagues'[25] work on rabbits confirms that, functionally, simple tenotomy is inferior to reinnervating a denervated muscle. However, nerve transfers cannot replace tendon transfers or nerve grafts on the reconstructive ladder. For certain problems, the best surgical strategy for a patient might be a combination of both nerve and tendon transfers; for example, a median to radial nerve transfer combined with a pronator teres to extensor carpi radialis brevis tendon transfer.[21]

GENERAL PRINCIPLES

Considerations in selecting a donor nerve for nerve transfer include[24,26]:

- If the goal is to achieve motor function, the donor nerve should be as purely motor as possible. The same is true for sensory function.
- The functional loss from transferring the donor nerve should be much less than the expected functional gain of the recipient nerve.
- The donor nerve should be sufficiently mobilized to achieve direct anastomosis with the recipient nerve.
- The donor and recipient nerves should have similar caliber.
- Postoperative reeducation is crucial for functional recovery.

- The donor nerve should ideally be uninjured.
- In cases that are not ideal, even injured and recovering nerves may still be used.
- In sensory nerve transfers, the denervated end should be anastomosed in an end-to-side fashion.
- There should be synergy between pretransfer donor nerve function and the intended recipient nerve function.

As an example of the last guideline regarding synergistic transfers, Ray and Mackinnon[27] have shown smoother postoperative reeducation after transferring the nerve to the flexor digitorum superficialis (FDS) to the nerve to the extensor carpi radialis brevis (ECRB) and the nerve to the flexor carpi radialis (FCR) to the posterior interosseous nerve (PIN), as opposed to FCR to ECRB and FDS to PIN transfers. Although the extensor muscles are still reinnervated, the antagonistic nerve transfers lead to poorer outcomes.

For motor recovery, surgical priority should be assigned first to elbow flexion before shoulder abduction and external rotation; for sensation, the priority is to restore sensation to the ulnar thumb and radial index finger for pinch.[22] As with any surgery, the patient should be able to tolerate the operation, general anesthesia, and should be mentally competent for rehabilitation. The wound should be clean with no active infection, and there should be enough soft tissue available for appropriate coverage.

Another important consideration is the timing of surgery. Even though nerve transfers have the advantage of requiring less time for reinnervation, the target muscles need to be reinnervated before they are irreversibly atrophied and replaced by fat cells, ideally before 12 to 18 months after injury, and certainly before 2 years.[20,21] With closed traction nerve injuries (neuropraxia), 3 months of observation is recommended because these injuries often recover spontaneously.[20]

Early reconstruction should be avoided in patients with neuritis for the same reason. In addition, if the intended target muscle is already irrecoverably deinnervated and atrophied, then traditional tendon transfers are indicated rather than nerve transfers. In cases with a narrow zone of injury, the nerves should be either primarily repaired or reconstructed with a nerve graft.[20]

With any nerve transfer, it is important to ensure a tension-free anastomosis. The mantra made famous by Mackinnon's group is "Donor distal, recipient proximal," which they recite before and during each nerve transfer they perform.[20,27,28] Besides the obvious advantage of enabling the patient to start on earlier motion and achieve better functional results from therapy, a tension-free anastomosis is also crucial for optimal nerve regeneration. Sunderland and colleagues'[29] study in rats showed that, once a critical state of tension was exceeded, nerve regeneration attempts resulted in decreased fiber count, nerve density, and percent nerve tissue.

For measuring recovery, most investigators report their sensory and motor recovery results based on Mackinnon and Dellon's[30] modifications to the British Medical Research Council's (MRC) report:

Sensory function

S0: Absence of sensibility
S1: Deep cutaneous pain sensation in the autonomous zone
S2: Some degree of superficial pain sensation and tactile sensibility
S2+: Same as S2, but with overresponse to stimuli
S3: Same as S2+ without over-reaction
S3+: good localization of stimuli and some return of 2-point discrimination
S4: complete recovery

Motor function

M0: no movement
M1: visible or palpable contraction
M2: muscle able to move joint when gravity eliminated
M3: contraction against gravity
M4: contraction against moderate resistance
M5: normal strength

SPECIFIC TRANSFERS

There are numerous nerve transfers that have been described in the literature, and therefore the discussion of all described nerve transfers is outside the scope of this article. This article focuses on a few classic nerve transfers to highlight the concepts and expected outcomes of these procedures.

As stated earlier, the resurgence of nerve transfers for brachial plexus reconstruction began with attempts to recover biceps function after injury. The nerve transfer published by Brandt and Mackinnon[16] (medial pectoral nerve to the musculocutaneous, lateral antecubital cutaneous directly to the biceps) showed promising results. Out of the 5 patients undergoing this transfer, 3 recovered elbow flexion against resistance, 1 had M3 recovery, and only 1 had no recovery at all. Oberlin and colleagues' technique, published shortly afterward, transferred a fascicle of the ulnar nerve (flexor carpi ulnaris [FCU]) to the motor nerve of the biceps. Of the 4 cases described, 3 recovered M4 strength and the other M3.[17]

Mackinnon's group further modified the Oberlin procedure by recruiting the brachialis muscle as an additional elbow flexor. In this so-called supercharged or Oberlin-plus technique, the FCU fascicle is transferred as before, but a branch of the median nerve (redundant fascicles to the flexor carpi radialis or flexor digitorum profundus/superficialis) is also transferred to a brachialis branch. The brachialis then fulfills its role as a primary elbow flexor, and the reinnervated biceps acts as both a supinator and elbow flexor. At the 6-month mark, 4 of these Oberlin-plus patients recovered MRC grade 4+ strength, and 2 patients had grade 4 strength.[19] Liverneaux and colleagues[31] also achieved superior results with the Oberlin-plus procedure, reporting a 100% recovery of MRC grade 4 in 10 cases.

In his single-surgeon retrospective review, Estrella[32] reported M4 elbow flexion recovery in 8 of 9 patients with either the Oberlin or Oberlin-plus, although he noted that the measured force of flexion was inferior to Liverneaux and colleagues'[31] results (2.7 kg compared with 3.7 kg). The Oberlin and Oberlin-plus transfers have been compared recently by Carlsen and colleagues,[33] who found no statistical difference between the two. They also observed that the patients who underwent the double nerve transfer had less severe injuries and higher preoperative DASH (Disabilities of Arm, Shoulder, and Hand) scores. As the investigators stated, this method of patient selection skews any superior results seen with the Oberlin-plus transfer.

Both the single and double nerve versions of the Oberlin transfer have proved so reliable that the indications have expanded over time. Although the best results are achieved with earlier reinnervation, Sedain and colleagues[34] performed the Oberlin transfer on 9 patients between 7 and 24 months following injury. All patients recovered useful biceps function, even the patient who was operated on 2 years after injury. On the other end of the spectrum, Shigematsu and colleagues[35] performed an Oberlin nerve transfer in an 8-month-old infant for obstetric brachial plexus palsy. Although this approach was aggressive compared with the typical watchful waiting period over 3 to 4 months, the investigators found full range of motion in elbow flexion and shoulder abduction. However, they noted that strength was still slightly less compared with the contralateral side.

Although more and more surgeons were beginning to use nerve transfers to successfully restore elbow function, it took longer for many to accept that the technique is as useful below the elbow. Skeptics doubted that nerve transfers could restore intrinsic muscle function and digital flexion.[36] However, even very distal nerve transfers have been performed and described with encouraging results. When discussing donor nerve selection for nerve transfers, Wood and Murray[26] eloquently point out that it is "limited only by human anatomy and human ingenuity." This observation applies not only to donor nerve selection but to nerve transfers. New techniques are continually being developed to treat a wide range of different problems.

As early as 1991, Mackinnon's group performed distal median to ulnar nerve transfers to restore ulnar intrinsic nerve function after high ulnar nerve injuries.[28] In this procedure, the anterior interosseus nerve is transferred to the deep motor branch of the ulnar nerve. Haase and Chung[37] presented 2 patients in whom this was performed. A nerve graft was used on the second patient because of excessive tension on the repair. In both patients, they described reinnervation of the intrinsics as seen on clinical examination and nerve conduction studies.[37]

A modification by Battiston and Lanzetta[38] also uses the transfer from the distal anterior interosseus nerve to the motor branch of the ulnar nerve, and adds a superficial sensory palmar branch of the median nerve to reinnervate the sensory ulnar nerve at Guyon's canal; in their own words, a surgically created Martin-Gruber anastomosis. For motor recovery, they reported 5 out of 7 patients with M4 strength after 2 years; 1 patient had M2 strength and the remaining patient had M5. Their sensory results were also encouraging, because 5 patients recovered S4 sensation and the others had S3+ recovery.[38] The 1 patient with M5 recovery was only 11 years old, but they still achieved good results with rest of their patients who ranged in age from their 20s to 50s.

To address sensory protection for the hypothenar aspect of the hand, Flores[39] adds a transfer of the superficial ulnar nerve to the third common palmar digital nerve. Although the sensation in the ring and small fingers does not contribute to fine manipulation of objects, Flores[39] aimed to prevent ulcerations from chronic anesthesia in that area. The anterior interosseous nerve to the motor branch of the ulnar nerve was performed as previously described, and resulted in 3 out of the 5 patients with M4 recovery compared with the preoperative baseline of complete ulnar palsy. With an end-to-side anastomosis of the superficial ulnar nerve to the third common palmar digital nerve, 2 patients achieved S4 sensory recovery, and the rest were graded at either S3 or S3+.

For high median nerve lesions, Bertelli and Ghizoni[40] described restoration of fingertip sensation by transferring very distal radial nerve branches to the palmar nerves at the level of the proximal phalanx. Similar to Flores'[39] rationale, the goal was to prevent cutaneous ulcers; in this case, on the fingertips. By transferring dorsal branches of the radial nerve from the index and thumb to the palmar nerves, they were able to show recovery of protective sensation in the thumb and index fingers. Locognosia was improved, with all 8 patients correctly localizing sensation in their thumbs. However, in half of their patients, stimuli to the index fingertip pulp were incorrectly localized to the dorsal proximal phalanx. Despite this, their work with nerve transfers show it is possible to restore at least some degree of sensation to the fingertips.[40]

A transfer from the median to the radial nerve can be applied as well. Redundant branches of the median nerve are typically transferred to branches of the radial nerve, such as the PIN and the nerve to the extensor carpi radialis brevis. Ray and Mackinnon[27] treated 19 patients with radial nerve palsy, and 11 achieved at least 4 out of 5 wrist and finger extension. An additional 5 patients had 4 out of 5 wrist extension but minimal finger extension. Only 1 patient failed to recover either wrist or finger extension to any degree. Nine of the patients additionally had a pronator teres to ECRB tendon transfer performed at the time of surgery to augment wrist extension. Although this would bias the nerve transfer results, it provides an example of a combination of nerve and tendon transfers being used as a treatment strategy. The other observation from this study is that the nerve to the FDS must be transferred to the ECRB and the nerve to the FCR to the PIN. If the FDS is transferred to the PIN and the FCR to the ECRB, the nerve transfers prove to be too antagonistic to achieve any meaningful motor function, even after tendon transfers are performed.

POSTOPERATIVE REHABILITATION

It has been widely published that the brain shows remarkable plasticity. Cortical reorganization has been shown not only in the acute setting but even long after nerve injury.[41] Results after nerve transfers are no exception. In their work with adult monkeys, Pons and colleagues[42] showed that the brain was able to reorganize its somatosensory cortical mapping to a greater degree than was previously thought. Merzenich and Jenkins[43] studied a variety of clinical situations in monkeys, such as denervation, nerve transection with repair, and behavioral training with varying stimuli. The somatosensory system was able to correct itself to properly localize stimulated sites, and this took place at the cortical level.[43] In addition, the most dramatic representational changes occurred with behavioral reinforcement.[43] This finding underscores the clinical importance of sensory rehabilitation. Imai and colleagues[44] confirmed that, after median nerve repairs, patients who underwent early sensory reeducation had less severe paresthesias and fared better with 2-point discrimination.

In addition to relearning sensory distribution, the brain is remarkable in its ability to relearn motor function. Malessy and colleagues[45] studied the cortical areas responsible for elbow flexion and showed remapping after intercostal to musculocutaneous nerve transfers. Anastakis and colleagues[46] confirmed the remapping process with functional MRI studies, and noted that reinforcement and repetition seemed to be the keys to successful motor learning following motor nerve transfers.

The early rehabilitation of nerve transfers is comparable with the rehabilitation of standard nerve repairs.[47] With no intraoperative tension at the anastomosis, the patient is generally immobilized for 7 to 10 days.[47] Unless nerve grafts are used, the patients are begun on range-of-motion exercises of the uninvolved adjacent joints as soon as 2 to 3 days after surgery. However, the patient should use a splint or sling to protect against excessive range of motion at the repair site.[48] In the case of the Oberlin transfer, the sling is worn for 2 to 3 weeks. After this time, the patient works on elbow range of motion and begins formal physical therapy at 6 weeks.[49] Early on, the goal is to maintain full passive range of motion by ensuring a balance in muscle pull. Resting splints can be applied to keep extensor tendons from overstretching and flexor tendons from overtightening; joint stiffness may be treated by stretching the muscles to prevent tightness.[48]

Muscle strength and endurance is crucial for restoration of function. In the case of motor nerve transfers, the patient must relearn how to contract the muscle. The patient must therefore initially co-contract both the donor muscle and new muscle, although eventually the patient should be able to contract the new muscle independently. For example, if the nerve to the FCU is transferred to the musculocutaneous nerve, the patient learns that the FCU must be flexed before he the elbow can be flexed; similarly, after an intercostal to musculocutaneous transfer, the patient starts with deep breathing exercises to initiate biceps flexion followed by abdominal strengthening exercises.[47] Relearning and motor rehabilitation is easier after transferring a synergistic donor nerve as opposed to an antagonistic nerve.[27,47] With any transfer, the keys to performance and improvement of a motor task are practice and repetition.[50]

Sensory reeducation can be broken down into early and late phases. During the early phase, only the specific distribution of the recovering nerve should be challenged. Otherwise, stimulation of multiple areas leads to competition over the same cortical region.[47] In addition, the stimulus should be delivered by an inanimate object as opposed to the patient's other hand to prevent cortical confusion. In protocol by Dellon and Jabaley,[51] the patient strokes the area with a pencil eraser, closes the eyes to focus on what they are feeling, and then opens the eyes to confirm and reinforce the sensation. As locognosia gradually improves, the patient is given increasingly discriminatory tasks to fine-tune the sensation.[48] This transition to the late phase may be several months after the transfer is performed, and it is during this time that the patient improves 2-point discrimination and learns to differentiate between common household objects.[51] Because the processes of cortical reactivation and reorganization continue long after injury, the late phase may continue many months or longer after surgery.[41,48]

SUMMARY

Many creative nerve transfers other than those listed have been attempted, and many more have yet to be performed and described. Even though it is beyond the scope of this article to list all the numerous transfers that have shown encouraging results, there is ample evidence to justify nerve transfers as a useful option in the hand surgeon's armamentarium. Also, nerve transfers and tendon transfers are not mutually exclusive. Different procedures are therefore best suited to different patients and patterns of injury. There are occasions when a nerve transfer would have the best results. There are also cases in which the patient would benefit most from a tendon transfer or a nerve graft instead. In some rare occasions, a combination of all 3 techniques might best serve the patient. When chosen for the appropriate situation, the nerve transfer is a time-tested procedure.

REFERENCES

1. Harris RI. The treatment of irreparable nerve injuries. Can Med Assoc J 1921;11:833–41.
2. Pollock LJ, Davis L. Peripheral nerve injuries. New York: PB Hoeber; 1933.
3. Turnbull F. Radial-median anastomosis. J Neurosurg 1948;5:562–6.
4. Turnbull F. Restoration of digital sensation after transference of nerves. J Neurosurg 1963;20:238–40.
5. Smith JW. Microsurgery of peripheral nerves. Plast Reconstr Surg 1964;33:317–29.
6. Sunderland S. The restoration of median nerve function after destructive lesions which preclude end-to-end repair. Brain 1974;97:1–14.
7. Chacha PB, Krishnamurti A, Soin K. Experimental sensory reinnervation of the median nerve by nerve transfer in monkeys. J Bone Joint Surg Am 1977;59:386–90.
8. Wong WC, Kanagasuntheram R. Early and late effects of median nerve injury on Meissner's and Pacinian corpuscles of the hand of the macaque (M. fascicularis). J Anat 1971;109:135–42.
9. Vij S, Kanagasuntheram R, Krishnamurti A. Enzymic changes in taste buds of monkey following transection of glossopharyngeal nerve. J Anat 1972;113:425–32.
10. Bedeschi P, Celli L, Balli A. Transfer of sensory nerves in hand surgery. J Hand Surg Br 1984;9:46–9.
11. Matloubi R. Transfer of sensory branches of radial nerve in hand surgery. J Hand Surg Br 1988;13:92–5.
12. Lurje A. Concerning surgical treatment of traumatic injury to the upper division of the brachial plexus (Erb's type). Ann Surg 1948;127:317–26.
13. Millesi H, Meissl G, Berger A. The interfascicular nerve-grafting of the median and ulnar nerves. J Bone Joint Surg Am 1972;54:727–50.
14. Millesi H, Meissl G, Berger A. Further experience with interfascicular grafting of the median, ulnar, and radial nerves. J Bone Joint Surg Am 1976;58:209–18.
15. Naff NJ, Ecklund JM. History of peripheral nerve surgery techniques. Neurosurg Clin North Am 2001;12:197–209, x.
16. Brandt KE, Mackinnon SE. A technique for maximizing biceps recovery in brachial plexus reconstruction. J Hand Surg 1993;18:726–33.
17. Oberlin C, Beal D, Leechavengvongs S, et al. Nerve transfer to biceps muscle using a part of ulnar nerve for C5-C6 avulsion of the brachial plexus: anatomical study and report of four cases. J Hand Surg 1994;19:232–7.
18. Brown JM, Shah MN, Mackinnon SE. Distal nerve transfers: a biology-based rationale. Neurosurg Focus 2009;26:E12.
19. Mackinnon SE, Novak CB, Myckatyn TM, et al. Results of reinnervation of the biceps and brachialis muscles with a double fascicular transfer for elbow flexion. J Hand Surg 2005;30:978–85.
20. Mackinnon SE, Colbert SH. Nerve transfers in the hand and upper extremity surgery. Tech Hand Up Extrem Surg 2008;12:20–33.
21. Tung TH, Mackinnon SE. Nerve transfers: indications, techniques, and outcomes. J Hand Surg 2010;35:332–41.

22. Dvali L, Mackinnon S. Nerve repair, grafting, and nerve transfers. Clin Plast Surg 2003;30:203–21.
23. Brenner MJ, Hess JR, Myckatyn TM, et al. Repair of motor nerve gaps with sensory nerve inhibits regeneration in rats. Laryngoscope 2006;116:1685–92.
24. Mackinnon SE, Humphreys DB. Nerve transfers. Operat Tech Plast Reconstr Surg 2002;9:89–99.
25. Guelinckx PJ, Carlson BM, Faulkner JA. Morphologic characteristics of muscles grafted in rabbits with neurovascular repair. J Reconstr Microsurg 1992;8:481–9.
26. Wood MB, Murray PM. Heterotopic nerve transfers: recent trends with expanding indication. J Hand Surg 2007;32:397–408.
27. Ray WZ, Mackinnon SE. Clinical outcomes following median to radial nerve transfers. J Hand Surg 2011; 36:201–8.
28. Brown JM, Yee A, Mackinnon SE. Distal median to ulnar nerve transfers to restore ulnar motor and sensory function within the hand: technical nuances. Neurosurgery 2009;65:966–77 [discussion: 977–8].
29. Sunderland IR, Brenner MJ, Singham J, et al. Effect of tension on nerve regeneration in rat sciatic nerve transection model. Ann Plast Surg 2004;53:382–7.
30. Mackinnon SE, Dellon AL. Surgery of the peripheral nerve. New York: Thieme; 1988. p. 118.
31. Liverneaux PA, Diaz LC, Beaulieu JY, et al. Preliminary results of double nerve transfer to restore elbow flexion in upper type brachial plexus palsies. Plast Reconstr Surg 2006;117:915–9.
32. Estrella EP. Functional outcome of nerve transfers for upper-type brachial plexus injuries. J Plast Reconstr Aesthet Surg 2011;64:1007–13.
33. Carlsen BT, Kircher MF, Spinner RJ, et al. Comparison of single versus double nerve transfers for elbow flexion after brachial plexus injury. Plast Reconstr Surg 2011;127:269–76.
34. Sedain G, Sharma MS, Sharma BS, et al. Outcome after delayed Oberlin transfer in brachial plexus injury. Neurosurgery 2011;69:822–7 [discussion: 827–8].
35. Shigematsu K, Yajima H, Kobata Y, et al. Oberlin partial ulnar nerve transfer for restoration in obstetric brachial plexus palsy of a newborn: case report. J Brachial Plex Peripher Nerve Inj 2006;1:3.
36. Rohde RS, Wolfe SW. Nerve transfers for adult traumatic brachial plexus palsy (brachial plexus nerve transfer). HSS J 2007;3:77–82.
37. Haase SC, Chung KC. Anterior interosseous nerve transfer to the motor branch of the ulnar nerve for high ulnar nerve injuries. Ann Plast Surg 2002;49: 285–90.
38. Battiston B, Lanzetta M. Reconstruction of high ulnar nerve lesions by distal double median to ulnar nerve transfer. J Hand Surg 1999;24:1185–91.
39. Flores LP. Distal anterior interosseous nerve transfer to the deep ulnar nerve and end-to-side suture of the superficial ulnar nerve to the third common palmar digital nerve for treatment of high ulnar nerve injuries: experience in five cases. Arq Neuropsiquiatr 2011;69:519–24.
40. Bertelli JA, Ghizoni MF. Very distal sensory nerve transfers in high median nerve lesions. J Hand Surg 2011;36:387–93.
41. Cusick CG, Wall JT, Whiting JH Jr, et al. Temporal progression of cortical reorganization following nerve injury. Brain Res 1990;537:355–8.
42. Pons TP, Garraghty PE, Ommaya AK, et al. Massive cortical reorganization after sensory deafferentation in adult macaques. Science 1991;252:1857–60.
43. Merzenich MM, Jenkins WM. Reorganization of cortical representations of the hand following alterations of skin inputs induced by nerve injury, skin island transfers, and experience. J Hand Ther 1993;6:89–104.
44. Imai H, Tajima T, Natsumi Y. Successful reeducation of functional sensibility after median nerve repair at the wrist. J Hand Surg 1991;16:60–5.
45. Malessy MJ, van der Kamp W, Thomeer RT, et al. Cortical excitability of the biceps muscle after intercostal-to-musculocutaneous nerve transfer. Neurosurgery 1998;42:787–94 [discussion: 794–5].
46. Anastakis DJ, Malessy MJ, Chen R, et al. Cortical plasticity following nerve transfer in the upper extremity. Hand Clin 2008;24:425–44, vi–vii.
47. Novak CB. Rehabilitation following motor nerve transfers. Hand Clin 2008;24:417–23, vi.
48. Mackinnon SE, Novak CB. Nerve transfers. New options for reconstruction following nerve injury. Hand Clin 1999;15:643–66, ix.
49. Toussaint CP, Zager EL. The double fascicular nerve transfer for restoration of elbow flexion. Neurosurgery 2011;68:64–7 [discussion: 67].
50. Duff SV. Impact of peripheral nerve injury on sensorimotor control. J Hand Ther 2005;18:277–91.
51. Dellon AL, Jabaley ME. Reeducation of sensation in the hand following nerve suture. Clin Orthop Relat Res 1982;163:75–9.

Suture-Button Suspensionplasty for the Treatment of Thumb Carpometacarpal Joint Arthritis

Jeffrey Yao, MD

KEYWORDS

- Thumb carpometacarpal arthritis • Suture button • Tightrope • Suspensionplasty
- Thumb arthroscopy

KEY POINTS

- Trapeziectomy alone has regained popularity for the treatment of thumb carpometacarpal joint arthritis, and the literature supports its use for this common problem.
- Suture button suspensionplasty eliminates the need for troublesome Kirschner wire fixation following trapeziectomy.
- Suture button suspensionplasty requires no soft tissue healing and therefore rehabilitation following this procedure may be begun as early as one week following surgery, thereby accelerating recovery.

INTRODUCTION

The thumb carpometacarpal (CMC) joint is a biconcave joint consisting of 2 saddle-shaped bones that articulate perpendicularly with each other. This unique biconcave configuration allows a wide range of motion essential for activities requiring pinch and grip. However, this increased range of motion comes at the expense of limited stability. Also, there are significant loads transmitted across this joint. A 1-kg pinch at the tip of the thumb translates into a 13-kg load at the base of the thumb.[1] As a result of such high loads during activities of daily living, the thumb CMC joint is the second most common site for the development of degenerative osteoarthritis in the upper limb.[1,2]

Osteoarthritis of the thumb CMC joint is initially treated nonoperatively with activity modification, splinting, antiinflammatory drugs, and intra-articular corticosteroid injections.[2] Surgical options are considered once these conservative measures have failed. There are numerous surgical techniques for treating thumb CMC arthritis. These techniques include volar ligament reconstruction,[3] first metacarpal osteotomy,[4–7] CMC joint arthrodesis,[8,9] total joint arthroplasty,[10] and trapeziectomy.[11,12] Partial or full trapeziectomy may be performed alone or with tendon interposition, ligament reconstruction, or ligament reconstruction combined with tendon interposition.[13–18] In addition, some of these techniques may be performed with an open technique or arthroscopically.[19–21] Comparative studies have shown no significant long-term differences in outcomes among these techniques,[22–25] except that trapeziectomy alone has the lowest incidence of complications[23,24] and the shortest intraoperative time.[18] Without appreciable long-term differences among methods, efforts have been made to find techniques that yield shorter recovery periods and better short-term outcomes.

Commonly, partial or full excision of the trapezium is accompanied by stabilization of the first metacarpal to prevent subsidence into the newly

Department of Orthopaedic Surgery, Stanford University, 450 Broadway Street, Suite C-442, Redwood City, CA 94063, USA
E-mail address: jyao@stanford.edu

Hand Clin 28 (2012) 579–585
http://dx.doi.org/10.1016/j.hcl.2012.08.013
0749-0712/12/$ – see front matter

created CMC space. In theory, this space is maintained for proper hematoma and scar tissue formation. Stabilization has been historically achieved by fixating the first metacarpal with a Kirschner wire (K-wire) to the second metacarpal, and maintaining the K-wire for the immediate postoperative period. However, K-wire fixation limits early recovery and mobilization of the thumb, because the wire is not removed until 4 weeks after surgery.

One alternative technique involves a suture-button (SB) suspensionplasty to overcome the limitations of K-wire fixation by using an SB implant to resist subsidence.[26] The SB device I use consists of braided polyester sutures (FiberWire, Arthrex, Naples FL) looped between 2 steel buttons: 1 button attaches to the base of the first metacarpal and the other button attaches to the second metacarpal (**Fig. 1**). This arrangement suspends the thumb ray from the second metacarpal and effectively prevents subsidence of the first metacarpal into the CMC space. Compared with K-wire fixation, SB suspensionplasty has been shown to achieve similar stability.[27] However, this suspensionplasty technique allows mobilization of the thumb as early as 10 days postoperatively because there is no implant left outside the skin. Early initiation of movement potentially leads to faster restoration of function and reduced recovery time. As a result, patients may return to work and engage in activities of daily living earlier, with increased satisfaction and quality of life.

INDICATIONS AND RATIONALE

The rationale for selecting the appropriate thumb CMC arthritis treatment is dependent on radiographic classifications defined by Eaton and Glickel.[28] The SB suspensionplasty technique may be performed with an arthroscopically assisted hemitrapeziectomy for patients presenting with Eaton stage II or III (see **Fig. 1**).[26] For Eaton stage IV, the procedure is performed after a traditional open technique of full trapeziectomy. My operative

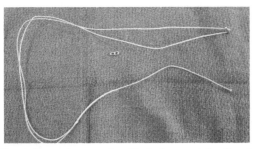

Fig. 1. Second-generation SB device used for thumb CMC suspensionplasty.

preferences and approaches based on Eaton stage are described in the next sections.

Eaton Stage I

This stage in the disease process is characterized by mild widening of the trapeziometacarpal joint as a result of some synovitis or effusion. Patients with Eaton stage I disease who are symptomatic despite nonoperative management may be treated with arthroscopic debridement, synovectomy, and electrothermal capsulorrhaphy.[29,30] Arthroplasty is generally not performed in this setting.

Eaton Stage II and III

Osteophyte formation, CMC joint-space destruction, and sclerotic bone development characterize Eaton stages II and III. These disease stages may be treated with any of the techniques mentioned earlier. My previous preference was to treat these patients with arthroscopic hemitrapeziectomy, with K-wire pinning across the CMC joint to prevent subsidence. However, as mentioned earlier, K-wire fixation immobilizes the thumb for 4 weeks postoperatively. This situation does not allow early range of motion and because of wire irritation or complications, this technique is a cause of considerable patient dissatisfaction. This article describes an alternative technique that leads to earlier mobilization of the thumb and provides effective resistance to subsidence.

Eaton Stage IV

Eaton stage IV is distinguished by pantrapezial spread of the disease; it is characterized by joint-space destruction at the CMC joint as well as at the scaphotrapeziotrapezoid joint. In this setting, a complete trapeziectomy through an open technique is indicated. A full trapeziectomy is appropriate to decrease the probability of continual pain from the scaphotrapeziotrapezoid joint. After excision of the trapezium, the CMC space is maintained with any of the techniques described earlier. My practice is to prevent subsidence of the thumb metacarpal with SB suspensionplasty after complete trapeziectomy.

SURGICAL TECHNIQUE
Arthroscopic Setup and Establishment of Portals

Arthroscopy is performed with either regional or general anesthesia. Regional anesthesia is preferred because it provides pain relief in the immediate postoperative period. A standard arthroscopy tower and a 2.3-mm arthroscope are needed for this procedure. To set up the operative field, the thumb is first placed in a finger trap and suspended from the arthroscopy tower (Linvatec, Largo, FL) at 5.44 to 6.8 kg (12 to 15 lbs) of longitudinal traction. The finger trap and hand are wrapped with a sterile elastic bandage (Coban [3M, St Paul, MN]) to stabilize it in the operative field (**Fig. 2**). The arm tourniquet is also positioned as proximal to the axilla as possible and inflated to 250 mm Hg.

The thumb CMC joint is located by palpating for a soft spot at the proximal end of the thumb metacarpal. The 1-U portal is named for its location ulnar to the extensor pollicis brevis (EPB). A syringe is used to inject normal saline solution into the thumb CMC space. The saline insufflates the joint to confirm the portal location and establish the appropriate angle of entry. Next, a number 11 scalpel is used to make a skin incision over the 1-U portal. The incision is gently spread using a blunt mosquito clamp to avoid injury to neighboring structures such as the abductor pollicis longus (APL), EPB, and extensor pollicis longus tendons, as well as the dorsal radial sensory nerve and radial artery. Once the level of the CMC joint capsule is reached, the previously injected saline solution should egress. A 2.3-mm arthroscope is then inserted into the joint, and fluoroscopy can be used to confirm the correct placement of the arthroscope in the CMC joint. A constant inflow of saline through the arthroscopy pump should

be set at 30 mm Hg to sufficiently distend the joint for proper visualization and clearing of debris.

Another portal (the working portal) is now established. Two choices are available for this portal: the 1-R or thenar portal. The 1-R portal is located radial to the APL at the same level as the 1-U portal, whereas the thenar portal is approximately 90° and 1 cm volar from the 1-R portal. In my opinion, the thenar portal is preferable over the 1-R portal because the thenar portal is farther away from structures vulnerable to injury, such as branches of the radial sensory nerve.[31] The perpendicular location of the thenar portal relative to the 1-U portal also enables better visualization during the arthroscopy and partial trapeziectomy because the instruments are orthogonal from each other (**Fig. 3**).

The proper location of the thenar portal is established by introducing an 18-gauge needle through the thenar musculature into the CMC joint. This procedure is performed under direct arthroscopic guidance. Once the proper position of the needle is confirmed, the thenar portal is established the same way the 1-U portal was established.

Arthroscopic Hemitrapeziectomy

A full-radius 3.5-mm shaver is introduced into the working portal. It is used to debride the joint of any remaining degenerative articular cartilage,

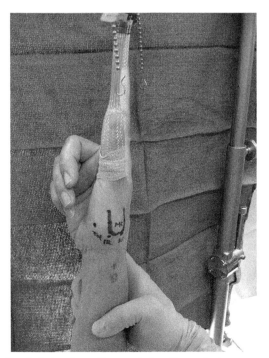

Fig. 2. Setup for arthroscopic hemitrapeziectomy.

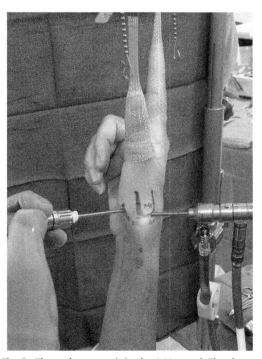

Fig. 3. The arthroscope is in the 1-U portal. The shaver is in the thenar portal.

articular debris, and synovitis. Frequently, loose bodies are encountered floating freely or fixed to soft tissue in the joint. These bodies should be removed. Once the debridement is complete, the 3.5-mm shaver is retracted and a 2.9-mm Vortex burr (Linvatec, Largo, FL) with a 3.5-mm sheath is introduced to perform the hemitrapeziectomy. Because the instrument is prone to becoming clogged, this arrangement of a smaller burr placed within a larger-sized sheath creates more space around the burr and minimizes the incidence of clogging. At least 3 to 5 mm of the distal trapezium should be removed for patients with Eaton stage II or III. During the procedure, alternating the instrument and the arthroscope between the 2 portals facilitates visualization and complete excision of the hemitrapezium. Fluoroscopy is also helpful in determining the level of resection and the amount of residual trapezium still present.

Next, a ballottement test is performed to establish a baseline level of subsidence before SB implantation. Alternating movements of pulling and compressing the thumb along the axis of the first metacarpal are visualized under spot or live fluoroscopy. The level of subsidence established at this point is later compared with the level of subsidence after SB device implantation (**Fig. 4**).

Open Trapeziectomy

Open trapeziectomy may be performed from a dorsoradial or volar (Wagner) approach. I prefer to

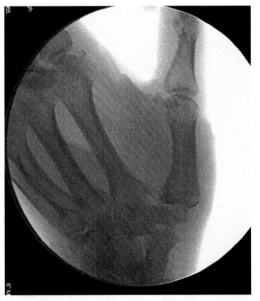

Fig. 4. Ballottement test shows complete subsidence of the thumb metacarpal with an axial load after complete trapeziectomy.

perform the trapeziectomy from a dorsoradial approach, with a 2.5-cm incision made directly over the tendons of the first dorsal extensor compartment and underlying CMC capsule. The APL and EPB tendons are then retracted and a longitudinal capsulotomy is performed, exposing the CMC joint. Full-thickness flaps of the capsule are elevated, and the underlying trapezium is dissected free from the rest of the capsule. With a combination of osteotomes and rongeurs, the trapezium is then removed, taking care to avoid injury to the flexor carpi radialis tendon deep within the wound. Similarly to the arthroscopic technique, a ballottement test is performed to establish a baseline level of subsidence before SB implantation.

SB Technique of Suspensionplasty

To place the SB device, a small incision is made immediately volar to the APL tendon, at the site of the 1-R portal. A blunt mosquito clamp is used to reach the dorsal radial aspect of the base of the first metacarpal. This placement promotes pronation of the thumb and also minimizes the chance of hardware prominence because it allows the SB to be placed beneath a portion of the APL tendon. When performed via an open approach, the dorsoradial aspect of the first metacarpal is also the location for the entry of the SB device.

A 1.1-mm SutureLasso guidewire (Arthrex, Naples, FL) is then introduced into the incision site and oriented in an oblique fashion from the base of the first metacarpal to the proximal diaphysis of the second metacarpal. In the first-generation technique, a 2.7-mm drill was then placed over the guidewire to drill the path for the suture button. However, because of concerns for fracture of the second metacarpal with this large drill, the second generation of this technique uses a newly engineered guidewire. This guidewire is specially designed to act as a suture passer by having a nitinol lasso attached to its proximal tip. An additional incision should be made immediately ulnar to the second metacarpal, and blunt dissection is used to reach down to the level of the bone. The second dorsal interosseous is elevated to allow for visualization of the ulnar aspect of the second metacarpal. Although the guidewire should be aimed towards the metadiaphyseal junction of the second metacarpal, the orientation of the guidewire is not important. Our unpublished data showed that an SB device placed with either a proximal or distal trajectory yields similar thumb ranges of motion, but that an SB device with a proximal trajectory is further away from the nerve to the first dorsal interosseous muscle than with a distal trajectory. There may therefore be no ideal trajectory of the SB device (from the thumb meta-carpal to the second metacarpal). The range of motion of the thumb in this cadaveric study was equivalent and full when the SB device traversed from the thumb to the diaphysis of the second metacarpal (distal trajectory) as well as a more horizontal (proximal trajectory) from the thumb to the metaphyseal area of the base of the second metacarpal. Therefore, our results suggest that the trajectory at which the SB device is placed is not crucial and does not adversely affect thumb range of motion.

The guidewire is drilled in a quadricortical fashion through both metacarpals. A C-clamp tar-geting guide may be useful to better control the placement and retrieval of the guidewire. The guidewire is then advanced fully through the center of the diaphysis to avoid iatrogenic fracture and retrieved out of the exit site (**Figs. 5** and **6**). As the guidewire is pulled through, the attached SB device is advanced with the guidewire. The prox-imal button is anchored on the base of the thumb metacarpal. The second button is placed over the sutures on to the second metacarpal, and the button is tensioned to sit flush against the dorsoul-nar cortex of the second metacarpal, with no inter-posed soft tissue.

At this point, correct tensioning should be set to prevent subsidence of the first metacarpal. Exces-sive tension should be avoided to prevent impingement between the first and second meta-carpal bases. One provisional knot is tied to the SB device and a repeat ballottement test is per-formed under fluoroscopy to assess adequate resistance to subsidence and to ensure there is no impingement (**Fig. 7**). The first ballottement test is used as a baseline. The thumb is also brought through a full range of motion to confirm

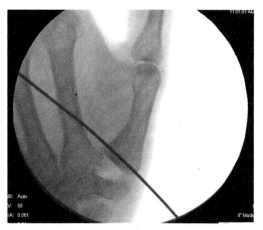

Fig. 6. Fluoroscopic view of the appropriate position of the guidewire.

that the implant has not been overtensioned. If necessary, adjustments to the tensioning may be made at this point. Once the tensioning is appro-priate, the remaining knots are securely tied and the suture ends are cut. The wounds are closed and the patient is placed in a short-arm thumb spica splint.

Aftercare

The patient returns for a follow-up visit within 2 weeks after surgery. The sutures are removed, radiographs are taken to display adequate mainte-nance of the thumb CMC space, and range-of-motion exercises are initiated with a hand therapist. At this time, a removable thermoplastic short-arm thumb spica splint is given to the patient to use as needed for comfort.

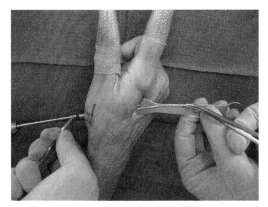

Fig. 5. Placement of the 1.1-mm guidewire from the thumb metacarpal to the diaphysis of the second metacarpal.

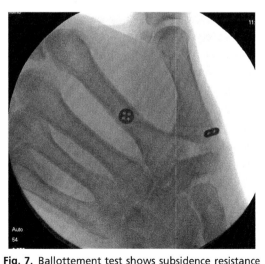

Fig. 7. Ballottement test shows subsidence resistance of the thumb metacarpal with an axial load after SB suspensionplasty.

RESULTS AND DISCUSSION

The arthroscopic technique is an effective and minimally invasive approach to treat thumb CMC arthritis. It may be combined with SB suspension-plasty to provide earlier mobilization of the thumb compared with conventional K-wire fixation, which requires at least 4 weeks of immobilization. For Eaton stage IV disease, I typically perform an open trapeziectomy and also use the SB suspension device and have also had excellent preliminary results.

I have performed the SB suspensionplasty on more than 40 patients, some of whom were more than 3 years postoperative (**Fig. 8**). I have had encouraging results, which are being prepared for publication. There have been 2 complications from this technique, both in the same patient. Six weeks postoperatively, this patient showed signs and symptoms of chronic regional pain syndrome with evidence of related disuse osteopenia. She subsequently fractured the second metacarpal. These complications occurred with the first-generation technique, and there have been no complications with the new second-generation

technique. Complications and inadequate fixation from the SB device have been reported in other areas of orthopedic surgery.[32–35] A recent report of a second metacarpal fracture was published with this technique.[36] This complication occurred with the first-generation technique.

Although the techniques currently available to treat thumb CMC arthritis deliver essentially equivalent results in the long-term, the usefulness of SB suspensionplasty after hemitrapeziectomy or full trapeziectomy may be its benefits in the short-term. Compared with K-wire fixation, SB suspensionplasty not only leads to earlier mobilization of the thumb but also avoids complications such as pin track infections, which may occur from K-wire fixation. We believe that faster overall recovery through earlier initiation of movement may increase patient satisfaction and enhance quality of life in the short-term. Further studies are necessary to validate the efficacy of the SB device, but preliminary results are encouraging.

REFERENCES

1. Cooney WP, Chao EY. Biomechanical analysis of static forces in the thumb during hand function. J Bone Joint Surg Am 1977;59(1):27–36.
2. Yao J, Park MJ. Early treatment of degenerative arthritis of the thumb carpometacarpal joint. Hand Clin 2008;24(3):251–61, v–vi.
3. Glickel SZ, Gupta S. Ligament reconstruction. Hand Clin 2006;22(2):143–51.
4. Wilson JN. Basal osteotomy of the first metacarpal in the treatment of arthritis of the carpometacarpal joint of the thumb. Br J Surg 1973;60(11):854–8.
5. Hobby JL, Lyall HA, Meggitt BF. First metacarpal osteotomy for trapeziometacarpal osteoarthritis. J Bone Joint Surg Br 1998;80(3):508–12.
6. Parker WL, Linscheid RL, Amadio PC. Long-term outcomes of first metacarpal extension osteotomy in the treatment of carpal-metacarpal osteoarthritis. J Hand Surg Am 2008;33(10):1737–43.
7. Tomaino MM. Basal metacarpal osteotomy for osteoarthritis of the thumb. J Hand Surg Am 2011; 36(6):1076–9.
8. Hartigan BJ, Stern PJ, Kiefhaber TR. Thumb carpometacarpal osteoarthritis: arthrodesis compared with ligament reconstruction and tendon interposition. J Bone Joint Surg Am 2001;83-A(10):1470–8.
9. Schröder J, Kerkhoffs GM, Voerman HJ, et al. Surgical treatment of basal joint disease of the thumb: comparison between resection-interposition arthroplasty and trapezio-metacarpal arthrodesis. Arch Orthop Trauma Surg 2002;122(1):35–8.
10. Badia A. Total joint arthroplasty for the arthritic thumb carpometacarpal joint. Am J Orthop 2008; 37(8 Suppl 1):4–7.

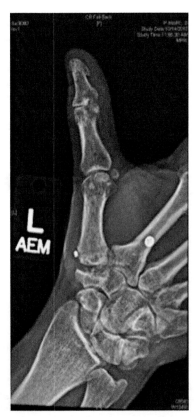

Fig. 8. Radiograph of a thumb 2 years after SB suspensionplasty. Note some subsidence has occurred, but the hemitrapeziectomy space is maintained.

11. Gervis WH. Excision of the trapezium for osteoarthritis of the trapezio-metacarpal joint. J Bone Joint Surg Br 1949;31B(4):537–9.

12. Fitzgerald BT, Hofmeister EP. Treatment of advanced carpometacarpal joint disease: trapeziectomy and hematoma arthroplasty. Hand Clin 2008;24(3): 271–6, vi.

13. Burton RI, Pellegrini VD. Surgical management of basal joint arthritis of the thumb. Part II. Ligament reconstruction with tendon interposition arthroplasty. J Hand Surg Am 1986;11(3):324–32.

14. Gerwin M, Griffith A, Weiland AJ, et al. Ligament reconstruction basal joint arthroplasty without tendon interposition. Clin Orthop Relat Res 1997;342:42–5.

15. Muermans S, Coenen L. Interpositional arthroplasty with Gore-Tex, Marlex or tendon for osteoarthritis of the trapeziometacarpal joint. A retrospective comparative study. J Hand Surg Br 1998;23(1):64–8.

16. Davis TR, Brady O, Barton NJ, et al. Trapeziectomy alone, with tendon interposition or with ligament reconstruction? J Hand Surg Br 1997;22(6):689–94.

17. Davis TR, Brady O, Dias JJ. Excision of the trapezium for osteoarthritis of the trapeziometacarpal joint: a study of the benefit of ligament reconstruction or tendon interposition. J Hand Surg Am 2004; 29(6):1069–77.

18. Park MJ, Lichtman G, Christian JB, et al. Surgical treatment of thumb carpometacarpal joint arthritis: a single institution experience from 1995-2005. Hand (N Y) 2008;3(4):304–10.

19. Adams JE, Merten SM, Steinmann SP. Arthroscopic interposition arthroplasty of the first carpometacarpal joint. J Hand Surg Eur Vol 2007; 32(3):268–74.

20. Earp BE, Leung AC, Blazar PE, et al. Arthroscopic hemitrapeziectomy with tendon interposition for arthritis at the first carpometacarpal joint. Tech Hand Up Extrem Surg 2008;12(1):38–42.

21. Sammer DM, Amadio PC. Description and outcomes of a new technique for thumb basal joint arthroplasty. J Hand Surg Am 2010;35(7):1198–205.

22. Martou G, Veltri K, Thoma A. Surgical treatment of osteoarthritis of the carpometacarpal joint of the thumb: a systematic review. Plast Reconstr Surg 2004;114(2):421–32.

23. Wajon A, Ada L, Edmunds I. Surgery for thumb (trapeziometacarpal joint) osteoarthritis. Cochrane Database Syst Rev 2005;(4):CD004631.

24. Wajon A, Carr E, Edmunds I, et al. Surgery for thumb (trapeziometacarpal joint) osteoarthritis. Cochrane Database Syst Rev 2009;(4):CD004631.

25. Vermeulen GM, Slijper H, Feitz R, et al. Surgical management of primary thumb carpometacarpal osteoarthritis: a systematic review. J Hand Surg Am 2011;36(1):157–69.

26. Cox CA, Zlotolow DA, Yao J. Suture button suspensionplasty after arthroscopic hemitrapeziectomy for treatment of thumb carpometacarpal arthritis. Arthroscopy 2010;26(10):1395–403.

27. Yao J, Zlotolow DA, Murdock R, et al. Suture button compared with K-wire fixation for maintenance of posttrapeziectomy space height in a cadaver model of lateral pinch. J Hand Surg Am 2010;35(12): 2061–5.

28. Eaton RG, Glickel SZ. Trapeziometacarpal osteoarthritis. Staging as a rationale for treatment. Hand Clin 1987;3(4):455–71.

29. Culp RW, Rekant MS. The role of arthroscopy in evaluating and treating trapeziometacarpal disease. Hand Clin 2001;17:315–9.

30. Furia JP. Arthroscopic debridement and synovectomy for treating basal joint arthritis. Arthroscopy 2010;26(1):34–40.

31. Walsh EF, Akelman E, Fleming BC, et al. Thumb carpometacarpal arthroscopy: a topographic, anatomic study of the thenar portal. J Hand Surg Am 2005; 30(2):373–9.

32. Willmott HJ, Singh B, David LA. Outcome and complications of treatment of ankle diastasis with tightrope fixation. Injury 2009;40(11):1204–6.

33. Kim ES, Lee KT, Park JS, et al. Arthroscopic anterior talofibular ligament repair for chronic ankle instability with a suture anchor technique. Orthopedics 2011;34(4):273.

34. Forsythe K, Freedman KB, Stover MD, et al. Comparison of a novel FiberWire-button construct versus metallic screw fixation in a syndesmotic injury model. Foot Ankle Int 2008;29(1):49–54.

35. Teramoto A, Suzuki D, Kamiya T, et al. Comparison of different fixation methods of the suture-button implant for tibiofibular syndesmosis injuries. Am J Sports Med 2011;39(10):2226–32.

36. Khalid M, Jones ML. Index metacarpal fracture after tightrope suspension following trapeziectomy: case report. J Hand Surg Am 2012;37(3): 418–22.

Advances in Upper Extremity Prosthetics

Dan A. Zlotolow, MD*, Scott H. Kozin, MD

KEYWORDS

- Prosthetic • Prosthesis • Upper extremity • Electrocorticography • Myoelectric

KEY POINTS

- Individually powered, myoelectrically controlled digits have opened the door to multifunctional, more lifelike prosthetic hands and partial hands.
- The future of prosthetic limb control may come from direct central nervous system control or from peripheral nervous system control via targeted reinnervation or neurointegration.
- The full potential of prosthetic limbs, no mater how powerful and nimble they become, will not be realized until the limbs can confer sensibility to their user.

INTRODUCTION

Lower extremity prosthetics have evolved to the point at which a bilateral below-the-knee amputee may be competitive with the best runners in the world.[1] The same success has not yet graced the upper extremity amputee. It was not long ago that the best we could offer a patient was a clumsy body-powered hook that provided one function: either active opening or closing (**Fig. 1**). Multiple task-specific terminal devices were required to accomplish simple daily tasks, requiring the patient to change these devices as needed.

Myoelectric devices offered more functionality and control because of active opening and closing, but the devices were heavy, limited to individuals with more proximal amputations (at least proximal to mid forearm), and short on battery life. The strength and speed of the limb is difficult to control and is limited by the properties of the sensors, motors, and bearings.

Another difficulty has been that neither myoelectric nor body-powered prostheses replicate the appearance of a normal hand. Passive or aesthetic prostheses may be worn for special occasions, but confer no function other than as an insensate extension of the residuum.

Innovations in prosthetics over the last several years have succeeded in improving several critical parameters: control, attachment, functionality, speed, size, weight, and power. Advances in motors, bearings, batteries, and materials have allowed for the development of devices that are easier to don, retain their charge longer, offer more control, are more versatile, and are more durable.

Better mechanics and materials have also advanced passive prostheses, which may now be made to have lockable, passively mobile joints. A posable hand is advantageous as a helper hand for performing simple tasks, and may be sufficient for a high-functioning unilateral amputee. Aesthetically, these limbs can be made to mirror the patient's intact arm, down to the hair and subcutaneous veins.

Patients will only use their prosthesis if they perceive an improvement from wearing it. Beyond improvements in function, patients also cite improved social integration, self-image, and perception by others. As prosthetics improve, not only functionally but also aesthetically, the threshold for acceptance will therefore be lowered. Patients who previously shunned prosthetic

Shriners Hospital for Children, Temple University School of Medicine, 3551 N. Broad St., Philadelphia, PA 19140, USA
* Corresponding author.
E-mail address: dzlotolow@yahoo.com

Hand Clin 28 (2012) 587–593
http://dx.doi.org/10.1016/j.hcl.2012.08.014
0749-0712/12/$ – see front matter © 2012 Elsevier Inc. All rights reserved.

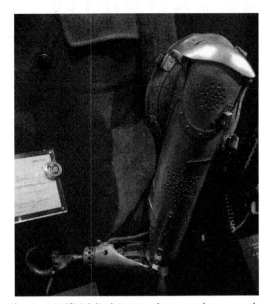

Fig. 1. "Artificial limb" worn by a gunlayer on the destroyer HMS Doon during World War I. Note the great attention to detail and the craftsmanship involved. However, the utility of the limb would have been limited by the simple hook terminal device and the weight of the materials (steel and leather). (*Courtesy of* Dan A. Zlotolow, MD.)

use are inquiring about cutting-edge prosthetics they have read about online or have seen on television.

These advances have not been inexpensive and likely would not have been possible so quickly without a commitment from the US Government. Improved front-line medical care combined with effective body armor in the Iraq and Afghanistan conflicts resulted in many soldiers returning home alive but with missing or severely compromised limbs. In 2006, the Defense Advanced Research Projects Agency (DARPA) responded with the Revolutionizing Prosthetics program. The Contineo Multi-Grasp Hand from Orthocare Innovations (Oklahoma City, OK) will be the first available commercial product resulting from this program.

MECHANICAL IMPROVEMENTS

The most advanced prosthetic upper limbs on, or soon to be on, the market are the i-Limb Ultra hand (Touch Bionics, Hillard, OH), the BeBionic V2 hand (RSL Steeper, Leeds, UK), the Contineo Multi-Grasp hand, and the Michelangelo hand (Otto Bock, Duderstadt, Germany). All offer much greater functionality than any previous single device. All also rely on myoelectric control with 1 or 2 sensors. Different grip, pinch, and other

functional patterns may be interchanged by a combination of myoelectric firing patterns (such as a short series of 2 or 3 contractions) or by manually adjusting the thumb position. The Contineo Multi-Grasp hand also features powered thumb abduction and adduction. Some offer a fully rotating forearm and wrist flexion/extension, whereas other terminal devices require manual wrist positioning.

The great advance that has allowed for the development of these hands has been the development of individually powered digits. Because the fingers are individually powered, a great variety of pinch and grasp patterns is possible. The user may now perform a 3-jaw chuck, power grip, tip pinch, key pinch, and many other patterns without the need to switch terminal devices. Also, individual finger torque control assures that the hand wraps around objects while providing equal pressure at each digit (**Fig. 2**). Variable pressure application allows the user to pick up an egg and a briefcase with the same terminal device, letting the user hold any object, regardless of contour, with the full grip of all the digits. It also assures a more natural-looking grasp pattern.

Aesthetically, the uncovered hands look like science fiction robot/cyborg hands (**Fig. 3**). Some users prefer to leave the components as exposed as possible, with only a grip-enhancing translucent silicone covering to showcase the cyborg look. For those who prefer discretion, silicone skin-colored coverings are also available in up to 10 different skin tones. Custom hand-painted "skins" are also available at a higher cost. Because the hands are all designed to simulate the positions of an intact hand, the hands look remarkably lifelike with a well-matched skin

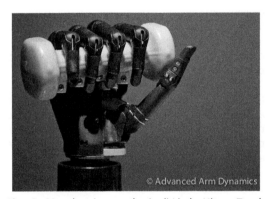

Fig. 2. Myoelectric prosthesis (i-Limb Ultra; Touch Bionics) showing the capability of each of the fingers to close around an object independently while applying the same amount of pressure. (*Courtesy of* Advanced Arm Dynamics, Redondo Beach, CA; with permission.)

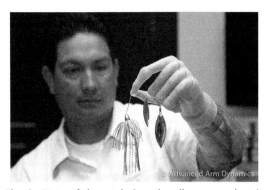

Fig. 3. State-of-the-art below-the-elbow myoelectric prosthesis with a grip-enhancing, translucent silicone skin. (*Courtesy of* Advanced Arm Dynamics, Redondo Beach, CA; with permission.)

covering. Hand movements remain slower and more determinate than for an intact hand, but are superior to the most prominent recent designs.

Some of the most exciting mechanical breakthroughs have been in partial hand prosthetics. The advent of self-powered digits also makes it possible to replace as many fingers as necessary for a partial hand amputee. The myoelectric sensors and battery can be placed locally, and concealed by the socket or a bracelet worn at wrist level (**Fig. 4**). A posable aesthetic partial hand device may be of great functional use if the thumb is present, allowing tip and key pinch as well as coarse grasp.

Above-the-elbow amputees and shoulder disarticulation patients are a difficult challenge for prosthetic design, because the loss of the elbow or shoulder adds more functional segments to the prosthesis. For these patients, the DARPA-funded Luke arm may soon be available (DEKA Research and Development Corp, Manchester, NH). Developed with Dean Kamen of Segway Inc (Bedford,

NH), the Luke uses both vibratory stimulation and pneumatic pressure pads for sensory feedback. It offers 16° of freedom and weighs less than 9 lb (4 kg) (50th percentile for a female arm).

For entire-limb replacement, the Johns Hopkins University Applied Physics Laboratory and the University of Pittsburgh are developing the Modular Prosthetic Limb (MPL). Funded largely by DARPA, the MPL allows 22° of freedom, with individual finger, thumb, wrist, forearm, and elbow control. Because it features brain interface control, the MPL may be useful not only for amputees but also for patients with spinal cord injuries.

IMPROVEMENTS IN CONTROL

The additional functionality of the new hands and limbs requires a more complex human-machine interface than that derived from 2 myoelectric sensors. Although the next-generation prosthetic hands use clever programming to multiply the number of possible grip patterns, switching between pinch and grasp modes is not intuitive and requires an extra step. Patients cannot transition smoothly from grasp to pinch, nor can they improvise new grasp and pinch patterns to meet their needs. The DEKA arm, for example, requires additional sensors for simultaneous control of its multiple functions.

The number of myoelectric sensor points may be increased by transferring distally innervating peripheral nerves from muscles that are no longer present or functional to more proximal available or functional musculature. Targeted reinnervation with nerves from the residual limb to more proximal musculature has enabled the creation of up to 6 sites for myoelectric control. In targeted reinnervation, nerves are transferred to the pectoralis major and minor according to the principal function of the donor nerve (**Fig. 5**). For example, the radial nerve may be used to signal elbow extension, the musculocutaneous branch to the brachialis for elbow flexion, the musculocutaneous branch to the biceps for supination, the median nerve for pronation, the ulnar nerve for finger flexion, and the posterior interosseous nerve for finger extension. The reinnervated muscle develops proprioception via the donor nerve, and the skin overlying the reinnervated muscle acquires the sensory territory of the transferred nerve.[2,3] This development not only allows the patient to be aware of the speed and force of contraction but may also be a source of sensory feedback in future devices.

Direct brain-wave control remains a long-term goal of research. Central control is ideal because it would be independent of the status of the

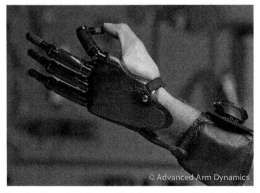

Fig. 4. Myoelectric partial hand prosthesis (i-Limb Ultra; Touch Bionics). (*Courtesy of* Advanced Arm Dynamics, Redondo Beach, CA; with permission.)

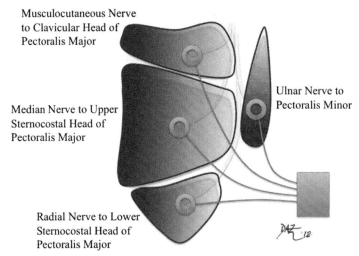

Musculocutaneous Nerve to Clavicular Head of Pectoralis Major

Median Nerve to Upper Sternocostal Head of Pectoralis Major

Ulnar Nerve to Pectoralis Minor

Radial Nerve to Lower Sternocostal Head of Pectoralis Major

Fig. 5. Schematic targeted reinnervation after shoulder disarticulation. Blue represents the myoelectric sensors (*circles*) and microprocessor box (*rectangle*) built into the suspension harness of the prosthesis. Red and yellow represent the muscles and their targeted reinnervation, respectively. (*Courtesy of* Dan A. Zlotolow, MD.)

peripheral nervous system in the residual limb. Moreover, minimal retraining would be necessary to operate complex, multifunctional prosthetics. All the patient would have to do is think about the motion, and the unique brain-wave pattern would be identified by an electroencephalogram and signal the limb to move. Experiments with primates and more recently with human volunteers have shown that this level of control may be achieved in the future.[4–8]

Neural control of prosthetics may be achieved by decoding target positions from the postparietal cortex (PPC) reach region. The PPC interprets sensory input, particularly visual, and generates a plan of action for the motor cortex. A computer then processes the signals to determine where and how to position the limb, bypassing the motor cortex entirely. One advantage of this more central control is that the prosthetic limb and processor would be able to optimize and coordinate individual movements of the limb to achieve the desired functional outcome without patients needing to concern themselves with controlling each individual joint. PPC control may be ideal for patients who have had strokes or others who have compromised motor cortices.

For patients with a functioning motor cortex, sensors overlying the brain may achieve more precise control. These sensors may be placed outside or inside the skull. Extradural but intracranial sensors have the advantage of minimizing distortion from the skull while also minimizing scar formation inside the brain itself (gliosis). Gliosis typically occurs within about 5 years after electrode implantation and limits or eliminates implant

sensitivity. Although gliosis does not develop in all patients, it does remain a major hurdle before intracranial implants become the standard of care for patients with spinal cord injury or limb deficiency.

In addition to gliosis, other limitations include the size of the processors required to decode the neural data, battery life, and stability of the recording devices. At present, the processing hardware is just small enough to fit into a backpack. Advances in miniaturization and application may come from the gaming industry. Video-game control systems are available today that offer electroencephalogram control and yet are only as cumbersome as wireless headphones (**Fig. 6**).

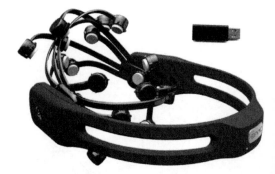

Fig. 6. Emotiv EPOC system (Emotiv Systems, Pyrmont, Australia) control device that sells for a few hundred dollars and may represent the near future of nonimplanted cortical control devices. (*Data from* Gomez-Gil J, San-Jose-Gonzalez I, Nicolas-Alonso LF, et al. Steering a tractor by means of an EMG-based human-machine interface. Sensors 2011;11:7110–26.)

Although not yet offering the same level of control as an electrocorticography (ECoG) system, these devices or their derivatives may have a role to play in the future of prosthetic control. Because of the wider application of this technology, these gaming devices retail for only a few hundred dollars (Emotiv Systems, Pyrmont, Australia).

Implantable brain electrodes and the process of ECoG were invented in the 1950s to identify the origins of epileptic seizures.[9] The DARPA prosthetics program achieved the first ECoG-controlled prosthetic arm in September 2011, fitted on a patient with tetraplegia. The patient, implanted with a CyberKinetics 96-electrode Brain Gate chip (CyberKinetics Neurotechnology Systems, Inc, Foxboro, MA), was able to control not only a robotic arm but also his lights and television.

Peripheral control options beyond myoelectric include neurointegration directly with artificial circuitry. As early as 2002, a 100-electrode array implanted into the median nerve of a volunteer was able to control a robot arm. Sensory feedback was provided by stimulating the first lumbrical.[10] The goal of creating an in-growth interface between peripheral nerves and inorganic sensors capable of detecting depolarization holds great promise and would allow specific functions to be directed by the nerve responsible for that function. However, unlike central control with external sensors, dissection of the target nerves and implantation of the sensors risk neuromas, local wound problems, and compromised limb/socket interface because of scarring or hypersensitivity.

IMPROVEMENTS IN ATTACHMENT

Most prosthetics are held on to the native limb by a combination of negative pressure and friction. A circumferential, closed-ended silicone liner serves as the interface between the prosthetic and native limb and provides the attachment point for the prosthesis. The residuum may develop skin problems, but a large sensate portion of the limb is shielded from the environment. Electric magnets may improve the ease and security of donning, wearing, and removing a prosthesis, but are still limited by the coverage of the residuum.

Osseointegration holds some promise for attaching prostheses to short-terminal segments and has been used for more than 20 years in Europe for lower and upper extremity amputees. The first osseointegration procedure was performed in 1990 for a short femoral segment, followed shortly thereafter by a thumb amputation (**Fig. 7**) and several transradial amputations.[11] Through a multistep process, a titanium bolt ("fixture") is fixed to the bone, allowing the prosthesis to be attached directly to the skeleton via a device known as an abutment. The skin at the interface of the abutment and the bone is attached directly to the end of the bone by removing any subcutaneous tissue over the bone end. A new implant design features attachment of defatted skin directly to a hydroxyapatite-coated flange on a unibody implant in an attempt to mimic the antler attachment to a deer skull (osseocutaneous integration).[12]

Because no socket is required and suspension of the device is unnecessary, the residuum is free from the typical skin complications of prosthetic wear and is also available for tactile feedback. Inclusion criteria for this procedure include difficulty with traditional prosthetic fitting, adequate bone stock to support the fixture, and an uncompromised immune system. Patients should be willing and able to perform routine implant care and adhere to the initial rehabilitation protocol.

Titanium is a well-tolerated, biocompatible metal, but concerns about superficial and deep

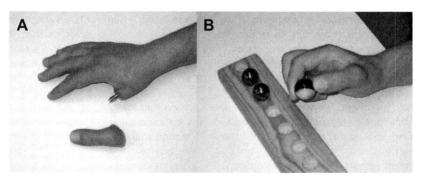

Fig. 7. Osseointegration of a passive thumb prosthesis for a partial amputation showing the device (*A*) and its function when donned (*B*). (*Reprinted from* Jönsson S, Caine-Winterberger K, Brånemark R. Osseointegration amputation prostheses on the upper limbs: methods, prosthetics and rehabilitation. Prosthet Orthot Int 2011;35:190–200; with permission.)

infections have limited broad acceptance of this technique. Dental and other implants around the face are commonly anchored directly to bone using titanium screw-in implants with minimal risk of infection.[13] The orthopedic experience with bone/implant interface difficulties in arthroplasties is cause for concern, but several important differences exist between osseointegration and ingrowth for arthroplasty implants: (1) osseointegration has no moving parts and, therefore, does not generate proinflammatory particulate debris; (2) the bolt in osseointegration is allowed to mature for 6 months before bearing weight; and (3) the bone and skin form an interface directly with the implant and the outside world analogous to bone and gums in the mouth. Nonetheless, much more needs to be known about the long-term and short-term consequences of osseointegration or osseocutaneous integration before they become viable treatment options.

THE CHALLENGES OF CONFERRING SENSIBILITY

The homunculus of children with congenital amputations does not include a space for the missing part. Attempts at creating a mental image of the missing part by early prosthetic fitting have been met with limited success.[14] The old adage of having to "fit" a child as soon as they can "sit" may no longer apply. Most children with one working limb reject their prosthesis because their own incomplete but sensate limb is more functional to them. Because the prosthetic limb has no sensation, children rarely incorporate it into their body image. They learn to accomplish their activities of daily living with 1 arm de novo.

By contrast, patients who suffer an amputation of their upper limb have not only well-established cortical representation for that limb but also have adapted to life in a bimanual way. Mastering activities of daily living with their residual limb requires relearning new techniques or adapting to their loss. These patients are more apt to embrace prosthetic wear, even without sensory feedback.

Nonetheless, without sensation, use of the prosthetic limb requires visual supervision. Modulating grip or pinch strength is also difficult even while observing the prosthetic, because there is currently no way of reliably conferring pressure sensation from the terminal device of the prosthetic.

Much of current research has focused on converting pressure readings from sensors in the terminal device to vibration motors at the end of the residuum. Volunteers have been able to detect gradations in force applied by the terminal device with an accuracy of 75% when both amplitude and frequency were varied in concert.[15] Pressure-generating pneumatically inflated pads are also in development.

ALTERNATIVES TO PROSTHETICS

For the patient with complete or partial loss of the upper extremity, nonprosthetic limb reconstruction options have been received with variable degrees of acceptance. The Krukenberg procedure is rarely performed today outside of the Third World and is typically restricted to visually impaired bilateral amputees. Separation of the radius and ulna may improve function, but aesthetic concerns have predominated. Several investigators have described transfer of the second toe to create sensate pinch at the limb terminus if no or only 1 digit remains.[16] The toe(s) may be placed on residual skeletal elements in the hand. For wrist or slightly more proximal amputations, a toe may be attached to the radius so that the radius itself may serve as a post against which to pinch. At present, these options have some advantage over prostheses in that they restore protective sensation to the prehensile function of the limb.

Allotransplantation is not yet ready for widespread use because of the risks associated with immunosuppression. Metabolic derangements, neoplasms, and death are known risk factors of arm or hand transplantation. The benefits of transplants over modern prosthetics are also unclear. Transplanted upper limb segments may be expected to recover protective sensation, but 2-point discrimination and proprioception are rare achievements. The limbs also develop variable degrees of joint contractures, limiting overall function. Restoration of preamputation function is not likely.

Giraux and colleagues[17] have found that after hand transplantation, the original sensorimotor cortex (SMC) map for hand activation is restored. The transplantation reverses the SMC loss after the initial hand amputation. Similarly, successful toe transfer produces temporal activation within the SMC, consistent with cortical plasticity.[18] Functional magnetic resonance imaging has shown that learning to use the toe transfer leads to an expansion in motor cortex representation. Practice magnifies the changes within the SMC. As the new motor skill is mastered, there is a subsequent decrease in the amount of cortical representation.[19,20] Functional magnetic resonance imaging studies have provided evidence that motor reorganization continues to evolve over time and may be modified by training and experience for a protracted time.[21] These findings suggest that prolonged therapy and training may be necessary to maximize cortical reorganization and functional outcome.

SUMMARY

The future of control mechanisms for upper limb prosthetics may follow 1 of 2 directions: direct peripheral nerve control via a neuroprosthetic interface or implantable ECoG with a low-power and miniaturized control processor concealed in the limb itself. Lighter materials, smaller and more powerful motors, sensory array capabilities, and reliable osseointegration have the potential to make prosthetics as functional as the native limb.

REFERENCES

1. Sokolove M. The fast life. What makes Oscar Pistorius run? The New York Times Magazine January 22, 2012;28–35.
2. Marasco PD, Schultz AE, Kuiken TA. Sensory capacity of reinnervated skin after redirection of amputated upper limb nerves to the chest. Brain 2009;132:1441–8.
3. Sensinger JW, Lock BA, Kuiken TA. Adaptive pattern recognition of myoelectric signals: exploration of conceptual framework and practical algorithms. IEEE Trans Neural Syst Rehabil Eng 2009;17:270–8.
4. Mulliken GH, Sam Musallam S, Anderson RA. Decoding trajectories from posterior parietal cortex. J Neurosci 2008;28:12913–26.
5. Velliste M, Perel S, Spalding MC, et al. Cortical control of a prosthetic arm for self-feeding. Nature 2008;19:1098–101.
6. Santucci DM, Kralik JD, Lebedev MA, et al. Frontal and parietal cortical ensembles predict single-trial muscle activity during reaching movements in primates. Eur J Neurosci 2005;22:1529–40.
7. Lebedev MA, Carmena JM, O'Doherty JE, et al. Cortical ensemble adaptation to represent velocity of an artificial actuator controlled by a brain-machine interface. J Neurosci 2005;25:4681–893.
8. Wessberg J, Stambaugh CR, Kralik JD, et al. Real-time prediction of hand trajectory by ensembles of cortical neurons in primates. Nature 2000;16:361–5.
9. Palmini A. The concept of the epileptogenic zone: a modern look at Penfield and Jasper's views on the role of interictal spikes. Epileptic Disord 2006; 8(Suppl 2):S10–5.
10. Warwick K, Gasson M, Hutt B, et al. The application of implant technology for cybernetic systems. Arch Neurol 2003;60:1369–73.
11. Jönsson S, Caine-Winterberger K, Brånemark R. Osseointegration amputation prostheses on the upper limbs: methods, prosthetics and rehabilitation. Prosthet Orthot Int 2011;35:190–200.
12. Kang NV, Pendegras C, Marks L, et al. Osseocutaneous integration of an intraosseous transcutaneous amputation prosthesis implant used for reconstruction of a transhumeral amputee: case report. J Hand Surg Am 2010;35:1130–4.
13. Albrektsson T, Brånemark PI, Hansson HA, et al. Osseointegrated titanium implants. Requirements for ensuring a long-lasting, direct bone-to-implant anchorage in man. Acta Orthop Scand 1981;52: 155–70.
14. James MA, Bagley AM, Brasington K, et al. Impact of prostheses on function and quality of life for children with unilateral congenital below-the-elbow deficiency. J Bone Joint Surg Am 2006;88:2356–65.
15. Cipriani C, D'Alonzo M, Carrozza MC. A miniature vibrotactile sensory substitution device for multifingered hand prosthetics. IEEE Trans Biomed Eng 2012;59:400–8.
16. Jones NF, Hansen SL, Bates SJ. Toe-to-hand transfers for congenital anomalies of the hand. Hand Clin 2007;23:129–36.
17. Giraux P, Sirigu A, Schneider F, et al. Cortical reorganization in motor cortex after graft of both hands. Nat Neurosci 2001;4:691–2.
18. Anastakis DJ, Malessy MJA, Chen R, et al. Cortical plasticity following nerve transfer in the upper extremity. Hand Clin 2008;24:425–44.
19. Manduch M, Bezuhly M, Anastakis DJ, et al. Serial fMRI assessment of the primary motor cortex following thumb reconstruction. Neurology 2002; 59:1278–81.
20. Friston KJ, Frith CD, Liddle PF, et al. Comparing functional (PET) images: the assessment of significant change. J Cereb Blood Flow Metab 1991;11: 690–9.
21. Gevins A, Leong H, Smith ME, et al. Mapping cognitive brain function with modern high-resolution electroencephalography regional modulation of high resolution evoked potentials during verbal and non-verbal matching tasks. Trends Neurosci 1995; 18:429–36.

Total Wrist Arthroplasty

Rowena McBeath, MD, PhD[a],*, A. Lee Osterman, MD[b]

KEYWORDS

- Wrist • Arthroplasty • Replacement • Implant • Radius • Hemiarthroplasty

KEY POINTS

- Total Wrist Arthroplasty is a treatment option for painful, nonfunctional wrists in disease states.
- Technologic advances in materials, wear properties, and manufacturing now account for increased implant longevity.
- Alternative surgical treatments such as distal radius hemiarthroplasty may serve as a treatment option for patients with higher activity levels and diffuse arthritis.
- With careful patient selection, soft tissue considerations, and novel implant designs, TWA may become a viable treatment staple for patients with functional wrist disability.

The importance of the wrist to human function cannot be underestimated. As Sterling Bunnell described, the wrist is the keystone to the hand.[1] Not only does the wrist augment fine motor control of the fingers, but it also aids in power grasp.[2] The versatility of wrist function is attributed to its range of motion, derived mainly from carpal bone shape and articulations, as well as its bodily position, serving as a fulcrum for crossing musculotendinous units. The normal wrist is not only flexible, but also stable, its strength derived from ligaments and capsule.[3]

ANATOMY AND KINESIOLOGY

Anatomically, the wrist is composed of 8 carpal bones and 3 joint articulations: radiocarpal, ulnocarpal, and midcarpal. Normal wrist flexion is 85° to 90°, with 65% of flexion occurring at the radiocarpal joint and 35% occurring at the midcarpal joint. Conversely, joint extension is 80° to 85°, with the radiocarpal joint contributing 35% and the midcarpal joint contributing 65% of extension.[4,5] Functional range of motion needed for most activities of daily living is 30° of flexion and extension, and 5° to 10° of radial and ulnar deviation.[6–8]

Historically, it was thought that the wrist is capable of motion only in 2 planes, radioulnar deviation and palmar flexion and extension.[9,10] The axis of motion is located within the head of the capitate, and rotational movement takes place through the proximal and distal radial ulnar joints.[3] Recently, however, cadaver studies examining wrist range of motion and stiffness in 24 positions revealed that the wrist mechanical axes are oriented obliquely to the anatomic axes, the primary direction being radial extension and ulnar flexion, along a path of a dart thrower's wrist motion.[11]

THE WRIST IN DISEASE STATES
Rheumatoid Arthritis

Wrist function is never more appreciated than when it is compromised, as in certain disease states. One disease that almost universally affects the wrist is rheumatoid arthritis. In rheumatoid arthritis, multiple joint involvement and upper extremity involvement are common, with the wrist joint being affected as well as small joints of the hand, elbow, and shoulder. Wrist involvement is common, affects up to 50% of patients within the first 2 years of disease onset, and affects

[a] The Philadelphia Hand Center, P.C., Thomas Jefferson University Hospital, 834 Chestnut Street, Suite G114, Philadelphia, PA 19107, USA; [b] Hand and Orthopaedic Surgery, The Philadelphia Hand Center, P.C., Thomas Jefferson University Hospital, 834 Chestnut Street, Suite G114, Philadelphia, PA 19107, USA
* Corresponding author.
E-mail address: rowena.mcbeath@gmail.com

Hand Clin 28 (2012) 595–609
http://dx.doi.org/10.1016/j.hcl.2012.08.015
0749-0712/12/$ – see front matter © 2012 Published by Elsevier Inc.

more than 90% of patients after 10 years, with bilateral involvement in 95% of patients.[12,13]

The mechanism of wrist degeneration in rheumatoid arthritis is via cartilage degradation, ligamentous laxity, and synovial expansion with erosion.[14] Synovial tissue hypertrophy subsequently involves all joints and tendon sheaths.[15] Early synovial infiltration and erosion of the distal ulna cause distal radioulnar joint instability.[15,16] Synovitis of the palmar wrist affects extrinsic and intrinsic ligaments, leading to carpal instability and collapse.[15] The proximal carpal row dislocates in the palmar and ulnar direction and supinates.[12] Coupled with caput ulnae, the extensor carpi ulnaris tendon changes its vector, becoming a wrist flexor without a stabilizing function.[17] Instability is exacerbated by tendon degeneration and subsequent attritional rupture, resulting in a catastrophic, unpredictable change in the center of rotation of the wrist and soft tissue balance. In late stages with volar subluxation, the radial wrist extensors are attenuated or ruptured, which is a contraindication for wrist replacement.

While early medical management may slow natural disease progression, many patients still have progressive and disabling disease.[15,18] Initial treatment consists of medical management via disease-modifying antirheumatic drugs (DMARDs). However, for persistent synovitis threatening tendon rupture and causing altered wrist joint function and mechanics, surgical options include tenosynovectomy and salvage procedures such as arthrodesis and arthroplasty. While wrist arthrodesis has long been considered the procedure of choice in the treatment of rheumatoid arthritis of the wrist, it is not without its disadvantages, primarily due to loss of wrist motion. Patients with an arthrodesis have difficulties with activities of daily living including fastening buttons, combing hair, writing, and perineal care.[19–21] Wrist arthrodesis also has a reported complication rate of 14% to 29%, with 65% of patients requiring plate removal.[22,23]

Osteoarthritis

Wrist osteoarthritis is common and results from nonunited or malunited fractures of the scaphoid or distal radius, disruption of the carpal ligaments such as resulting in Scapho Lunate Advanced Collapse (SLAC) arthritis, avascular necrosis of the carpus, crystal deposition diseases, or developmental abnormalities. It is often bilateral. Unlike rheumatoid arthritis the osteoarthritis disease process is usually limited to the wrist, and the functional demands often include unrestricted activities. The current concern is that total wrist arthroplasty will not hold up to these use loads.

TOTAL WRIST ARTHROPLASTY

An alternative surgical procedure to provide pain relief and retain motion and function in patients with destructive wrist arthritis is total wrist arthroplasty (TWA). Indications for TWA are pancarpal advanced arthritis in a patient willing to accept a low-demand lifestyle, who desires the ability to perform activities that require wrist motion.[24] A controversial indication is the older active patient with osteoarthritis. Even a few degrees of wrist motion greatly increase the reach of fingers in space, and may have enormous functional consequences for patients with multilevel disease of the upper extremity.[25] Also, when bilateral wrist disease exists, arthroplasty of the nondominant side and arthrodesis on the dominant side have been favored.[26–28] Interestingly, multiple studies have shown patients with TWA on 1 side and arthrodesis on the other side to prefer the TWA.[1,29–32]

While TWA is an innovative alternative to wrist arthrodesis, controversy exists over its widespread use. Cavaliere and Chung performed a systematic review of 18 TWA studies representing approximately 500 procedures, and 20 total wrist fusion studies representing over 800 procedures.[33] When outcomes were compared, they found high patient satisfaction in both groups; however, TWA complication and revision rates were higher, while total wrist fusion seemed to provide more reliable relief.[33] While this initial data questioned whether there was substantial advantage of TWA over wrist fusion, subsequent studies using cost-utility analysis demonstrated the following:

> TWA has only an incrementally higher cost over wrist fusion.
> Patients with rheumatoid arthritis place emphasis on maintaining wrist motion.
> Patients who place emphasis on maintaining wrist motion would prefer TWA over wrist fusion and nonoperative management.[34,35]

This analysis showed that even with higher complication rates, TWA is a cost-effective and important surgical option for patients with rheumatoid arthritis.

Patients with debilitating post-traumatic arthritis and osteoarthritis also have a need for salvage procedures. While wrist arthrodesis is the gold standard for manual laborers with post-traumatic arthritis, few studies have examined the role of TWA in these patient populations. In a study of 25 patients with post-traumatic arthritis treated with TWA (age range 56–75 years), Levadoux and Legre found 84% of their patients demonstrated increased range of motion and grip strength.[36] There were four postoperative complications, including two infections. Two patients who had undergone prior proximal row carpectomy developed severe postoperative pain and were revised to total wrist arthrodesis.[36] This finding led the authors to conclude prior proximal row carpectomy to be a contraindication to TWA. Also, the 4 youngest patients in the study group ultimately required TWA revision to wrist arthrodesis, which was thought to be due to high activity and stress on the prosthesis.[36] Although patients with post-traumatic arthritis and osteoarthritis are typically young, active, and thus not ideal TWA candidates,[37] TWA may provide an alternative salvage procedure for low-demand patients with the ability to adhere to strict activity limitations.[38]

Given that TWA may provide an acceptable alternative for a certain patient population, it is not a viable treatment option for everyone. Contra-indications to TWA include a history of bone infection, ligamentous laxity or nonfunctional radial wrist extensors, poor bone stock as evidenced by resorption of the distal carpal row, and the need to bear weight as in the use of walking aides.[24] As with many novel devices, TWA implants have evolved over generations, with concomitant discovery of technical pearls and pitfalls. The most salient points in TWA development will be chronicled.

HISTORY OF TWA
The First Implants

The first total wrist implant was performed by Themistocles Gluck (1853–1942, **Fig. 1**), a German doctor whose early experimental work and interests concerned organ resection and transplantation.[39] In particular, Gluck used guide rails for tissue regeneration after nerve and tendon replacement, and subsequently used ivory intramedullary pegs and nails for fracture fixation.[40,41] As ivory would be incorporated into the bone with minimal inflammatory response, Gluck decided that it would be the most suitable material for implantation.[42] In 1890, Gluck performed the first total wrist implant in a 19-year old man with a 21-month history of tuberculosis of his right wrist. The implant was made of ivory and composed of a ball-and-socket articulation with forks at both ends, one to fit the ulna and radius, and the other in the metacarpal medullary canals.[41] The device incorporated without shortening, and the patient's pain was ameliorated; however, a chronic fistula persisted due to the original disease process.[39]

Research into other biologically inert materials was continued by Swanson, who developed

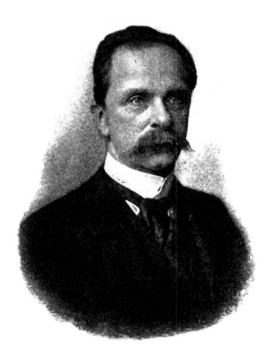

Fig. 1. Themistocles Gluck (1853–1942), inventor of first total wrist implant. (*From* Pagel JL. Biographisches Lexikon hervorragender Ärzte des neunzehnten Jahrhunderts. Berlin-Wien: Urban & Schwarzenberg, 1901.)

a double-stemmed, flexible-hinge implant for the radiocarpal joint made of silicone elastomer in 1967 (**Fig. 2**).[25,43–45] It was essentially an enlarged version of his popular Meta Carpal Phalangeal Joint implant. Indications for a silicone wrist implant included cases of rheumatoid arthritis, osteoarthritis, or post-traumatic arthritis resulting in severe wrist instability, deformity, and ankylosis.[46]

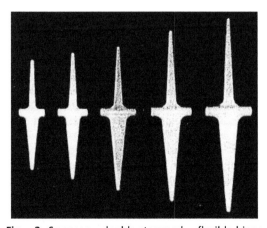

Fig. 2. Swanson double-stemmed, flexible-hinge radiocarpal joint implant. (*From* Swanson AB, Swanson GD, Maupin BK. Flexible implant arthroplasty of the radiocarpal joint: surgical technique and long-term study. Clin Orthop Relat Res 1984; 187:94–106; with permission.)

Contraindications included open epiphyses, inadequate skin, bone or neurovascular status, absent wrist extensor function, patient lack of cooperation, and heavy manual labor.[46] A retrospective study of 170 wrists in 129 patients who underwent silastic wrist implants revealed complete pain relief in 90% of patients, 7% of patients with mild pain, and 3% of patients with moderate pain after an average of 4 years follow-up.[46] At this time, average post-op flexion (34°) and extension (26°) provided a 60° arc of motion, which was maintained throughout the follow-up period. Complications requiring revision surgery existed in 25 wrists (14%); nine wrists underwent revision for implant fracture (5%). Four wrists underwent revision for tendon imbalance, and five for concomitant tendon imbalance and recurrent synovitis. Implants were removed and replaced in 22 cases (12%).[46] Later, metal grommets were added to protect the silicone prosthesis from breakage, wear, and subsidence.

Several other retrospective series of silastic radiocarpal implants have noted other complications, including implant subsidence, silicone synovitis, and prosthesis fracture.[47,48] Rossello and colleagues[49] examined 32 silastic implants with titanium grommets in 29 patients from 2.5 to 8 years follow-up and noted 20% implant subsidence but no revisions. Jolly and colleagues[47] examined the outcomes of 28 silastic implants (without grommets) at an average of 44 months follow-up and noted a 52% implant fracture rate; 26% of prostheses underwent revision. The pathology from two of the revision cases demonstrated a foreign body reaction to silicone. Overall implant survival at 77 months was 42%, leading the authors to conclude that silastic radiocarpal implants should only be used in the low-demand patient with poor bone stock.[47]

Ball-and-socket Designs

The first TWA with the goal to recreate functional joint motion was created by Hans Christoph Meuli in 1970. To imitate normal wrist motion, Meuli considered the normal wrist a biaxial joint with center of motion at the capitate, and developed an implant with a ball-and-socket design (**Fig. 3**).[50] With this design, his implants were completely unconstrained and largely uncemented, permitting motion in all planes as well as slight distraction.[50] Initial implants had balls made of polyester, which were soon abandoned for ultrahigh molecular weight polyethylene due to immunogenicity. Also, the early designs would tend to ulnar deviate if the prosthesis was not perfectly centered. Early outcomes noted that extensor deficits resulted in prosthesis subluxation, while inadequate bone

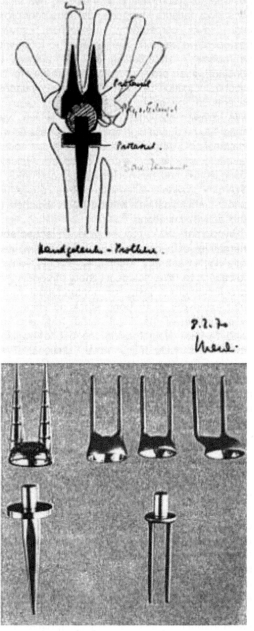

Fig. 3. (*Top*) Blueprint for Meuli's first total wrist prosthesis. (*Bottom*) Evolution of designs of Meuli's total wrist prosthesis. ([*Top and Bottom*] *From* Meuli HC. Meuli total wrist arthroplasty. Clin Orthop Relat Res 1984;187:107–11; with permission.)

stock led to early loosening.[50] These observations refined the implant indications, which had to take into account pain, disability, and local findings such as individual center of rotation and extensor deficits. Contraindications for wrist arthroplasty included heavy manual labor and reliance on walking aids, as well as insufficient bone stock.

Subsequent retrospective studies performed by Meuli and others revealed persistent rates of revision and implant loosening despite advanced surgical designs. In a review of 50 Meuli Wrist Prosthesis-III prostheses in 45 patients performed predominantly for rheumatoid arthritis after an average of 4.5 years follow-up (range 2–6 years), Meuli and Fernandez reported excellent results in 24 wrists, good results in 12 wrists, fair results in 5 wrists, and poor results in 8 wrists.[51] Eleven of 49 prostheses had faulty positioning of the carpal component, of which 8 prostheses were associated with radiographic signs of loosening and needed surgical revision. The authors attributed the 15 complications of these 50 prostheses to incorrect surgical technique and malalignment, 13 of which occurred on the carpal side.[51] However, analysis of 140 Meuli prostheses performed at the Mayo Clinic revealed a reoperation rate of 33% for major complications, including dislocations (8.6%), loosening (2.9%), and soft-tissue contracture (12.1%).[52] The authors also noted progressive volar displacement of the cup component with distal component loosening, causing increased wrist dorsiflexion, subsequent flexor tendon wear, and ensuing tendon rupture and carpal tunnel syndrome.[52] These observations led Cooney and colleagues[52] to identify factors responsible for implant failure to be prosthesis alignment, fixation, and soft tissue balance, and to no longer recommended the Meuli prosthesis for clinical use.

Shortly after the debut of the Meuli prosthesis, an alternative design for TWA was revealed by Robert G. Volz.[3] In his analysis of wrist kinematics, Volz emphasized that the wrist has little inherent bony stability, which is instead conferred from the dorsal and palmar ligamentous structures and capsule.[3] Also, Volz noted that the wrist withstands significant forces of distraction during certain activities, such as heavy lifting, and that the application of 40 pounds of distractive force at the wrist can widen the distance between the carpals and the distal radial articulating surface by five-eighths of an inch.[3] Taking these observations into account, the Volz/Arizona Medical Center (AMC) prosthesis had a hemispherical design with radii of 2 different dimensions and a polyethylene interface, to achieve motion in 2 planes without rotation, providing 90° of flexion and extension, and 50° of radial ulnar deviation (**Fig. 4**).[3] Proximal and distal component cementation further enhanced prosthesis stability.

Early results of 50 Volz/AMC semiconstrained, cemented prostheses in 45 patients, predominantly with rheumatoid arthritis, revealed no cases of loosening, infection, increased pain, or recurrent

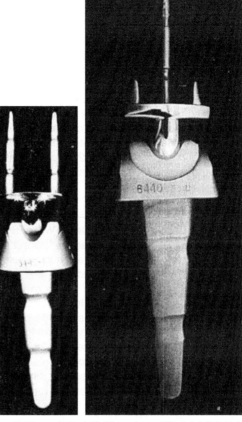

Fig. 4. The original (*left*) and modified (*right*) Volz/AMC prosthesis. ([*Left*] *From* Volz RG. The development of a total wrist arthroplasty. Clin Orthop Relat Res 1976;116:209–14; with permission; and [*right*] *From* Volz RG. Total wrist arthroplasty: a clinical review. Clin Orthop Relat Res 1984;187:112–20; with permission.)

dislocation over a follow-up of 6 to 34 months.[53] There were two cases of immediate postoperative dislocation, thought to be due to contracted volar wrist capsule.[53] However, the most frequent complication was a tendency for the wrist to drift into ulnar deviation, which occurred in 7 of the 21 patients included in the study. This was thought to be due to the radialward shift of the prosthesis' axis of rotation, and transfer of the Extensor Carpi Ulnaris (ECU) to the base of the fourth metacarpal was recommended.[53] Results of 25 prostheses in 22 patients with a modified design (see **Fig. 4**, right) revealed no cases of loosening, dislocation, radio-ulnar imbalance, dislocation, or infection over a follow-up of 6 months to 6.7 years.[1] However, Menon reviewed his results of 18 modified Volz prostheses in 16 patients over a follow-up of 24 to 66 months (average 40 months), and demonstrated a 44% complication rate. Two dislocations occurred in the immediate postoperative period; five cases of muscle imbalance causing flexion and ulnar deviation deformities with eventual implant migration and cortical penetration were reported, and there were three cases of loosening and one case of infection, resulting in an overall reoperation rate of 33%.[54] Menon attributed the complication rate primarily to muscle imbalance, loosening, and dislocation, and deemed this complication rate unacceptable. In a smaller but more recent study, Gellman and colleagues[55] evaluated 14 prostheses in 13 patients over an average 6.5-year follow-up and noted a 27% complication rate, composed of 2 dislocations and 2 infections.

Third-Generation Designs

There have been many subsequent TWA designs. For example, Figgie and colleagues[56] described the trispherical wrist prosthesis, a semiconstrained implant that consists of metacarpal and radial components articulating with a polyethylene bearing and an axle restraint. In a retrospective study of 35 trispherical prostheses in 34 patients over an average follow-up of 9 years (range 5–11 years), Figgie and colleagues[32] reported 6 patients with postoperative tendon attrition, 7 patients with radiographic signs of implant loosening, 3 instances of implant malposition and subsequent metacarpal stem migration, and 2 revisions for loosening and pain, respectively. Of note, the authors stressed the need to restore wrist center of rotation; otherwise an ulnar deviation deformity would result from tendon imbalance.

Another design, the biaxial total wrist prosthesis, was developed and in use at the Mayo Clinic since the early 1980s. This prosthesis has a nonconstrained, convex–concave ellipsoid articulating surface, thought to be more physiologic in nature (**Fig. 5**). Cobb and Beckenbaugh performed a retrospective review of 46 biaxial total wrist prostheses in rheumatoid arthritis patients over an average follow-up of 6.5 years (range 5–9.9 years). The authors reported significant improvements in pain, range of motion (extension and radial deviation), and grip strength (preoperative 4.1 kg–6.5 kg postoperative). While the biaxial total wrist prosthesis had an overall 5-year survival of 83% (67% without cement), there was radiographic loosening in 14 cases (22%), all of which had subsidence and 8 of which were revised. Eleven failures were reported, including 8 loosenings of the distal implant (13%, 5 of which were attributed to technical difficulties) and 6 intraoperative complications (perforation of the third metacarpal [4 cases], soft tissue imbalance [1 case], and radial deviation [1 case]).[57] Interestingly, the authors

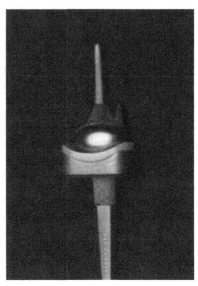

Fig. 5. Biaxial total wrist prosthesis. (*From* Cobb TK, Beckenbaugh RD. Biaxial total wrist arthroplasty. J Hand Surg Am 1996;21:1011–21; with permission.)

found significant effects of preoperative radial deformity on implant survival, as soft tissue imbalance resulting in radial deformity resulted in only 25% survivorship free of revision, compared with 87% for those patients without radial deformities.[57] Given the percentage of distal implant loosening, the authors recommended that the biaxial total wrist prosthesis be reserved for low-demand patients with rheumatoid arthritis unable to compensate for wrist fusion.

Other investigators have also noted complications with the biaxial total wrist prosthesis. Stegemen and colleagues[58] performed a retrospective review of 16 uncemented biaxial total wrist prostheses in 16 patients with rheumatoid arthritis over an average of 25 months (range 5–60 months). While 63% of patients noted improvement and increased range of motion, four patients experienced early dislocations and underwent component revision. In a larger study, Krukhaug and colleagues[59] examined outcomes of 90 biaxial total wrist prostheses and noted 5-year survival of 77%, with the most common reasons for revision being distal component loosening and pain. Most recently however, van Harlingen and colleagues[60] performed a retrospective review of 32 biaxial total wrist prostheses at average of 6 years follow-up (range 5–8 years), and although they noted a 7-year survival rate of 81%, there were 31 complications, including 22 wrists (67%) with radiographic signs of loosening and 8 revisions (25%). While the biaxial total wrist prosthesis has been withdrawn from the market in some areas, the authors recommend close follow-up of these patients given the high complication rate. As with other designs of this era, wrist imbalance and erosion of the metacarpal fixation continued to plague these designs (**Fig. 6**).

In 1998, Jay Menon described the Universal total wrist implant (KMI, San Diego, California), which was conceived by taking into account the failures of previous total wrist prosthetic designs. The Universal total wrist implant is a nonconstrained prosthesis; its radial articular surface has a 20° articulation, and its concavity provides stability when the components are tensioned (**Fig. 7**).[61] The carpal component is ovoid in shape, supports the first and fifth ray, thus preventing proximal migration, and is secured via screw fixation.[61] Also, particular to the Universal total wrist implant is its ability to deal with bone shortage or excess; carpal bone height can be restored via insertion of bone graft. An oblique osteotomy removes less bone from the radius, and intercarpal fusion decreases carpal component toggle, thereby reducing loosening.[61,62]

Indications for the Universal total wrist implant included chronic wrist pain or deformity. Contraindications included history of infection, systemic lupus erythematosus, extensor tendon ruptures, and heavy labor.[61] Menon, in his early retrospective review of 37 Universal total wrist implants in 31 patients at a follow-up of 6.7 years (range 48–120 months), revealed significant increases in range of motion (dorsiflexion and radial deviation).[61] However, there was a 32% complication rate, the most common complication being volar wrist dislocation (5 cases), followed by radial-sided loosening (2 cases).[61] Volar dislocation was attributed to excessive bone resection. Subsequent prospective studies performed by Divelbiss and colleagues[63] of 22 implants in 19 patients with rheumatoid arthritis over a follow-up period of 1 to 2 years reported increased range of motion, Disabilities of the Arm, Shoulder and Hand (DASH), scores and pain relief; there was a 14% complication rate due to component instability attributed to ligamentous laxity in patients with active disease. Midterm results of 21 patients with Universal total wrist implants revealed no dislocations or surgical revisions at an average follow-up of 5.5 years (range 3–8 years); only 2 patients exhibited radiographic findings of loosening.[64] However, recent long-term follow-up of 19 Universal total wrist implants in 15 patients with rheumatoid arthritis over an average follow-up of 7.3 years (range 5–10 years) was significant for 5-year survival rates of 75% and 7-year survival rates of 60%; 50% of the prostheses underwent revision, while 45% of prostheses were revised for loosening[65].

Current Designs

There are currently 3 US Food and Drug Administration (FDA)-approved TWA designs: Universal 2 total wrist implant (KMI, San Diego, California), ReMotion total wrist arthroplasty (SBI, Morrisville, Pennsylvania), and Maestro Wrist Reconstructive System (Biomet, Warsaw, Indiana). Recent preliminary results of the Universal 2 total wrist implant are promising; a retrospective review of 17 wrist arthroplasties in 15 patients over a follow-up period from 20 to 74 months revealed decreased pain and increased range of motion and DASH scores.[66] Importantly, only 1 patient had carpal loosening, and 1 patient had early postoperative dislocation.[66]

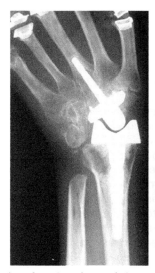 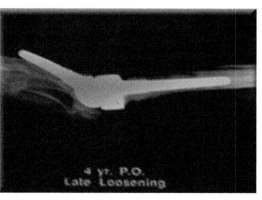

Fig. 6. Examples of modes of TWA failure, including imbalance (*left*) and metacarpal loosening (*right*).

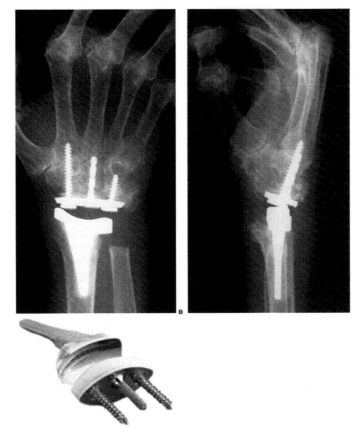

Fig. 7. (*Top*) radiographs of universal total wrist implant in a patient with rheumatoid arthritis. (*Bottom*) Universal 2 total wrist implant. ([*Top*] *From* Divelbiss BJ, Sollerman C, Adams BD. Early results of the universal total wrist arthroplasty in rheumatoid arthritis. J Hand Surg Am 2002;27:195–204; with permission; and [*bottom*] *Courtesy of* KMI, San Diego, California.)

The ReMotion TWA was released for general use in 2002; its unique design features include an ultrahigh density polythylene ellipse that rotates on the carpal plate, avoiding torque transmission to the metal carpus component (**Fig. 8**).[67] The proximal component is an elliptical cup and intramedullary stem with 10° palmar tilt and 10° of radioulnar inclination.[67] Carpal fixation is provided by a central press-fit stem with 2 screws compressing the plate to the hamate on 1 side and the scaphoid, trapezoid, and second metacarpal base on the other.[67] Short-term results of the ReMotion TWA in 20 wrists at an average of 32 months follow-up revealed 41% clinical score improvement in rheumatoid patients, and 27% clinical score improvement in nonrheumatoid patients.[68] One carpal and one radial loosening were observed in rheumatoid patients.[68]

There have not yet been outcomes studies of the Maestro implant (see **Fig. 8**), and the following section presents the authors' experience with the Maestro Wrist Reconstructive System.

CASE EXAMPLE AND SURGICAL TECHNIQUE: MAESTRO

The patient had severe end-stage rheumatoid arthritis with complete destruction of her carpus and distal radial ulnar joint. There was marked extensor and flexor tenosynovitis, and she had median neuropathy at the carpal tunnel level. She was admitted to address each of the problems with a total wrist replacement, interpositional arthroplasty of the distal radial ulnar joint, stabilization of the distal ulnar stump, and median nerve decompression along with flexor and extensor tenosynovectomy. The extensive nature of the surgery, expected outcomes, risks, complications, and alternatives were discussed.

Following the induction of anesthesia, a well-padded tourniquet was applied to the right upper arm. The arm and hand were prepared and draped in the standard fashion. Loupe magnification was used for all dissection. Examining the wrist under anesthesia showed marked swelling with extensor

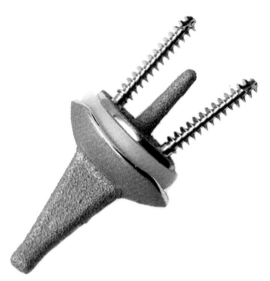

Fig. 8. ReMotion total wrist implant. (*Courtesy* of Small Bone Innovations, Inc., Morrisville, PA.)

tenosynovitis and marked swelling volarly. The distal radial ulnar joint was markedly proud dorsally. Under fluoroscopy, there was complete carpal disruption with ulnar translocation. The distal radial ulnar joint was dislocated dorsally, consistent with caput ulna syndrome. Both the radiocarpal and distal radial ulnar joints were completely disrupted **(Fig. 9)**.

An Esmarch bandage was used to exsanguinate the limb, and a tourniquet was inflated to 250 mm Hg. The carpal tunnel release was performed in standard fashion. As expected, there was flexor tendon synovitis consistent with rheumatoid arthritis, and a full flexor tenosynovectomy from the musculotendinous junction to the lumbrical junction was done of all the tendons. All tendons were intact.

Attention was now turned to the wrist replacement. A longitudinal incision was made from the middle of the long finger metacarpal to 2 cm proximal to Lister's tubercle. The dorsal radial and dorsal ulnar sensory nerves were carefully identified and protected. The Extensor Pollicis Longus (EPL) was released and radialized.

Extensor tenosynovectomy was performed in all involved compartments. Once the tenosynovectomies were complete, it was noted that the tendons were all intact. Attention was then turned to the distal radial and ulnar joints. The distal radio-ulnar joint capsule was opened in an anatomic fashion. It was markedly dilated. The ulna was not only subluxed but also had end-stage arthritic disease. A site for the distal ulnar resection was located and using a saw, osteotomes, and rongeurs, the distal ulna was excised and all synovitis removed.

At this point, the authors now turned attention to the radial carpal joint. Through a longitudinal capsular splitting incision based on the third metacarpal, capsular flaps were elevated. As expected, there was marked undercutting and erosion of the radius. There was complete arthritic change of the radiocarpal joint. The authors then proceeded to perform the carpal resection. The guide was placed parallel to the longitudinal axis of the long finger metacarpal and stabilized with two 0.062-in K-wires. The proximal carpal row, edge of the hamate, and 3 mm of the proximal capitate head were resected. The carpal component was then trialed.

The wrist was then palmarflexed and a K-wire was driven down the center of the distal radius medullary canal; a fully centered position was confirmed using fluoroscopy. The radius was reamed. The radial resection guide was attached, and the distal radius articular surface was resected. The radius was then broached, trials inserted, the wrist reduced, and range of motion as well as stability examined clinically and fluoroscopically. Once in place, the range of motion obtained was 45° of extension to 25° of flexion, 4° of radial and 20° of ulnar deviation with excellent stability. The authors had full pronation and supination. The trials were then exchanged for final implants and fixation performed to the second metacarpal shaft and hamate. The authors then performed a capsular repair to the radius using a suture anchor.

Attention was then turned to the distal radial ulnar joint. Volar sutures were placed. With this done, the prosthesis was seated, and the authors imbricated the distal radial ulnar joint capsule, performing an interposition-type arthroplasty. The authors then relocated the ECU, leaving it to stabilize the distal ulnar stump; it was woven through the distal ulnar stump with multiple drill holes in the bone and passed through bone. When the authors were finished, the stump was stable; pronation and supination were full with excellent tracking of the distal ulnar stump.

The wound was then copiously irrigated, the EPL radialized, and extensor retinaculum repaired. The tourniquet was let down and the dorsal and volar wounds closed in a layered fashion. Radiographs of the wrist showed good implant alignment (see **Fig. 9**).

FAILED TWA: REVISION ARTHROPLASTY VERSUS ARTHRODESIS

Surgical options for failed total wrist arthroplasty include revision arthroplasty and arthrodesis. In a study of 9 failed total wrist arthroplasties (8 Trispherical, 1 Volz), Lorei and colleagues[69] noted that the most common cause for failure was metacarpal loosening with dorsal perforation of the

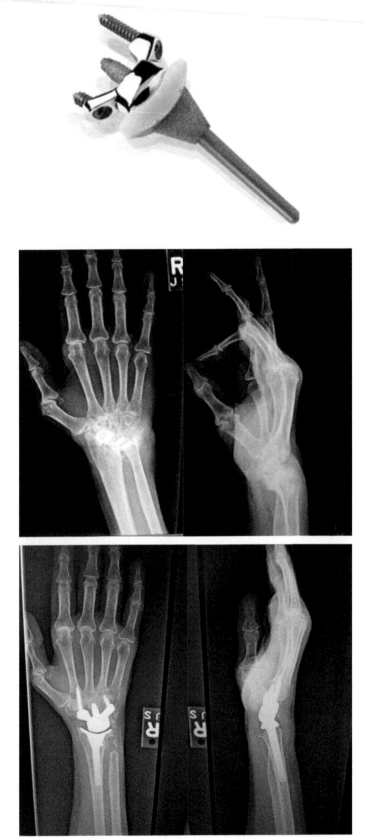

Fig. 9. (*Top*) Maestro TWA (Biomet, Warsaw Indiana). (*Middle*) Preoperative wrist radiographs of patient with rheumatoid arthritis. (*Bottom*) radiographs of Maestro TWA in this patient with rheumatoid arthritis.

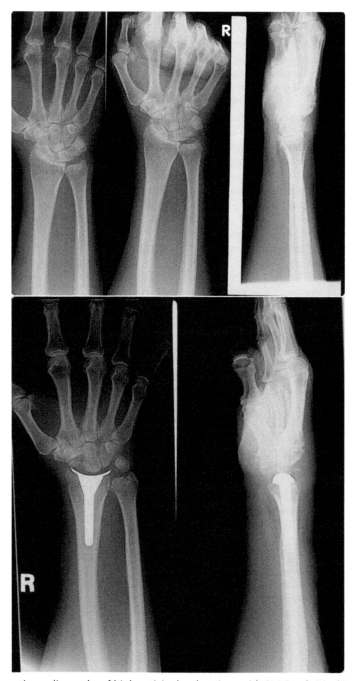

Fig. 10. (*Top*) Preoperative radiographs of high-activity level patient with SLAC arthritis. (*Bottom*) postoperative radiographs of patient 2 years after distal radius hemiarthroplasty.

stem. Three patients underwent revision TWA with custom components; 5 patients had conversion to wrist arthrodesis, and 1 patient underwent resection arthroplasty. After average follow-up of 3.3 years, those patients treated with revision arthroplasty were pain free, and functional with no evidence of implant loosening; those who

underwent arthrodesis demonstrated fusion after an average of 4.8 months.[69] The authors concluded that failed TWA could be salvaged to fusion or revision arthroplasty in most patients.

Vogelin and Nagy also retrospectively reviewed outcomes after revision TWA or arthrodesis after failed TWA.[70] Sixteen Meuli wrist prostheses in

13 patients were revised for failure due to mechanical and/or soft tissue problems. Eleven revision arthroplasties in 10 wrists, 3 arthrodeses and 2 primary soft tissue reconstructions were performed. Five of the 11 revision arthroplasties were converted to arthrodeses after an average of 5 (range 3–8 years) years; salvage arthrodesis was difficult to achieve in 2 of 9 cases. The authors concluded that revision arthroplasty may be useful; however, complications and reoperations are possible after both revision arthroplasty and arthrodesis.[70]

Beer and Turner examined arthrodesis as a salvage procedure for failed TWA.[71] Thirteen arthroplasties were performed for 8 silicone implants (Dow Corning Wright, Arlington, TN), 2 Meuli total wrist implants (DePuy, Warsaw, IN), 1 Volz (Howmedica, Rutherford, NJ) and 1 BIAX (DePuy, Warsaw, IN) total wrist implant. At an average follow-up of 28 months, 17 complications occurred in 9 patients, with 5 developing pseudoarthroses and 4 patients with symptomatic migrating pins. Due to the high incidence of pseudoarthroses, the authors recommended more rigid fixation techniques be used for arthrodesis after failed TWA.[71] More recently, another retrospective study of arthrodesis performed for 21 failed TWAs (12 Biaxial, 4 Meuli, 3 silicone, and 2 KMI) in 17 patients revealed adequate fusion in 11 wrists and nonunion in 10 wrists.[72] Complications occurred in 8 wrists and consisted of: pin migration (4 wrists), hardware failure (2 wrists), and painful hardware (2 wrists). Although arthrodesis is a viable salvage option for failed TWA, technical difficulties arise from osteoporotic and poor bone stock.[72]

A New Alternative: Distal Radius Hemiarthroplasty

Notwithstanding the technical challenges that remain to ensure TWA longevity in the low-demand patient with pancarpal arthritis, surgical treatment options for patients with widespread arthritis and high activity levels are limited. For such patients, prior surgical options included salvage procedures such as limited intercarpal arthrodesis or proximal row carpectomy. However, multiple authors have shown that outcomes of such salvage procedures suffer when arthritis affects the articulating joint surface: lunate involvement in scaphoid excision 4-corner arthrodesis, and capitate/lunate fossa involvement in proximal row carpectomy.[73,74]

Recently, investigators[75] have performed distal radius hemiarthroplasty coupled with proximal row carpectomy in lieu of TWA in those patients who have higher activity demands and yet widespread disease (see **Fig. 9**). In these cases, a proximal row carpectomy is performed, and the distal radius resurfaced with the radial component of the TWA. Boyer and Adams have reported two cases of distal radius hemiarthroplasty with the Universal 2 distal radius implant with good patient satisfaction thus far.[75] The authors have performed distal radius hemiarthroplasty using the Maestro distal radius implant, and have also observed high patient satisfaction and good return of function (**Fig. 10**). Although the outcomes are still short-term and anecdotal, the authors feel that distal radius hemiarthroplasty may serve as an intermediate arthroplasty option for those patients with diffuse arthritis yet higher activity levels.

SUMMARY

In reviewing the history of total wrist arthroplasty as a treatment option for painful, nonfunctional wrists in disease states, certain observations can be made:

- It is worthwhile to preserve wrist joint motion in patients with multiple joint involvement and fairly low demand.
- The diseased wrist joint has a drastically altered center of rotation, kinematics, and soft tissue balance compared with the normal wrist.
- It is difficult to predict and account for the effects of the disease state on implant mechanics and wear.
- Current long-term results of TWA designs are not ideal, with frequent reoperation rates for loosening and instability.
- Salvage options such as revision wrist arthroplasty and arthrodesis are not without complications.

Although the studies examined have overall been small and retrospective, it is clear that total wrist replacement designs and surgical techniques that result in consistently improved patient function have not yet been achieved.

Despite these difficulties, modern discovery has the capacity to improve the role of total wrist replacement in the surgical armamentarium for the diseased wrist. Recent analysis of wrist kinematics reveals that the traditional axis of rotation may in actuality be oblique to the anatomic axis, which may improve future implant designs.[11] Also, technologic advances in materials, wear properties, and manufacturing now account for increased implant longevity. Use of DMARDs reduces the severity of many diseased wrists at presentation, making preoperative tendon rupture and poor soft tissue balance less frequent now as compared with decades earlier. All of these advances may improve total wrist replacement design, survival, and hence patient function. Also, alternative surgical treatments such as distal radius hemiarthroplasty may serve as a treatment option for patients with higher activity levels and diffuse arthritis. The authors believe that with careful patient selection, soft tissue considerations, and novel implant designs, TWA will become a viable treatment staple for patients with functional wrist disability.

REFERENCES

1. Volz RG. Total wrist arthroplasty: a clinical review. Clin Orthop Relat Res 1984;187:112–20.
2. Straub LR, Ranawat CS. The wrist in rheumatoid arthritis: surgical treatment and results. J Bone Joint Surg Am 1969;51(1):1–20.
3. Volz RG. The development of a total wrist arthroplasty. Clin Orthop Relat Res 1976;116:209–14.
4. Landsmeer JM. Studies in the anatomy of articulation, The equilibrium of the 'intercalated' bone. Acta Morphol Scand 1961;3:287–303.
5. MacConaill MA. The mechanical anatomy of the carpus and its bearings on some surgical problems. J Anat 1941;75:166–75.
6. Ryu JY, Cooney WP 3rd, Askey LJ, et al. Functional ranges of motion of the wrist joint. J Hand Surg Am 1991;16(3):409–19.
7. Brumfeld RH, Champoux JA. A biomechanical study of normal functional wrist motion. Clin Orthop 1984;187:23–5.
8. Palmer AK, Werner FW, Murphy D, et al. Functional wrist motion: a biomechanical study. J Hand Surg Am 1985;10(1):39–46.
9. Gardner G, Gray DJ, O'Rahilly R. Anatomy. 3rd edition. Philadelphia: W. B. Saunders Co; 1969.
10. Hollingsworth WH. Textbooks of anatomy. 2nd edition. Philadelphia: Hoeber; 1967.
11. Crisco JJ, Heard WM, Rich RR, et al. The mechanical axes of the wrist are oriented obliquely to the anatomical axes. J Bone Joint Surg Am 2011; 93(2):167–77.
12. Trieb K. Treatment of the wrist in rheumatoid arthritis. J Hand Surg Am 2008;33:113–23.
13. Hamalainen M, Kammonen M, Lehtimaki M, et al. Epidemiology of wrist involvement in rheumatoid arthritis. Rheumatol 1992;17:1–7.
14. Shapiro JS. The wrist in rheumatoid arthritis. Hand Clin 1996;12:477–95.
15. Papp SR, Athwal GS, Pichora DR. The rheumatoid wrist. J Am Acad Orthop Surg 2006;14:65–77.
16. Wilson RL, DeVito MC. Extensor tendon problems in rheumatoid arthritis. Hand Clin 1996;12:551–9.
17. Adams BD, Divelbiss BJ. Reconstruction of the post-traumatic unstable distal radioulnar joint. Orthop Clin North Am 2001;32:353–63.

18. Breedveld FC. Current and future management approaches for rheumatoid arthritis. Arthritis Res 2002;4(Suppl 2):S16–21.
19. Hastings H II. Total wrist arthrodesis for post-traumatic conditions. Indiana Hand Center Newsletter 1993;1:14.
20. Millender LH, Nalebuff EA. Arthrodesis of the rheumatoid wrist. J Bone Joint Surg Am 1973;55: 1026–34.
21. Carroll RE, Dick HM. Arthrodesis of the wrist for rheumatoid arthritis. J Bone Joint Surg Am 1971; 53:1365–9.
22. Field J, Herbert TJ, Prosser R. Total wrist fusion. J Hand Surg Br 1996;21:429–33.
23. Clendenin MB, Green DP. Arthrodesis of the wrist—complications and their management. J Hand Surg 1981;6:253–7.
24. Ilan DI, Rettig ME. Rheumatoid arthritis of the wrist. Bull Hosp Jt Dis 2003;61(3&4):179–85.
25. Swanson AB. Flexible implant arthroplasty for arthritic disabilities of the radiocarpal joint: a silicone rubber intramedullary stemmed flexible hinge implant for the wrist joint. Orthop Clin North Am 1973;4:383–94.
26. Courtman NH, Sochart DH, Trail IA, et al. Biaxial wrist replacement. Initial results in the rheumatoid patient. J Hand Surg Br 1999;24(1):32–4.
27. Figgie HE, Inglis AE, Straub LR, et al. A critical analysis of alignment factors influencing functional results following trispherical total wrist arthroplasty. J Arthroplasty 1986;1(3):149–56.
28. Radmer S, Andresen R, Spearman M. Wrist arthroplasty with a new generation of prostheses in patients with rheumatoid arthritis. J Hand Surg Am 1999;24:935–43.
29. Kobus RJ, Turner RH. Wrist arthrodesis for the treatment of rheumatoid arthritis. J Hand Surg Am 1990; 15(4):541–6.
30. Vicar AJ, Burton RI. Surgical management of the rheumatoid wrist: fusion or arthroplasty. J Hand Surg Am 1986;11(6):790–7.
31. Goodman MJ, Millender LH, Nalebuff ED, et al. Arthroplasty of the rheumatoid wrist with silicone rubber: an early evaluation. J Hand Surg Am 1980; 5(2):114–21.
32. Figgie MP, Ranawat CS, Inglis AF, et al. Trispherical total wrist arthroplasty in rheumatoid arthritis. J Hand Surg Am 1990;15:217–23.
33. Cavaliere CM, Chung KC. A systematic review of total wrist arthroplasty compared with total wrist arthrodesis for rheumatoid arthritis. Plast Reconstr Surg 2008;122:813–25.
34. Cavaliere CM, Oppenheimer AJ, Chung KC. Reconstructing the rheumatoid wrist: a utility analysis comparing total wrist fusion and total wrist arthroplasty from the perspectives of rheumatologists and hand surgeons. Hand (N Y) 2010;5:9–18.

35. Cavaliere CM, Chung KC. A cost utility analysis of non-operative management, total wrist arthroplasty, and total wrist fusion in rheumatoid arthritis. J Hand Surg Am 2010;35(3):379–91.

36. Levadoux M, Legre R. Total wrist arthroplasty with destot prostheses in patients with post-traumatic arthritis. J Hand Surg Am 2003;28:405–13.

37. Adams B. Complications of wrist arthroplasty. Hand Clin 2010;26:213–20.

38. Kamal R, Weiss AP. Total wrist arthroplasty for the patient with non-rheumatoid arthritis. J Hand Surg Am 2011;36:1071–2.

39. Ritt MJ, Stuart PR, Naggar L, et al. The early history of arthroplasty of the wrist. J Hand Surg Br 1994;19:778–82.

40. Gluck T. Autoplastik-transplantation-implantation von Fremdkörpern. In: Vorstand der, Gesellschaft, editors. Verhandlungen der Berliner medicinischen Gesellschaft aus dem Gesellschaftsjahre, 21. Berlin: Schumacher; 1890. p. 79–98.

41. Gluck T. Referat uber die durch das moderne chirurgische Experiment gewonnenen positiven Resultate, betreffend die Naht und den Ersatz von Defecten höherer Gewebe, sowie über die Verwehrtung resorbirbarer und lebendiger Tampons in der Chirurgie. Archiv fur Klinische Chirurgie 1890;41:187–239.

42. Levay D. The history of orthopaedics. Casterton Hall (United Kingdom): The Parthenon Publishing Group; 1990.

43. Swanson AB. Silicone rubber implants for replacement of arthritic or destroyed joints in the hand. Surg Clin North Am 1968;48:1113.

44. Swanson AB. Flexible implant arthroplasty for arthritic finger joints—rationale, technique and results of treatment. J Bone Joint Surg Am 1972;54:435.

45. Swanson AB. Flexible implant arthroplasty in the hand. Clin Plast Surg 1976;3:141.

46. Swanson AB, Swanson GD, Maupin BK. Flexible implant arthroplasty of the radiocarpal joint: surgical technique and long-term study. Clin Orthop Relat Res 1984;187:94–106.

47. Jolly SL, Ferlic DC, Clayton ML. Swanson silicone arthroplasty of the wrist in rheumatoid arthritis: a long-term follow-up. J Hand Surg Am 1992;17:142–9.

48. Smith RJ, Atkinson RE, Jupiter JB. Silicone synovitis of the wrist. J Hand Surg Am 1985;10(1):47–60.

49. Rossello MI, Costa M, Pizzorno V. Experience of total wrist arthroplasty with silastic implants plus grommets. Clin Orthop Relat Res 1997;342:64–70.

50. Meuli HC. Meuli total wrist arthroplasty. Clin Orthop Relat Res 1984;187:107–11.

51. Meuli HC, Fernandez DL. Uncemented total wrist arthroplasty. J Hand Surg Am 1995;20:115–22.

52. Cooney WP III, Beckenbaugh RD, Linscheid RL. Total wrist arthroplasty: problems with implant failures. Clin Orthop Relat Res 1984;187:121–8.

53. Volz RG. Total wrist arthroplasty: a new approach to wrist disability. Clin Orthop Relat Res 1977;128:180–9.

54. Menon J. Total wrist replacement using the modified Volz prosthesis. J Bone Joint Surg Am 1987;69(7):998–1006.

55. Gellman H, Hontas R, Brumfield RH Jr. Total wrist arthroplasty in rheumatoid arthritis: a long term clinical review. Clin Orthop Relat Res 1997;342:71–6.

56. Figgie HE III, Ranawat CS, Inglis AE, et al. Preliminary results of total wrist arthroplasty in rheumatoid arthritis using the trispherical total wrist arthroplasty. J Arthroplasty 1988;3:9–15.

57. Cobb TK, Beckenbaugh RD. Biaxial total wrist arthroplasty. J Hand Surg Am 1996;21:1011–21.

58. Stegeman M, Rijnberg WJ, van Loon CJ. Biaxial total wrist arthroplasty in rheumatoid arthritis. Satisfactory functional results. Rheumatol Int 2005;25:191–4.

59. Krukhaug Y, Lie SA, Havelin LI, et al. Results of 189 wrist replacements: a report from the Norwegian Arthroplasty Register. Acta Orthop 2011;82(4):405–9.

60. van Harlingen D, Heesterbeek PJ, deVos MJ. High rate of complications and radiographic loosening of the biaxial total wrist arthroplasty in rheumatoid arthritis. Acta Orthop 2011;82(6):721–6.

61. Menon J. Universal total wrist implant: experience with a carpal component fixed with three screws. J Arthroplasty 1998;13(5):515–23.

62. Adams BD. Total wrist arthroplasty. Tech Hand Upper Extrem Surg 2004;8(3):130–7.

63. Divelbiss BJ, Sollerman C, Adams BD. Early results of the universal total wrist arthroplasty in rheumatoid arthritis. J Hand Surg Am 2002;27:195–204.

64. Ferreres A, Lluch A, del Valle M. Universal total wrist arthroplasty: midterm follow-up study. J Hand Surg Am 2011;36:967–73.

65. Ward CM, Kuhl T, Adams BD. Five- to ten-year outcomes of the universal total wrist arthroplasty in patients with rheumatoid arthritis. J Bone Joint Surg Am 2011;93(10):914–9.

66. van Winterswijk PJ, Bakx PA. Promising clinical results of the universal total wrist prosthesis in rheumatoid arthritis. Open Orthop J 2010;4:67–70.

67. Gupta A. Total wrist arthroplasty. Am J Orthop 2008;37(Suppl 8):12–6.

68. Herzberg G. Prospective study of a new total wrist arthroplasty: short term results. Chir Main 2011;30(1):20–5.

69. Lorei MP, Figgie MP, Ranawat CS, et al. Failed total wrist arthroplasty: analysis of failures and results of operative management. Clin Orthop Relat Res 1997;342:84–93.

70. Vogelin E, Nagy L. Failed Meuli total wrist arthroplasty. J Hand Surg Br 2003;28(1):61–8.

71. Beer TA, Turner RH. Wrist arthrodesis for failed wrist implant arthroplasty. J Hand Surg Am 1997;22:685–93.

72. Rizzo M, Ackerman DB, Rodrigues RL, et al. Wrist arthrodesis as a salvage procedure for failed implant arthroplasty. J Hand Surg Eur Vol 2011;36: 29–33.

73. Culp RW, McGuigan FX, Turner MA, et al. Proximal row carpectomy: a multicenter study. J Hand Surg Am 1993;18:19–25.

74. Kwon BC, Choi SJ, Shin J, et al. Proximal row carpectomy with capsular interposition arthroplasty for advanced arthritis of the wrist. J Bone Joint Surg Br 2009;91(12):1601–6.

75. Boyer JS, Adams B. Distal radius hemiarthroplasty combined with proximal row carpectomy: case report. Iowa Orthop J 2010;30:168–73.

Distal Ulna Arthroplasties

Mark Rekant, MD

KEYWORDS

- Ulnar arthroplasty • Distal radioulnar joint • Wrist replacement • Triangular fibrocartilage complex

KEY POINTS

- Understanding the complex distal radioulnar joint (DRUJ) and distal ulnar anatomy is key to success.
- Treatment options for degenerative ulnar head problems are ever evolving.
- DRUJ implant arthroplasty is a useful and viable option for ongoing wrist pain.

The distal radioulnar joint (DRUJ) is the distal link between the radius and the ulna, and forms a pivot for forearm pronation and supination. The DRUJ is half of a bicondylar forearm joint, with its condyle, the head of the ulna, articulating with the sigmoid notch of the radius. The DRUJ provides 2 functions: transmission of force with lifting and grip from the carpus to the forearm, and facilitation of forearm rotation. After years of study, it has become clear this bony articulation is inherently incongruent, and little stability at this joint is provided from the bony architecture.[1–3] The articular congruity between the ulna and the radius through the DRUJ has been shown to account for approximately 30% of the total constraint of the DRUJ.[3] The surrounding soft tissues about the DRUJ play a substantial role in guiding and restraining the joint. The soft-tissue constraints of the DRUJ include static and dynamic stabilizers. The primary stabilizers of the DRUJ, the dorsal and palmar radioulnar ligaments, are components of the triangular fibrocartilage complex (TFCC). These ligaments attach to the radius at the margins of the sigmoid notch and converge to form a single attachment at the fovea and base of the ulnar styloid. There are several different interpretations of the specific roles of each of these ligaments, but it is clear that the integrity of both ligaments is necessary for a stable DRUJ.[1–3] The DRUJ joint capsule is an important stabilizer of the DRUJ, most evident in positions of extreme pronation and supination. The entire soft-tissue envelope of the ulnar side of the distal forearm and wrist (including the volar extrinsic ligaments, retinaculum and the extensor carpi ulnaris subsheath) forms an important secondary stabilizer, as does the interosseous membrane.[1–3]

As well as being susceptible to idiopathic arthritis, any injury or deformity of the DRUJ involving the radius or ulna can alter the function of this joint.

Over the last 30 years, various treatment options have been explored for treating DRUJ pain, instability, and degeneration. Treatment options for irreparable destruction of this joint have ranged from fusion of the DRUJ joint to a variety of excision techniques with soft-tissue reconstructions.[4–7]

Historically, debilitating symptoms relating to the DRUJ have been treated with surgical techniques performed with partial or complete ulnar head resections. Common surgical interventions over the last 30 years include the Darrach procedure, Sauvé-Kapandji procedure, or hemi-resection interposition of tendon (HIT), also referred to as the Bower procedure.[4–7] As these customary practices do not yield desirable results for all patients, surgeons and device manufacturers have sought to develop alternative treatment modalities in recent years.

The Darrach procedure is considered to be the traditional approach to excising the arthritic surface of the DRUJ. This procedure was first illustrated in 1913.[4] William Darrach described a volar approach to the DRUJ followed by distal

Department of Orthopaedic Surgery, Thomas Jefferson University, PA, USA
E-mail address: mrekant@comcast.net

Hand Clin 28 (2012) 611–615
http://dx.doi.org/10.1016/j.hcl.2012.08.016
0749-0712/12/$ – see front matter © 2012 Elsevier Inc. All rights reserved.

ulnar head resection to alleviate ulnar-sided wrist pain. While this is a widely performed practice, potential complications include distal forearm instability and convergence. The primary cause of these complications is the removal of the ulnar head and destabilization of the remaining distal ulna, which ironically is also commonly the basis of patients' pain relief. Subsequently, there have been several modifications to his procedure that entail limited or partial excision of the distal ulnar head, with interposition of soft tissue to stabilize the remaining distal ulna and to prevent distal ulnar convergence and impingement with the radius.[8–12]

The HIT was formulated by William Bowers.[6] Many variations of this concept have also been described. The general concept of the procedure involves a partial resection of the distal ulna in an oblique fashion to match the slope of the sigmoid notch of the radius with preservation of the TFCC origin/insertion on the remaining distal ulnar styloid. Tendons (either the palmaris longus, flexor carpi ulnaris, or extensor carpi ulnaris), joint capsule, or pronator quadratus muscle has been used as an interposition spacer placed into the newly established void. This custom has shown good success in younger patients; however, the clinical outcomes still leave patients with reduced grip strength among other potential complications, as previously mentioned.[13–15]

While excision procedures are well documented, each of them relies on permanently altering the wrist anatomy by removal of bone mass with no replacement or substitution of the excised bone. As described by Berger in 2008,[16] when the ulnar head is removed the stability of the DRUJ is altered. The radius and ulna are uncoupled and the radius is no longer in contact with the ulna at the wrist level, creating an intrinsically unstable construct. In addition, there is loss of the soft-tissue attachments of the TFCC and DRUJ joint capsule to the distal ulnar head, as in the case of a Darrach resection arthroplasty. The dynamic stabilizers in this region are then unopposed, and pull the radius and ulna together. This process results in convergence of the ulnar stump and distal radius as well as loss of tension in the interosseous membrane, further destabilizing the forearm.[17]

To offset these prospective occurrences, fusion of the DRUJ was proposed by Sauvé and Kapandji.[5] This procedure involves the resection of a wafer of ulnar bone several centimeters proximal to the DRUJ. However, the ulnar head itself remains intact. The ulnar head is then fused to the distal radius after denuding the remaining articular cartilage of the DRUJ. The presence of the distal ulna stabilizes the joint and provides a buttress from ulnar and proximal translocation of the carpus. While this procedure may effectively alleviate DRUJ arthritic pain, there remains potential for complications including nonunion as well as osteosynthesis across the pseudoarthrosis site, convergence of the proximal ulnar stump, reduced grip strength, and reduced rotational range of motion.[18–21]

In recent years, new approaches for treating patients suffering from DRUJ instability and arthritis of the distal ulna have emerged, including various implants and techniques for DRUJ implant arthroplasty. Surgical indications include patients with debilitating pain, deformity, weakness, and/or diminished hand function from any of a multiple of underlying ailments including osteoarthritis, rheumatoid arthritis, ulnar impaction or impingement, failed Darrach procedures, and failed matched resections or HIT procedures. Additional indications also include failed fracture management of the distal ulna. Over the last several years, numerous orthopedic manufacturers have developed ulnar arthroplasty products. The benefits to patients who have received an ulnar head implant include pain relief (as was the case with the Darrach procedure), good stability of the DRUJ (an advantage of the Sauvé-Kapandji procedure), and better forearm stability by diminishing convergence while improving form and function.

Attempts to use soft-tissue procedures alone to stabilize the DRUJ after ulnar head resection have been found to be mechanically ineffective because of the inability to create a soft-tissue stabilizing procedure based on a vector that holds the radius and ulna apart.[22] Therefore, attempts to counter such instability with soft-tissue procedures have been largely unsuccessful.

Silicone ulnar head replacements, described by Swanson[23] in 1973, have largely been abandoned in recent years because of the potential for the development of silicone synovitis.[24] Subsequent studies have reported poor results, with cases demonstrating postoperative fractures 15% of the time, angulation 40%, and bony resorption 100% of the time.[25] A second study of 45 patients noted migration or breakage 63% of the time, and all developed silicone synovitis.[24]

Recent advancements in technologies and understanding of the ulnar aspect of the wrist have permitted more attractive options of replacement/reconstruction of the ulnar head and DRUJ. As an alternative to silicone, Herbert and van Schoonhoven[26] designed a ceramic ulnar head endoprosthesis. Although avoiding the dilemma of silicone synovitis and implant breakdown, the ceramic implant also demonstrated limited successes, as there are limited opportunities for soft-tissue reconstruction or stabilization of the implant.[26]

Emerging technologies have provided additional options including nonconstrained ulnar head replacement or semiconstrained total DRUJ replacement, with the rationale of preventing impingement and improving stability of the DRUJ while providing pain relief and increasing hand and wrist function. This next generation of endoprostheses allows for a closer anatomic reconstruction of the bony and joint anatomy while allowing for maintenance and repair of important soft-tissue constraints. The surgeon and implant designers must be cognizant of the importance for implant success relying not only on implant design and position but also on the surrounding DRUJ stabilizers, with primary restraint coming from the TFCC and secondary stabilizers.

The rationale for implantation of an endoprosthetic ulnar head is based on the need for direct contact between the distal ulna and the radius, which completes the distal mechanical link of the forearm joint while providing restoration of soft-tissue tension and preventing impingement.

One recent option is the uHead (Small Bone Innovations, Morrisville, PA). This endoprosthesis offers the surgeon the opportunity to manage DRUJ disease with a tailored approach to anatomic restoration. The implant, made of cobalt chrome with a plasma-coated stem, permits modularity with multiple ulnar head and stem sizes to best match the patient's anatomy. The stem design allows for a press fit with minimal soft-tissue disruption. The uHead also provides eyelet holes for reattachment of the TFCC and adjacent soft tissues directly to the implant head. A study regarding outcomes of 19 wrists from 17 patients performed for impingement after Darrach and painful arthrosis of the DRUJ with 2-year follow-up was published recently.[27] The investigators reported pain scores decreased by 50%, functional scores improved 3-fold, and grip strength improved by 4 kg (16%). All wrists were clinically stable, with patients describing 100% "improvement," and stating they would have the surgery again. Complications noted were ulna fracture (1) that healed with screw fixation, neuroma formation (1) that led to chronic pain, instability (1) that resolved with a tendon stabilization procedure, progressive degeneration of the sigmoid notch (1) that was treated with resurfacing of sigmoid notch, and 2 cases of stem loosening.

Another study examined the results of 22 wrists in 20 patients with painful DRUJ arthrosis or failed resection arthroplasty at an average of 4.5 years' follow-up, with an average Mayo Wrist Score of 73 (good).[28] The investigators reported complications in 4 patients with recurrent instability (2 symptomatic, 2 asymptomatic) and 3 patients who underwent revisions; 2 for instability (stabilized successfully) and 1 replacement of the implant due to breakage after a fall.

More recently, a partial ulnar head replacement implant was designed to minimize the ulnar resection and to optimize the functional results of implant arthroplasty for the treatment of distal radioulnar arthritis. This implant option, the Ascension partial ulnar head replacement (Ascension Orthopedics, Austin, TX), involves replacement of all articular surfaces of the ulnar head while the ligaments and other bony anatomy responsible for DRUJ stability are maintained. This endoprosthesis allows retention of the ulnar neck, ulnar styloid, extensor carpi ulnaris groove, ulnocarpal ligament attachments, extensor carpi ulnaris sheath, and the TFCC attachments to the ulnar styloid, in an effort to minimize risk of DRUJ instability, implant prominence, soft-tissue irritation, and ulnocarpal instability. As this implant requires less bone removal, there is greater potential for preservation of the DRUJ soft tissues with potentially less alteration of joint mechanics.[29]

The results of the first 10 patients treated by 3 surgeons were reviewed to assess this implant's clinical efficacy. Plain radiographs demonstrated a good match (within 7%) between the size and shape of the natural ulna and after implant replacement, as well as for ulnar variance, ulnar offset, and ulnar height at the DRUJ. DRUJ stability was maintained by subjective assessment, and there was no loss of forearm rotation. Of the 10 clinical patients, 7 were treated for osteoarthritis and 3 for posttraumatic arthritis. In a retrospective chart review at an average 6 months' follow-up, there were no intraoperative or postoperative complications. Pain relief was good in all patients; however, none were completely pain free. Motion was also improved in all, with patients achieving at least 75° of pronation and 65° of supination. Wrist flexion and extension were unaffected. There were no cases of DRUJ instability.[29,30]

With a similar intent to minimize bony resection, a pyrocarbon spacer, Eclypse (Orthopedic Solutions, Tornier SAS, Montbonnot, France), has been developed to substitute the articular portion of the damaged ulnar head in patients with isolated DRUJ degenerative arthritis. This implant uses a pyrocarbon head fitted onto a titanium stem to attempt restoration of the arthritic joint. Early results have been reported as promising, with good pain relief and return to function.[31]

The most complex option for a problematic DRUJ is a total DRUJ replacement endoprosthesis as presented by Luis Scheker (Aptis Medical, Louisville, KY). This device is a bipolar, self-stabilizing implant and is also modular. This implant offers to ability to replace the ulnar head and sigmoid notch with the capacity to preserve the TFCC and joint stabilizers. The Aptis DRUJ arthroplasty affords longitudinal migration of the radius during pronation and supination of the forearm and also reestablishes lifting capability by reconstructing the ulnar support of the distal radius.[32] This implant for total replacement arthroplasty of the DRUJ also enables the surgeon to salvage the DRUJ following failed ulnar head resection arthroplasty or ulnar head endoprosthesis. Similar to other implant concepts, this implant may also be used effectively for the primary treatment of rheumatoid, degenerative, or posttraumatic arthritis presenting with pain and weakness of the wrist joint not improved by nonoperative treatment. Instability of the distal ulna with radiographic evidence of dislocation or erosive changes of the DRUJ is also an appropriate indication for this procedure.

Surgical outcomes were evaluated in a recent study of 31 wrists in 31 patients.[32] Pain levels were noted, with patients reporting an average preoperative pain score of 4.2 followed by a postoperative pain score of 1.0. Forearm rotation postoperatively was reported with pronation 79° and supination 72°. Grip strength improved from 11 kg preoperatively to 22 kg postoperatively. Complications included 1 case with a wound infection and 1 patient who developed chronic regional pain syndrome. There was no evidence of radiographic loosening. There were 2 cases of implant failure that reportedly occurred subsequent to motor vehicle accidents postoperatively.

In summary, our commitment to improving patient function and outcomes is enhanced with an increasing knowledge and understanding of newer, and perhaps superior surgical implant options to complement techniques such as the Darrach distal ulnar excisional arthroplasty, Sauvé-Kapandji arthroplasty, or hemi-resection arthroplasty.

Ulnar head replacement arthroplasty prevents impingement, retensions the DRUJ stabilizers, and may effectively treat patients' pain. However, these endoprostheses rely on adequate soft-tissue stabilization. If stability is not possible, total DRUJ replacement as described by Scheker may be a viable option.

To date, these enhanced implant options have been shown to be promising. However, the caveat remains that high-volume long-term studies are currently lacking.

REFERENCES

1. Haugstvedt JR, Berger RA, Berglund LJ, et al. An analysis of the constraint properties of the distal radioulnar ligament attachments to the ulna. J Hand Surg Am 2002;27(1):61–7.
2. Haugstvedt JR, Berger RA, Nakamura T, et al. Relative contributions of the ulnar attachments of the triangular fibrocartilage complex to the dynamic stability of the distal radioulnar joint. J Hand Surg Am 2006;31(3):445–51.
3. Stuart PR, Berger RA, Linscheid RL, et al. The dorsopalmar stability of the distal radioulnar joint. J Hand Surg Am 2000;25(4):689–99.
4. Darrach W. Partial excision of lower shaft of ulna for deformity following Colles's fracture. Ann Surg 1913; 57:764–5.
5. Sauvé L, Kapandji M. Nouvelle technique de traitement chirurgical des luxations récidivantes isolées de l'extrémité inférieure du cubitus. J Chir 1936;7:589.
6. Bowers WH. Distal radioulnar joint arthroplasty: the hemiresection interposition technique. J Hand Surg 1985;10A:169–78.
7. Watson HK, Ryu JY, Burgess RC. Matched distal ulnar resection. J Hand Surg 1986;11A:812–7.
8. Breen TF, Jupiter JB. Extensor carpi ulnaris and flexor carpi ulnaris tenodesis of the unstable distal ulna. J Hand Surg 1989;14:612–7.
9. Tsai TM, Shimizu H, Adkins P. A modified extensor carpi ulnaris tenodesis with the Darrach procedure. J Hand Surg 1993;18(4):697–702.
10. Ruby LK, Ferenz CC, Dell PC. The pronator quadratus interposition transfer: an adjunct to resection arthroplasty of the distal radioulnar joint. J Hand Surg 1996;21:60–5.
11. Johnson RK. Stabilization of the distal ulna by transfer of the pronator quadratus origin. Clin Orthop Relat Res 1992;275:130–2.
12. Bain GI, Heptinstall RJ, Webb JM, et al. Hemiresection of the distal ulna by means of pronator quadratus interposition and volar stabilization. Tech Hand Up Extrem Surg 2007;11(1):83–6.
13. Bain GI, Pugh DM, MacDermid JC, Roth JH. Matched hemiresection interposition arthroplasty of the distal radioulnar joint. J Hand Surg 1995;20(6):944–50.
14. Bowers WH. Distal radioulnar arthroplasty: the hemiresection-interposition technique. J Hand Surg 1985;10A:169–78.
15. Faithfull K, Kwa S. A review of ulnar hemiresection arthroplasty. J Hand Surg 1992;17B:408–10.
16. Berger RA. Indications for ulnar head replacement. Am J Orthop (Belle Mead NJ) 2008;37:17–20.
17. Sauerbier M, Hahn ME, Fujita M, et al. Analysis of dynamic distal radioulnar convergence after ulnar head resection and endoprosthesis implantation. J Hand Surg 2002;27(3):425–34.
18. Taleisnik J. The Sauvé-Kapandji procedure. Clin Orthop 1992;275:110–24.
19. Sanders RA, Frederick HA, Hontas RB. The Sauvé-Kapandji procedure: a salvage operation for the distal radioulnar joint. J Hand Surg 1991;16A:1125–9.

20. Nakamura R, Tsunoda K, Watanabe K, et al. The Sauvé-Kapandji procedure for chronic dislocation of the distal radio-ulnar joint with destruction of the articular surface. J Hand Surg 1992;17B:127–32.

21. Minami A, Suzuki K, Suenaga N, et al. The Sauvé-Kapandji procedure for osteoarthritis of the distal radioulnar joint. J Hand Surg 1995;20A:602–8.

22. Sauerbier M, Berger RA, Fujita M, et al. Radioulnar convergence after distal ulnar resection—mechanical performance of two commonly used soft tissue stabilizing procedures. Acta Orthop Scand 2003; 74(4):420–8.

23. Swanson AB. Implant arthroplasty for disabilities of the distal radioulnar joint. Orthop Clin North Am 1973;4(2):373–82.

24. Sagerman SD, Seiler JG, Fleming LL, et al. Silicone rubber distal ulnar replacement arthroplasty. J Hand Surg Br 1992;17(6):689–93.

25. Stanley D, Herbert TJ. The Swanson ulnar head prosthesis for post-traumatic disorders of the distal radio-ulnar joint. J Hand Surg Br 1992;17(6):682–8.

26. Herbert TJ, van Schoonhoven J. Ulnar head prostheses: a new solution for problems at the distal radioulnar joint. In: Simmen BR, Allieu Y, Lluch A, et al, editors. Hand arthroplasties. London: Martin Dunitz; 2000. p. 145–9.

27. Willis A, Berger R, Cooney W. Arthroplasty of the distal radioulnar joint using a new ulnar head endoprosthesis: preliminary report. J Hand Surg 2007; 32A:177–89.

28. Shipley N, Dion G, Bowers W. Ulnar head implant arthroplasty: an intermediate term review of 1 surgeon's experience. Tech Hand Up Extrem Surg 2009;13:160–4.

29. Adams B. White paper, Ascension Orthopaedics.

30. Conaway DA, Kuhl TL, Adams BD. Comparison of the native ulnar head and a partial ulnar head resurfacing implant. J Hand Surg 2009;34(6): 1056–62.

31. Garcia-Elias M. Eclypse: partial ulnar head replacement for the isolated distal radio-ulnar joint arthrosis. Tech Hand Up Extrem Surg 2007;11(1):121–8.

32. Laurentin-Perez L, Goodwin A, Babb A, et al. A study of functional outcomes following implantation of a total distal radioulnar joint prosthesis. J Hand Surg 2008;33E(1):18–28.

Index

Hand Clin 28 (2012) 617–620
http://dx.doi.org/10.1016/S0749-0712(12)00136-9
0749-0712/12/$ – see front matter © 2012 Elsevier Inc. All rights reserved.

hand.theclinics.com

United States Postal Service

Statement of Ownership, Management, and Circulation
(All Periodicals Publications Except Requestor Publications)

1. Publication Title	2. Publication Number									3. Filing Date
Hand Clinics	0	0	0	-	7	0	9			9/14/12

4. Issue Frequency	5. Number of Issues Published Annually	6. Annual Subscription Price
Feb, May, Aug, Nov	4	$368.00

7. Complete Mailing Address of Known Office of Publication *(Not printer) (Street, city, county, state, and ZIP+4®)*

Elsevier Inc.
360 Park Avenue South
New York, NY 10010-1710

Contact Person
Stephen R. Bushing

Telephone *(Include area code)*
215-239-3688

8. Complete Mailing Address of Headquarters or General Business Office of Publisher *(Not printer)*

Elsevier Inc., 360 Park Avenue South, New York, NY 10010-1710

9. Full Names and Complete Mailing Addresses of Publisher, Editor, and Managing Editor *(Do not leave blank)*

Publisher *(Name and complete mailing address)*

Kim Murphy, Elsevier, Inc., 1600 John F. Kennedy Blvd. Suite 1800, Philadelphia, PA 19103-2899

Editor *(Name and complete mailing address)*

David Parsons, Elsevier, Inc., 1600 John F. Kennedy Blvd. Suite 1800, Philadelphia, PA 19103-2899

Managing Editor *(Name and complete mailing address)*

Barbara Cohen-Kligerman, Elsevier, Inc., 1600 John F. Kennedy Blvd. Suite 1800, Philadelphia, PA 19103-2899

10. Owner *(Do not leave blank. If the publication is owned by a corporation, give the name and address of the corporation immediately followed by the names and addresses of all stockholders owning or holding 1 percent or more of the total amount of stock. If not owned by a corporation, give the names and addresses of the individual owners. If owned by a partnership or other unincorporated firm, give its name and address as well as those of each individual owner. If the publication is published by a nonprofit organization, give its name and address.)*

Full Name	Complete Mailing Address
Wholly owned subsidiary of	1600 John F. Kennedy Blvd., Ste. 1800
Reed/Elsevier, US holdings	Philadelphia, PA 19103-2899

11. Known Bondholders, Mortgagees, and Other Security Holders Owning or Holding 1 Percent or More of Total Amount of Bonds, Mortgages, or Other Securities. If none, check box ☐ None

Full Name	Complete Mailing Address
N/A	

12. Tax Status *(For completion by nonprofit organizations authorized to mail at nonprofit rates) (Check one)*
The purpose, function, and nonprofit status of this organization and the exempt status for federal income tax purposes:
☐ Has Not Changed During Preceding 12 Months
☐ Has Changed During Preceding 12 Months *(Publisher must submit explanation of change with this statement)*

PS Form **3526**, September 2007 (Page 1 of 3 (Instructions Page 3)) PSN 7530-01-000-9931 **PRIVACY NOTICE:** See our Privacy policy in www.usps.com

13. Publication Title		14. Issue Date for Circulation Data Below
Hand Clinics		August 2012

15. Extent and Nature of Circulation			Average No. Copies Each Issue During Preceding 12 Months	No. Copies of Single Issue Published Nearest to Filing Date
a. Total Number of Copies *(Net press run)*			1308	1175
b. Paid Circulation (By Mail and Outside the Mail)	(1)	Mailed Outside-County Paid Subscriptions Stated on PS Form 3541 *(Include paid distribution above nominal rate, advertiser's proof copies, and exchange copies)*	804	737
	(2)	Mailed In-County Paid Subscriptions Stated on PS Form 3541 *(Include paid distribution above nominal rate, advertiser's proof copies, and exchange copies)*		
	(3)	Paid Distribution Outside the Mails Including Sales Through Dealers and Carriers, Street Vendors, Counter Sales, and Other Paid Distribution Outside USPS®	245	261
	(4)	Paid Distribution by Other Classes Mailed Through the USPS (e.g. First-Class Mail®)		
c. Total Paid Distribution *(Sum of 15b (1), (2), (3), and (4))*		►	1049	998
d. Free or Nominal Rate Distribution (By Mail and Outside the Mail)	(1)	Free or Nominal Rate Outside-County Copies Included on PS Form 3541	51	63
	(2)	Free or Nominal Rate In-County Copies Included on PS Form 3541		
	(3)	Free or Nominal Rate Copies Mailed at Other Classes Through the USPS (e.g. First-Class Mail)		
	(4)	Free or Nominal Rate Distribution Outside the Mail (Carriers or other means)		
e. Total Free or Nominal Rate Distribution *(Sum of 15d (1), (2), (3) and (4))*		►	51	63
f. Total Distribution *(Sum of 15c and 15e)*		►	1100	1061
g. Copies not Distributed *(See instructions to publishers #4 (page #3))*		►	208	114
h. Total *(Sum of 15f and g)*		►	1308	1175
i. Percent Paid *(15c divided by 15f times 100)*			95.36%	94.06%

16. Publication of Statement of Ownership
If the publication is a general publication, publication of this statement is required. Will be printed ☐ Publication not required
in the November 2012 issue of this publication.

17. Signature and Title of Editor, Publisher, Business Manager, or Owner	Date
[signature] Stephen R. Bushing – Inventory Distribution Coordinator	September 14, 2012

I certify that all information furnished on this form is true and complete. I understand that anyone who furnishes false or misleading information on this form or who omits material or information requested on the form may be subject to criminal sanctions (including fines and imprisonment) and/or civil sanctions (including civil penalties).

PS Form **3526**, September 2007 (Page 2 of 3)

Moving?

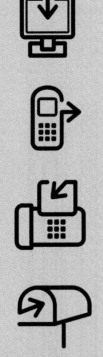

Make sure your subscription moves with you!

To notify us of your new address, find your **Clinics Account Number** (located on your mailing label above your name), and contact customer service at:

Email: journalscustomerservice-usa@elsevier.com

800-654-2452 (subscribers in the U.S. & Canada)
314-447-8871 (subscribers outside of the U.S. & Canada)

Fax number: 314-447-8029

Elsevier Health Sciences Division
Subscription Customer Service
3251 Riverport Lane
Maryland Heights, MO 63043

*To ensure uninterrupted delivery of your subscription, please notify us at least 4 weeks in advance of move.

Printed and bound by CPI Group (UK) Ltd, Croydon, CR0 4YY

03/10/2024

01040344-0011